HANDBOOK OF
ENDOCRINOLOGY
Second Edition
VOLUME II

EDITED BY
George H. Gass
Harold M. Kaplan

CRC Press
Boca Raton   New York   London   Tokyo

Publisher: Robert B. Stern
Project Editor: Albert W. Starkweather, Jr.
Marketing Manager: Becky McEldowney
Cover Design: Denise Craig
PrePress: Carlos Esser
Manufacturing: Sheri Schwartz

Library of Congress Cataloging-in-Publication Data

Handbook of endocrinology / edited by George H. Gass, Harold M. Kaplan. -- 2nd ed.
     p. cm.
     Rev. ed. of: CRC handbook of endocrinology / editors, George H. Gass and Harold M.
Kaplan, c1982.
     Includes bibliographical references and index.
     ISBN 0-8493-9429-5 (v. 1 : alk. paper), -- ISBN 0-8493-9430-9 (V. 2 : alk. paper)
     1. Endocrinology--Handbooks, manuals, etc. I. Gass, George H. II. Kaplan, Harold
Morris, 1908- . III. CRC handbook of endorcinology.
     [DNLM: 1. Endocrine Glands--physiology. 2. Hormones--physiology.
3. Endocrine Diseases. 4. Endocrinology. WK 100 H236 1996]
QP187.C73 1996
612′.4--dc20
DNLM/DLC
for Library of Congress   96-13983
                                            CIP

No claim to original U.S. Government works
International Standard Book Number 0-8493-9430-9
Library of Congress Card Number 96-13983
Printed in the United States of America 1 2 3 4 5 6 7 8 9 0
Printed on acid-free paper

PREFACE

This *Handbook of Endocrinology, Volumes I and II,* presents a review of selected topics by 36 authors. Each topic is broad in scope and intensive in approach. The endocrine literature is now so extensive that it would take several volumes to encompass it.

The present book is a general reference source for the academic endocrinologist, teacher, and researcher, for graduate students working in current areas of the field, and for biologists interested in the chemical control of bodily systems, adjunctive to neural regulation. Physicians with special interests in endocrinology will find chapters that have considerable relevance to their work. The references provided herein are numerous and updated. The descriptions of the endocrine processes provide data in the fields of anatomy, histology, physiology, and pathophysiology.

Overall, the reader will have access to a comprehensive survey of the chemical nature of hormones, their synthesis, secretion and transport, their actions and mechanisms of action, and their degradation and excretion, in mammals and man.

The editors fully appreciate the expertise and the large amount of time spent by the contributors. This book is their work.

George H. Gass
Harold M. Kaplan

THE EDITORS

George H. Gass, M.D., is the retired Chairman of the Department of Basic Medical Sciences of the Oklahoma State University College of Osteopathic Medicine (formerly the Oklahoma College of Osteopathic Medicine and Surgery). Previously he held the position of Director, Endocrinologic Pharmacology Research Laboratory at Southern Illinois University, during which time he also held the positions of Professor of Physiology and Professor of Medicine. He has had a very diverse career, including industry (Lederle Laboratories) and government (Food and Drug Administration).

Dr. Gass was awarded his doctorate at The Ohio State University. Following graduation Dr. Gass served in the Endocrine Branch of the Food and Drug Administration in Washington, D.C., where he performed biological assay procedures, biostatistics, and endocrine research for four years before leaving to enter higher education. Dr. Gass' best known work in the Food and Drug Administration was in the co-development of the uterine weight method for estrogen assay and detection. Dr. Gass assumed his duties at Southern Illinois University, Department of Physiology, in the fall of 1959 and immediately upon arrival set up the Endocrinologic Pharmacology Research Laboratory. A number of students obtained their research experience under Dr. Gass in that laboratory, where it was first discovered that a quantitative measure of a chemical carcinogen (diethylstilbestrol)-dose response of mammary tumors existed. This research has become a classic and, although published in 1964, has more recently been repeated by the Center for Toxicological Research with Dr. Gass consulting.

Dr. Gass, as a member of the staff of Southern Illinois University, received a number of honors and served on numerous occasions as a consultant for government and industry. Dr. Gass is a fellow of the American Association of Science, an Alexander von Humboldt fellow, and a Fullbright alumnus.

He was requested to serve as a consultant for the National Center for Toxicology, Food Administration, to help determine the carcinogenicity and estrogenicity of female sex hormones, both naturally occurring and synthetic. During his 18 years at Southern Illinois University he taught physiology and pharmacology. His last position as Chairman of the Department of Basic Medical Sciences allowed him intimate contact with the basic scientists in the college, including those in human anatomy, histology, pharmacology, physiology, behavior, and biochemistry.

Harold M. Kaplan, Ph.D., is Visiting Professor in the Medical Preparatory Program in the School of Medicine at Southern Illinois University (SIU) at Carbondale. Dr. Kaplan received the A.B. degree at Dartmouth College in 1930, the A.M. degree at Harvard University in 1931, and the Ph.D. degree at Harvard in 1933. He was an Assistant Instructor at Harvard, 1933–1934, and Instructor to Professor of Physiology at Middlesex University Medical School in Massachusetts, 1934–1945, as well as Department Chairman for many years. He was Professor of Veterinary Physiology and Department Chairman at Brandeis University from 1945 to 1947. He was Associate Professor of Physiology at the University of Massachusetts at Fort Devens from 1947 to 1949, serving as Department Chairman in 1948–1949. Dr. Kaplan was Associate Professor at SIU in 1949 and became Professor of Physiology and Department Chairman in 1971. He was simultaneously a professor in the SIU School of Medicine from 1974 to the present. He was Director of the SIU Animal Quarters (Vivarium) intermittently from 1950 to 1982.

Dr. Kaplan was President of the Illinois State Academy of Science, 1969–1970, and is both a life member and honorary member. He was President of the American Association for Laboratory Animal Science, 1966–1967, and is a life member and honorary member. He was on the Board of Directors of the Institute of Laboratory Animal Resources, 1965–1969, and the Illinois Society for Medical Research, 1962–1986. He was on the Science Advisory Committee at Illinois Wesleyan University, 1970–1976. He was President of Sigma Xi (National Honor Society) SIU chapter, 1989–1990, as well as Phi Kappa Phi (National Honor Society), SIU chapter, 1976–1977 and 1983–1984. He was an editorial advisor for the National Forum, 1986–1989. He was President of the Emeritus Faculty Organization at SIU, 1993–1995. Dr. Kaplan has served as Science Consultant for the Applied Research and Development Laboratory in Mt. Vernon, IL, since 1983. He is a fellow of the AAAS. He was Chairman of the Editorial Board, Laboratory Animal Science, 1963–1974.

Dr. Kaplan is the co-author of about 200 research papers and has written 10 books. He is a contributor to five chapters in an accepted biological laboratory text.

CONTRIBUTORS

Iain Anderson
Department of Biochemistry
University of Wisconsin
Madison, Wisconsin

Joachim Braun
Gynaekologische und Ambulatorische
  Tierklinik
Ludwig-Maximilans-Universität
Munich, Germany

George M. Brenner
Oklahoma State University
College of Medicine
Tulsa, Oklahoma

Varadaraj Chandrashekar
Department of Physiology
Southern Illinois University
  School of Medicine
Carbondale, Illinois

David E. C. Cole
Department of Clinical Biochemistry
Banting Institute
University of Toronto
Toronto, Ontario, Canada

Theresa Duello
Department of Obstetrics and Gynecology
University of Wisconsin
Madison, Wisconsin

Jack Gorski
Department of Biochemistry
University of Wisconsin
Madison, Wisconsin

Wesley Gray
Department of Biochemistry
University of Wisconsin
Madison, Wisconsin

Tamara Greco
Department of Human Genetics
University of Michigan
Ann Arbor, Michigan

Qunfang Hou
Cellular and Developmental Biology
Harvard University
Cambridge, Massachusetts

Julio Licinio
National Institutes of Health
CNE
NIMH
Bethesda, Maryland

Scott Lundeen
Women's Health Research Institute
Wyeth-Ayerst Research
Radnor, Pennsylvania

John E. Morley
Division of Geriatric Medicine
St. Louis University Health Science Center
St. Louis, Missouri

John J. Peluso
Department of Obstetrics and Gynecology
University of Connecticut Health Center
Farmington, Connecticut

Béla E. Piacsek
Department of Biology
Marquette University
Milwaukee, Wisconsin

Raj Purushothaman
Geriatric Research, Education,
  and Clinical Center
St. Louis University Health Sciences Center
St. Louis, Missouri

Alexander J. Rouch
Department of Physiology and Pharmacology
College of Osteopathic Medicine
Tulsa, Oklahoma

Phyllis W. Speiser
Division of Pediatric Endocrinology
North Shore University Hospital–Cornell
  University Medical College
Manhasset, New York

Esther M. Sternberg
National Institutes of Health
CNE
NIMH
Bethesda, Maryland

Rudolf Stolla
Gynaekologische und Ambulatorische
  Tierklinik
Ludwig-Maximilans-Universität
Munich, Germany

Reinhold Vieth
Department of Pathology and Laboratory
  Medicine
Mount Sinai Hospital
Toronto, Ontario, Canada

Perrin C. White
Department of Pediatrics
University of Texas
Southwestern Medical Center
Dallas, Texas

Corinne G. Wong
Department of Ophthalmology/Center for
  Occupational and Environmental Health
University of California at Irvine
Irvine, California

Leon J. Yoder
Department of Internal Medicine
Broken Arrow Medical Center
Broken Arrow, Oklahoma

TABLE OF CONTENTS

Chapter 1

ADRENAL MEDULLA: CHROMAFFIN CELL FUNCTION AND TRANSPLANTATION

George M. Brenner

CONTENTS

The sympathoadrenal neuroendocrine system consists of the sympathetic nervous system and the adrenal medulla. The functional endocrine cells of the medulla are called chromaffin cells because of their affinity for chromium salts during histologic staining and are embryologically derived from neuroectodermal cells of the neural crest. Chromaffin cells share with postganglionic sympathetic fibers the ability to synthesize, store, and secrete catecholamines. Preganglionic sympathetic nerve fibers enter the adrenal medulla through the splanchnic nerves and synapse directly on chromaffin cells. When the sympathetic nervous system is activated, chromaffin cells release catecholamines, primarily epinephrine, into venous sinusoids that drain into the adrenal vein and eventually into the inferior vena cava.

The adrenal medulla complements the sympathetic nervous system in several ways. For example, the effects of catecholamines released from the medulla can last five to ten times longer than those released from postganglionic sympathetic nerves and can reach tissues via the circulation that are not innervated by the sympathetic nervous system. The functional anatomy and physiology of the adrenal medulla, including the synthesis, storage, and degradation of catecholamines, has been reviewed by Tsapatsaris and Breslin.[1] In this chapter, the focus will be on recent findings concerning catecholamine synthesis and secretion, and adrenal medulla transplantation.

SYNTHESIS OF CATECHOLAMINES

The amino acid tyrosine is converted to epinephrine in a four-step biosynthetic pathway that is sequentially catalyzed by tyrosine hydroxylase (TH), aromatic-L-amino-acid (DOPA) decarboxylase, dopamine-β-hydroxylase (DBH), and phenylethanolamine N-methyltransferase (PNMT) as shown in Figure 1. In these reactions, tyrosine is hydroxylated to form DOPA, DOPA is decarboxylated to form dopamine, dopamine is hydroxylated to form norepinephrine, and norepinephrine is methylated to form epinephrine. The full-length cDNAs for all four enzymes have now been cloned, and the genetic aspects of these enzymes have been reviewed.[2] Recent advances in the molecular biology and genetics of these enzymes should lead to a greater understanding of the pathogenesis of Parkinson's disease and other neurologic disorders[3,4] and improve the utilization of adrenal transplantation in the treatment of Parkinson's disease.

0-8493-9430-9/96/$0.00+$.50
© 1996 by CRC Press, Inc.

Tyrosine[1] $\rightarrow$ DOPA[2] $\rightarrow$ Dopamine[3] $\rightarrow$ Norepinephrine[4] $\rightarrow$ Epinephrine

1. Tyrosine hydroxylase

2. aromatic-L-amino-acid decarboxylase

3. Dopamine-β-hydroxylase

4. Phenylethanolamine *N*-methyltransferase

FIGURE 1. Biosynthesis of epinephrine

TH is the rate-limiting enzyme in catecholamine synthesis and is affected by several regulatory factors. The human TH gene produces four mRNAs through splicing, and these multiple forms may participate in regulation of TH activity under physiologic and pathologic conditions.[5] It was recently shown that TH binds iron reversibly and that its catalytic activity is strictly dependent on this metal, whereas other ions were inhibitory.[6] A number of regulatory factors affect the synthesis or activity of TH and the regulatory mechanisms have been reviewed.[7,8] PNMT activity is induced by the adrenal corticosteroids, providing a functional basis for the anatomical association of cortex and medulla.[9] The regulation of biosynthetic enzymes is summarized in Table 1.

TABLE 1
Regulation of Catecholamine Biosynthetic Enzymes

Factor	Mechanism/Effect	References
Nerve growth factor	Induces transcription of TH gene; involves c-fos	10
GABA	Modulates expression of TH gene	11
cAMP-dependent protein kinases	Phosphorylation increases TH activity	12
Nicotine	Increased TH gene transcription via nicotinic receptor activation and other mechanisms	13
Secretin, VIP, atrial natriuretic peptide	Increase TH activity via cAMP-mediated phosphorylation	14, 15
VIP	Induces TH in PC12 cells	16
Ferrous ion	Activates the less active form of TH	17
Bioflavanoids	Quercetin inhibits TH activity *in vitro*	18
Bradykinin	Increases phosphorylation and activity of TH	19
Glucocorticoids	Regulates levels of TH and PNMT via cAMP	20
Glucocorticoids, nicotine	Brief pulse elevates PNMT after lag period	21
Angiotensin	Induces TH and PNMT mRNA via Ca-mediated activation of protein kinase C	22
Prolactin	Inhibits TH activity in cultured bovine chromaffin cells	23
Cytoskeletal G-actin	Increases TH activity *in vitro*	24
Cold stress	Increases TH mRNA and TH levels	25
Hypothyroidism	Decreases TH activity in developing rats	26

GABA, γ-aminobutyric acid; cAMP, cyclic adenosine monophosphate; VIP, vasoactive intestinal peptide; TH, tyrosine hydroxylase; PC12, pheochromocytoma (rat); PNMT, phenylethanolamine *N*-methyltransferase.

STIMULUS-SECRETION COUPLING

Chromaffin cells store catecholamines in membrane-bound organelles called chromaffin granules or vesicles. Stimulation of chromaffin cells with acetylcholine or nicotine induces a series of events leading to secretion of chromaffin granule contents in a process called exocytosis. These events include receptor activation, calcium entry, dissolution of the actin

Summary of Chromaffin Cell Exocytosis

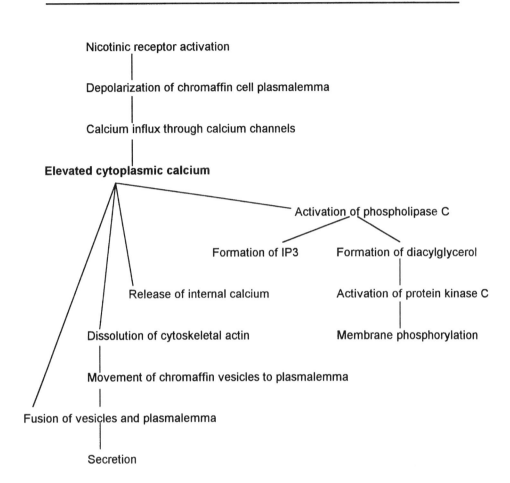

FIGURE 2.   Summary of chromaffin cell exocytosis. IP3, inositol-1,4,5-triphosphate.

network in the subplasmalemmal space, fusion of granule and cell membranes, and the release of granule contents into the extracellular space.[27] These events are summarized in Figure 2.

RECEPTORS

The cholinergic nicotinic receptor has long been regarded as the principal receptor mediating exocytosis in adrenal chromaffin cells,[28] although recent evidence suggests that the receptor may possess mixed nicotinic and muscarinic characteristics.[29] Although evidence gathered in the last decade has revealed that a number of other receptors on chromaffin cells mediate catecholamine secretion or modify nicotine-induced secretion, it is clear that nicotine stimulation releases a larger percentage of stored catecholamine than any other agonist. $GABA_B$ agonists,[30] histamine,[31] and glycine also produce a substantial secretory response,[2,32] whereas other agonists stimulate considerably less catecholamine secretion.[33] Glycine has been shown to preferentially release epinephrine from chromaffin cells.[30]

Aside from inducing basal catecholamine secretion, some agonists modulate nicotine-induced secretion. Atrial natriuretic peptide[34] and insulin growth factor[35] enhance nicotinic-mediated secretion, whereas chromostatin,[36] dopamine D_2,[37] $GABA_B$,[30] opioid,[38] prostaglandin

E_2 (PGE_2),[39] somatostatin,[40] and substance P[41] reduce nicotine-induced secretion. Substance P is believed to modulate the nicotinic receptor, possibly sequestering receptors so that they cannot respond to agonists.[42]

SECOND MESSENGERS: CALCIUM

The various receptors that mediate chromaffin cell catecholamine secretion via exocytosis appear to be linked with increased intracellular calcium. Secretion evoked by nicotinic stimulation can be abolished by removal of external calcium, thereby demonstrating that it is calcium entry, not release, from internal stores that primarily activates exocytosis.[28] Calcium accumulation is very rapid, precedes catecholamine secretion, and terminates earlier than exocytosis.[43] Calcium entry is also involved in the secretory effect of histamine and angiotensin II.[33] There is some evidence that intracellular calcium levels control the influx of calcium during the secretory process by modulating the activity of calcium channels.[44]

Calcium is believed to gain access to chromaffin cells mainly through L-type dihydropyridine-sensitive, voltage-dependent calcium channels, because entry is inhibited by calcium channel antagonists such as nifedipine and enhanced by calcium ionophores such as Bay-K-8644.[44,45] However, dihydropyridine antagonists do not completely inhibit nicotine-stimulated catecholamine secretion, and it has been found that chromaffin cells also possess dihydropyridine-insensitive, omega-conotoxin-sensitive calcium channels which contribute to the influx of calcium when cells are depolarized.[46,47] Angiotensin-induced secretion also involves an omega-conotoxin-sensitive pathway.[48] Video imaging of fura-2 loaded cells has revealed that the increased intracellular calcium due to calcium influx is initially localized to the subplasmalemmal space, then spreads into the interior to give a uniform elevation of calcium throughout the cytoplasm. Thereafter, the release of calcium from intracellular stores contributes to a second wave of intracellular calcium elevation.[49,50]

The release of calcium from internal stores after nicotinic stimulation is believed to be mediated by calcium itself (calcium-induced calcium release) and by inositol-1,4,5-triphosphate (IP_3), which is generated in chromaffin cells by the calcium-dependent activation of phospholipase C.[51] There is some evidence that the IP_3-sensitive store is associated with the endoplasmic reticulum, whereas the calcium-sensitive store is colocalized with a calcium-sequestering protein, calsequestrin, which is distributed throughout the cytoplasm.[52] These two calcium stores have been distinguished using caffeine and thapsigargin, which selectively release calcium from the calcium- and IP_3-sensitive stores, respectively.[53,54]

Histamine can stimulate chromaffin cell catecholamine secretion through activation of both H_1 and H_2 histamine receptors. H_1 receptor activation is accompanied by the accumulation of inositol triphosphates,[55] whereas H_2 activation elevates cyclic adenosine monophosphate (cAMP) levels.[56] In contrast to nicotinic stimulation, histamine H_1 receptor-mediated secretion appears to be dependent on the release of intracellular calcium at low histamine concentrations.[57] At higher histamine concentrations, both intracellular and extracellular calcium contributes to the secretory response.

EXOCYTOSIS

Although calcium is responsible for initiating exocytosis, the sequence of events that follow the entry of calcium into chromaffin cells has been unclear. Evidence has been gathered that suggests that calcium alters the subplasmalemmal cytoskeleton, whereby chromaffin granules gain access to exocytotic sites on the plasma membrane.[27] Chromaffin cells are particularly rich in cytoskeletal actin filaments, which form a continuous network connecting the secretory granules and the plasma membrane. Several calcium-regulated actin-binding proteins have been localized in the chromaffin cell periphery, suggesting that the organization of the actin network may be controlled by changes in intracellular calcium. These proteins include fodrin[58] and caldesmon,[59] which cross-link actin filaments into networks, and gelsolin,[60] which severs actin filaments. It has been proposed that calcium may inactivate fodrin and activate gelsolin so that the peripheral cytoplasm undergoes solation and the movement of secretory granules to the plasmalemma is facilitated.[27]

Other calcium-binding proteins localized in chromaffin cells include the annexins such as calpactin and synexin. These membrane-associating proteins are believed to have a role in the fusion of vesicle and plasma membranes during exocytosis. The roles of various calcium-binding proteins in exocytosis have been reviewed[61] and are summarized in Table 2.

TABLE 2
Calcium-Binding Proteins in Chromaffin Cell Exocytosis

Protein	Description	Mechanism	Proposed Effect(s)	References
Actin	Cytoskeletal protein	Calcium, protein kinase C promote disassembly	Cytoskeletal actin impedes exocytosis; F-actin disassembled during exocytosis	62, 63
Adseverin, gelsolin	Actin-binding proteins	Calcium-activated	Sever actin filaments, prevent actin gel formation	60, 64–66
Kinesin	Translocator protein	Requires adenosine triphosphate	Transports chromaffin vesicles on microtubules	67
Fodrin	Membrane protein		Membrane retrieval after exocytosis?	58, 68
p65, synaptophysin	Calmodulin-binding proteins of vesicles	Site of vesicle-membrane interaction	Mediate exocytosis	69, 70
Calmodulin	Calcium-binding protein	Mediates effects of calcium on exocytosis	Possible role in vesicle transport and membrane fusion	71
Annexins: calpactin, synexin, and others	Membrane-associating proteins	Calcium-mediated aggregation with membranes	Membrane fusion during exocytosis; regulation of cytoskeleton	72–76

There is some evidence that chromaffin cell stimulation leads to disassembly of actin filaments following calcium entry. Bader et al.[27] used fluorescent antibody techniques to visualize actin filaments and the inner membranes of secretory granules. They observed that chromaffin cell stimulation caused a complete loss of actin fluorescence accompanied by the appearance of granule membrane fluorescence on cell surfaces.

The sequence of morphologic changes associated with exocytosis has been studied with Normarski microscopy in living chromaffin cells using a video camera and image processor.[77] This technique revealed fusion of chromaffin granules and the plasma membrane, extrusion of granule contents, plasma membrane retrieval, and other events during exocytosis. Whereas the initial events of exocytosis occurred in less than 16 ms, membrane retrieval required more than 60 s. Another study used deep-etch electron microscopy and immunocytochemistry to provide evidence that calpactin I changes conformation so as to cross-link secretory granules and the plasma membrane during chromaffin cell stimulation.[78]

It has been possible to quantify catecholamine secretion produced by single exocytotic events in individual cultured bovine chromaffin cells using voltammetric microelectrodes.[79] This permitted secretion to be resolved into discrete packets of attomole quantities of catecholamines that were temporally localized in the millisecond range, and it was found that the secretory action of nicotine continued for a longer time period than that of other secretagogues.

The final phase of chromaffin cell catecholamine secretion is called endocytosis. Whereas exocytosis involves the incorporation of vesicular membrane into the plasma membrane, endocytosis reverses this process. Recent studies have begun to examine the role of calcium and nucleotide triphosphates in endocytosis. The results suggest that once exocytosis has begun, endocytosis can proceed in the absence of calcium or magnesium adenosine triphosphate (ATP).[80] Thus, endocytosis may be driven by exocytosis.

OTHER SECOND MESSENGERS

Although calcium has been established as the primary second messenger mediating catecholamine secretion in chromaffin cells, other messengers may have a secondary or modulating role. Cholinergic stimulation increases the levels of both cAMP and cyclic guanosine monophosphate (cGMP) in chromaffin cells. Although cAMP is a major activator of exocytosis in a number of cell types, some studies show that it inhibits nicotine-induced secretion in chromaffin cells.[81]

The GABA$_B$ agonist, baclofen, affects both basal and nicotine-induced catecholamine secretion. It induced a dose-dependent increase in basal chromaffin cell catecholamine secretion with a parallel increase in cAMP and calcium, whereas it markedly reduced catecholamine secretion and the intracellular calcium evoked by nicotinic stimulation.[82] The ability of cAMP to inactivate cholinergic nicotinic receptors by phosphorylation[83] may explain the inhibition of evoked catecholamine secretion by GABA$_B$ agonists. Cyclic GMP does not stimulate secretion but appears to potentiate secretion induced by low doses of nicotine.[56] The mechanism of this effect is unclear because cGMP did not affect intracellular calcium levels in chromaffin cells.

Other second messengers involved in chromaffin cell secretion include protein kinase C (PKC) and nitric oxide. PKC may have a modulatory role in regulating catecholamine secretion but does not appear to be required for secretion.[84,85] It is translocated from cytosol to membranes following cholinergic[86] or angiotensin II[48] activation of chromaffin cells, and there is evidence that it may phosphorylate membrane proteins that attenuate secretion.[87]

It has been reported recently by Moro et al. (see Ref. 93) that a variety of secretagogues activate the L-arginine:nitric oxide pathway in adrenal cells resulting in activation of cGMP, and it was postulated that cGMP may play a role in controlling local blood flow and the access of catecholamines to the systemic circulation. The role of various second messengers in chromaffin cell stimulus-secretion coupling is summarized in Table 3.

TABLE 3
Second Messengers in Chromaffin Cell Stimulus-Secretion Coupling

Receptors	Second Messenger	Mechanism/Effect	References
Nicotinic, histamine H$_1$, angiotensin II, bradykinin, methacholine, prostaglandin E$_2$	Inositol triphosphate	Releases internal calcium	88
Muscarinic, angiotensin II, bradykinin, natriuretic peptides	cGMP	Affects nicotinic-induced secretion, vasodilation	89, 90
Various	Protein kinase C	Inhibits histamine- and muscarine-evoked secretion; potentiates bradykinin secretion	91
Histamine H$_2$, nicotinic	cAMP	Facilitates or inhibits catecholamine release	92
Methacholine, DMPP	Nitric oxide	Activates guanylate cyclase	93

DMPP, dimethylphenylpiperazinium.

Cholinergic stimulation of chromaffin cells evokes the release of catecholamines, chromogranins, peptides, and other components of the chromaffin granules. A study of the relative magnitude of the secretion of several catecholamines and peptides from canine adrenal medulla indicates that epinephrine and dopamine secretion is much greater than norepinephrine under resting conditions, whereas dopamine secretion is much greater than epinephrine and norepinephrine during nicotinic stimulation.[94] This finding may have significant implications for the use of chromaffin cell transplantation as a means of replacing the dopamine deficiency associated with Parkinson's disease. It may be possible to use transdermal nicotine administration to augment the release of dopamine from adrenal tissue transplanted to the striatum.

ADRENAL MEDULLA TRANSPLANTATION

There has been an explosion of research on neural and adrenal medullary transplantation over the last 10 years. Much of the impetus for this research derives from studies showing that the motor deficits of animal models of Parkinson's disease could be improved by intracerebral grafting of neural[95] or adrenal medullary tissue.[96] The principal objective of transplantation has been to restore brain function in degenerative diseases, but other potential applications of adrenal medullary transplantation have also been investigated (Table 4).

TABLE 4
Novel Applications of Adrenal Medullary Transplantation

Application	Source of AM	Site Implanted	Effects Observed	Comment	References
Antidepressant activity	Rat, adult	Rat frontal cortex	Increased NE levels	Grafts survived and produced monoamines	97
Terminal cancer pain	Human	Spinal subarachnoid space	Increased CSF enkephalin and catecholamines	Decreased pain scores; reduced opioid intake	98
Motor impairment in aging	Rat, adult	Rat, caudate	Improved motor coordination	Used uphill beam test	99

AM, adrenal medulla; NE, norepinephrine; CSF, cerebrospinal fluid.

Animal and human studies have examined the functional mechanisms underlying the recovery of motor function in experimental or idiopathic parkinsonism, and much information has been obtained concerning factors that enhance graft viability. Nishino[100] recently reviewed studies on intracerebral grafting of catecholamine-producing cells, including the sequence of functional changes that contribute to the restoration of deteriorated brain function, and these are summarized in Table 5. The initial survival and growth of grafts is one of the most crucial factors leading to functional improvement. Yet, several postmortem analyses of brains of patients who received adrenal medullary grafts found that most of the graft tissue was necrotic and only a few adrenal medullary cells had survived.[101,102] In other postmortem studies, TH staining was negative[103] or sparse.[104,105]

TABLE 5
Stages of Graft Survival and Function

Stage	Functions
I—Survival and growth	Catecholamine synthesis and release; receptor up-regulation normalized; reuptake transporters expressed
II—Reconstruction of neural networks	Neural regulation and feedback regulation established
III—Grafts release trophic substances	Neurite outgrowth; enhanced regeneration and survival
IV—Expression of substrate molecules	Provide guidance, footing, or bridge for extended axonal growth

These findings have provided indirect support for the trophic hypothesis for the behavioral recovery produced by adrenal medullary grafts in Parkinsonian patients. This hypothesis proposes that neurotrophic factors produced by adrenal cells enhance the survival and regeneration of host neurons and is directly supported by evidence that adrenal grafts to the striatum

TABLE 6
Factors Affecting Adrenal Medulla Graft Survival

Factor	Source of AM Cells	Site Implanted	Results	Comments	References
Immunoisolation of AM cells	Bovine, encapsulated cells	Rat, spinal cord	Prevented graft rejection	Cells released catecholamines and opioid peptides	108
Chromaffin cell isolation	Bovine, cells isolated *in vitro*	Rat, intrastriatal	Isolated chromaffin cell grafts survived up to 2 months	Nonchromaffin cells appeared to decrease chromaffin cell survival	109
Peripheral nerve cograft	Mouse	Mouse, striatum	Enhanced recovery of nigrostriatal function	Striatal dopamine increased	110
Intercostal nerve cograft	Human, autologous	Human, striatum	Motor scores improved for up to 12 months	Longer follow-up needed	111
NGF injection	Mouse	Mouse, putamen	Increased graft survival and volume	Some chromaffin cells transformed into neurons	112
Precavitaton surgery	Human, autologous	Human, caudate	Patients improved more than those without precavitation	Transplanted cells responded to NGF	113
Intermediate transplantation to the omentum	Rat, autologous	Rat, great omentum	Cells survived and produced catecholamines for 16 weeks	All grafts became densely vascularized	114
Presurgical perfusion and dissection of AM	Human, autologous	Human, caudate	Improvement stabilized at 7 months with decreased L-DOPA dosage required	Improvement maintained up to 18 months	115

AM, adrenal medulla; NGF, nerve growth factor.

of Parkinsonian mice and monkeys increases TH immunoreactivity and catecholamine fluorescence in tissue surrounding the grafts.[106] Moreover, the adrenal tissue used for grafting in a Parkinsonian patient was found to express β-NGF (nerve growth factor) mRNA, suggesting that β-NGF may have a role in the clinical improvement that follows grafting.[107]

Several techniques have been studied to improve the survival and function of adrenal medullary grafts, including the transplantation of isolated chromaffin cells, the encapsulation of transplanted cells, and the cografting of peripheral nerve tissue to provide a source of NGF (Table 6). Some of these studies suggest that nonchromaffin cells may reduce chromaffin survival by stimulating immunologic mechanisms leading to graft rejection, and that isolation of chromaffin cells before transplantation or by encapsulating transplanted cells may prevent rejection. The putative role of NGF after peripheral nerve cografts is supported by a recent study showing that NGF injection at the time of adrenal medulla transplantation increased the survival rate and volume of adrenal grafts and enhanced the transformation of chromaffin cells into neurons.

Several surgical techniques also show promise of enhancing graft viability. These include surgical precavitation and intermediate transplantation to the omentum.

REFERENCES

1. **Tsapatsaris, N. P. and Breslin, D. J.,** Physiology of the adrenal medulla, *Urol. Clin. North Am.*, 16, 439, 1989.
2. **Weinshilboum, R. M.,** Catecholamine biochemical genetics, in *Catecholamines II: Handbook of Experimental Pharmacology, Vol. 90/II*, Trendelenburg, U. and Weiner, N., Eds., Springer-Verlag, Berlin, 1989, 391.
3. **Nagatsu, T.,** Genes for human catecholamine-synthesizing enzymes, *Neurosci. Res.*, 12, 315, 1991.
4. **Nagatsu, T.,** Tyrosine hydroxylase in relation to Parkinson's disease: a historical overview and future prospect, in *Parkinson's Disease: From Clinical Aspects to Molecular Basis*, Nagatsu, T., Narabayashi, H., and Yoshida, M., Eds., Springer-Verlag, Berlin, 1991, 1.
5. **Nagatsu, T.,** The human tyrosine hydroxylase gene, *Cell. Mol. Neurobiol.*, 9, 313, 1989.
6. **Haavik, J., Le Bourdellès, Martínez, A, Flatmark, T., and Mallet, J.,** Recombinant human tyrosine hydroxylase isozymes: reconstitution with iron and inhibitory effect of other metal ions, *Eur. J. Biochem.*, 199, 371, 1991.
7. **Zigmond, R. E.,** A comparison of the long-term and short-term regulations of tyrosine hydroxylase activity, *J. Physiol. (Paris)*, 83, 267, 1988.
8. **Zigmond, R. E., Schwarzschild, M. A., and Rittenhouse, A. R.,** Acute regulation of tyrosine hydroxylase by nerve activity and by neurotransmitters via phosphorylation, *Annu. Rev. Neurosci.*, 12, 415, 1989.
9. **Carmichael, S. W.,** What is a ganglion doing inside a gland? *IBRO News*, 17, 6, 1989.
10. **Gizang-Ginsberg, E. and Ziff, E. B.,** Nerve growth factor regulates tyrosine hydroxylase gene transcription through a nucleoprotein complex that contains c-fos, *Genes Dev.*, 4, 477, 1990.
11. **Strong, R., Hale, C., Moore, M. A., Wessels-Reiker, M., Armbrecht, H. J., and Richardson, A.,** GABA receptor modulation of tyrosine hydroxylase gene expression in the rat adrenal gland, *Neurosci. Lett.*, 117, 175, 1990.
12. **Mena, M. A., Casavejos, M. J., Bonin, A., Ramos, J. A., and Garcia-Yebenes, J.,** Effects of dibutyryl cyclic AMP and retinoic acid on the differentiation of dopamine neurons: prevention of cell death by dibutyryl cyclic AMP, *J. Neurochem.*, 65, 2612, 1995.
13. **Fossom, L. H., Carlson, C. D., and Tank, A. W.,** Stimulation of tyrosine hydroxylase gene transcription rate by nicotine in rat adrenal medulla, *Mol. Pharmacol.*, 40, 193, 1991.
14. **Roskoski, R., Jr., White, L., Knowlton, R., and Roskoski, L. M.,** Regulation of tyrosine hydroxylase activity in rat PC12 cells by neuropeptides of the secretin family, *Mol. Pharmacol.*, 36, 925, 1989.
15. **Yanagihara, N., Okazaki, M., Terao, T., Uezono, Y., Wada, A., and Izumi, F.,** Stimulatory effects of brain natriuretic peptide on cyclic GMP accumulation and tyrosine hydroxylase activity in cultured bovine adrenal medullary cells, *Naunyn-Schmied. Arch. Pharmacol.*, 343, 289, 1991.
16. **Wessels-Reiker, M., Haycock, J. W., Howlett, A. C., and Strong, R.,** Vasoactive intestinal polypeptide induces tyrosine hydroxylase in PC12 cells, *J. Biol. Chem.*, 266, 9347, 1991.
17. **Ishii, A., Kiuchi, K., Matsuyama, M., Satake, T., and Nagatsu, T.,** Ferrous ion activates the less active form of human adrenal tyrosine hydroxylase, *Neurochem. Int.*, 16, 59, 1990.
18. **Morita, K., Teraoka, K., Oka, M., and Azuma, M.,** Effect of hypoglycemic sulfonylurea, glibenclamide, on the rate of catecholamine synthesis in cultured adrenal chromaffin cells, *Biochem. Pharmacol.*, 39, 976, 1990.
19. **Houchi, H., Masserano, J. M., Bowyer, J. F., and Weiner, N.,** Regulation of tyrosine hydroxylase activity in pheochromocytoma PC12 cells by bradykinin, *Mol. Pharmacol.*, 37, 104, 1990.
20. **Stachowiak, M. K., Hong, J.-S., and Viveros, O. H.,** Coordinate and differential regulation of phenylethanolamine N-methyltransferase, tyrosine hydroxylase and proenkephalin messenger RNAs by neural and hormonal mechanisms in cultured bovine adrenal medullary cells, *Brain Res.*, 510, 277, 1990.
21. **Betito, K., Diorio, J., and Boksa, P.,** Brief cortisol exposure elevates adrenal phenylethanolamine N-methyltransferase after a necessary lag period, *Eur. J. Pharmacol.*, 238, 273, 1993.
22. **Stachowiak, M. K., Jiang, H.-K., Poisner, A. M., Tuominen, R. K., and Hong, J.-S.,** Short and long term regulation of catecholamine biosynthetic enzymes by angiotensin in cultured adrenal medullary cells: molecular mechanisms and nature of second-messenger systems, *J. Biol. Chem.*, 265, 4694, 1990.
23. **Hernández, M. L., de Miguel, R., Ramos, J. A., and Fernández-Ruiz, J. J.,** Prolactin inhibits the activity of tyrosine hydroxylase in cultured bovine adrenal chromaffin cells in a dose-dependent manner, *Brain Res.*, 528, 175, 1990.
24. **Morita, K., Nakanishi, A., and Oka M.,** In vitro activation of bovine adrenal tyrosine hydroxylase by rabbit skeletal muscle actin: evidence for a possible role of cytoskeletal elements as an activator for cytoplasmic enzymes, *Biochim. Biophys. Acta*, 993, 21, 1989.
25. **Baruchin, A., Weisberg, E. P., Miner, L. L., Ennis, D., Nisenbaum, L. K., Naylor, E., Stricker, E. M., Zigmond, M. J., and Kaplan, B. B.,** Effects of cold exposure on rat adrenal tyrosine hydroxylase: an analysis of RNA, protein, enzyme activity and cofactor levels, *J. Neurochem.*, 54, 1769, 1990.
26. **Blouquit, M. F., Valens, M., Bagayoko, A., and Gripois, D.,** Adrenal tyrosine hydroxylase activation in the developing rat: influence of the thyroid status, *J. Dev. Physiol.*, 14, 325, 1990.

27. **Bader, M.-F., Simon, J.-P., Sontag, J.-M., Langley, K., and Aunis, D.,** Role of calcium in the secretion and synthesis in bovine adrenal chromaffin cells, *Adv. Exp. Med. Biol.*, 269, 93, 1990.

28. **Burgoyne, R. D.,** Control of exocytosis in adrenal chromaffin cells, *Biochim. Biophys. Acta*, 1071, 174, 1991.

29. **Shirvan, M. H., Pollard, H. B., and Heldman, E.,** Mixed nicotinic and muscarinic features of cholinergic receptor coupled to secretion in bovine chromaffin cells, *Proc. Natl. Acad. Sci. U.S.A.*, 88, 4860, 1991.

30. **Castro, E., Oset-Gasque, M. J., and González, M. P.,** GABA_A and GABA_B receptors are functionally active in the regulation of catecholamine secretion by bovine chromaffin cells, *J. Neurosci. Res.*, 23, 290, 1989.

31. **Noble, E. P., Bommer, M., Liebisch, D., and Herz, A.,** H1-histaminergic activation of catecholamine release by chromaffin cells, *Biochem. Pharmacol.*, 15, 37, 1988.

32. **Yadid, G., Maor, G., Youdim, M. B. H., Silberman, M., and Zinder, O.,** Autoradiographic localization of strychnine-sensitive glycine receptor in bovine adrenal medulla, *Neurochem. Res.*, 18, 1051, 1993.

33. **O'Sullivan, A. J. and Burgoyne, R. D.,** A comparison of bradykinin, angiotensin II and muscarinic stimulation of cultured bovine adrenal chromaffin cells, *Biosci. Rep.*, 9, 243, 1989.

34. **O'Sullivan, A. J. and Burgoyne, R. D.,** Cyclic GMP regulates nicotine-induced secretion from cultured bovine adrenal chromaffin cells: effects of 8-bromo-cyclic GMP, atrial natriuretic peptide, and nitroprusside (nitric oxide), *J. Neurochem.*, 54, 1805, 1990.

35. **Dahmer, M. K. and Perlman, R. L.,** Bovine chromaffin cells have insulin-like growth factor-I (IGF) receptors: IGF-I enhances catecholamine secretion, *J. Neurochem.*, 51, 321, 1988.

36. **Galindo, E., Rill, A., Bader, M.-F., and Aunis, D.,** Chromostatin, a 20-amino acid peptide derived from chromogranin A, inhibits chromaffin cell secretion, *Proc. Natl. Acad. Sci. U.S.A.*, 88, 1426, 1991.

37. **Bigornia, L., Suozzo, M., Ryan, K., Napp, D., and Schneider, A. S.,** Dopamine receptors on adrenal chromaffin cells modulate calcium uptake and catecholamine release, *J. Neurochem.*, 51, 999, 1988.

38. **Lemaire, S., Livett, B. G., Tseng, R., Mercier, P., and Lemaire, I.,** Studies on the inhibitory action of opiate compounds in isolated bovine adrenal chromaffin cells: noninvolvement of stereospecific opiate binding sites, *J. Neurochem.*, 36, 886, 1981.

39. **Karapalis, A. C., Funk, C. D., and Powell, W. S.,** Binding of prostaglandin E2 to cultured bovine adrenal chromaffin cells and its effect on catecholamine secretion, *Biochim. Biophys. Acta*, 1010, 369, 1989.

40. **Mizobe, F., Kozousek, V., Dean, D. M., and Livett, B. G.,** Pharmacological characterization of adrenal paraneurons: substance P and somatostatin as inhibitory modulators of the nicotinic response, *Brain Res.*, 178, 555, 1979.

41. **Role, L. W., Leeman, S. E., and Perlman, R. L.,** Somatostatin and substance P inhibit catecholamine secretion from isolated cells of guinea-pig adrenal medulla, *Neuroscience*, 6, 1813, 1981.

42. **Kent-Baun, J. A., Lyford, L. K., Gross, D. J., and Westhead, E. W.,** Effects of substance P on secretion of catecholamines from populations of bovine chromaffin cells and on calcium transients in individual cells, *Ann. N.Y. Acad. Sci.*, 632, 241, 1991.

43. **Artalejo, C. R., Bader, M. F., Aunis, D., and Garcia, A. G.,** Inactivation of the early calcium uptake and noradrenaline release evoked by potassium in cultured chromaffin cells, *Biochem. Biophys. Res. Commun.*, 134, 1, 1986.

44. **Artalejo, C. R., Garcia, A. G., and Aunis, D.,** Chromaffin cell calcium channel kinetics measured isotopically through fast calcium, strontium, and barium fluxes, *J. Biol. Chem.*, 262, 915, 1987.

45. **Ceña, V., Stutzin, A., and Rojas, E.,** Effects of calcium and Bay K-8644 on calcium currents in adrenal medullary chromaffin cells, *J. Membr. Biol.*, 112, 255, 1989.

46. **Bansal, M. K., Philips, J. H., and Van Heyningen, S.,** The inhibition by pertussis and tetanus toxins of evoked catecholamine release from intact and permeabilized bovine adrenal chromaffin cells, *FEBS Lett.*, 276, 165, 1990.

47. **Rosario, L. M., Soria, B., Feuerstein, G., and Pollard, H. B.,** Voltage-sensitive calcium flux into bovine chromaffin cells occurs through dihydropyridine-sensitive and dihydropyridine- and omega-conotoxin-insensitive pathways, *Neuroscience*, 29, 735, 1989.

48. **McMillian, M. K., Hudson, P. M., Suh, H. H., Ye, H., Tuominne, R. K., and Hong, J. S.,** Role of omega-conotoxin GVIA-sensitive calcium entry in angiotensin II-stimulated [^{3}H]phorbol 12, 13-dibutyrate binding in bovine adrenal medullary cells, *J. Neurochem.*, 61, 93, 1993.

49. **Cheek, T. R., Jackson, T. R., O'Sullivan, A. J., Moreton, R. B., Berridge, M. J., and Burgoyne, R. D.,** Simultaneous measurements of cytosolic calcium and secretion in single bovine adrenal chromaffin cells by fluorescent imaging of fura-2 in cocultured cells, *J. Cell Biol.*, 109, 1219, 1989.

50. **Burgoyne, R. D.,** Control of exocytosis in adrenal chromaffin cells, *Biochim. Biophys. Acta*, 1071, 174, 1991.

51. **Eberhard, D. A. and Holz, R. W.,** Cholinergic stimulation of inositol phosphate formation in bovine adrenal chromaffin cells: distinct nicotinic and muscarinic mechanisms, *J. Neurochem.*, 49, 1634, 1987.

52. **Vilmart-Seuwen, J., Kersken, H., Stürzl, R., and Plattner, H.,** ATP keeps exocytosis sites in a primed state but is not required for membrane fusion: an analysis of Paramecium cells in vitro and in vivo, *J. Cell Biol.*, 103, 1279, 1986.

53. **Cheek, T. R., O'Sullivan, A. J., Moreton, R. B., Berridge, M. J., and Burgoyne, R. D.,** The caffeine-sensitive Ca2+ store in bovine adrenal chromaffin cells: an examination of its role in triggering secretion and Ca2+ homeostasis, *FEBS Lett.*, 266, 91, 1990.

54. **Robinson, I. A. and Burgoyne, R. D.,** Characterisation of distinct inositol 1,4,5-triphosphate-sensitive and caffeine-sensitive calcium stores in digitonin-permeabilised adrenal chromaffin cells, *J. Neurochem.*, 56, 1587, 1991.

55. **Noble, E. P., Bommer, M., Leibisch, D., and Herz, A.,** H_1-histaminergic activation of catecholamine release by chromaffin cells, *Biochem. Pharmacol.*, 37, 221, 1988.

56. **Marley, P. D., Thomson, K. A., Jachno, K., and Johnston, M. J.,** Histamine-induced increases in cyclic AMP levels in bovine adrenal medullary cells, *Br. J. Pharmacol.*, 104, 839, 1991.

57. **Borges, R.,** Ionic mechanisms involved in the secretory effects of histamine in the rat adrenal medulla, *Eur. J. Pharmacol.*, 241, 189, 1993.

58. **Langley, O. K., Perrin, D., and Aunis, D.,** Alpha-fodrin in the adrenal gland: localization by immunoelectron microscopy, *J. Histochem. Cytochem.*, 34, 517, 1986.

59. **Burgoyne, R. D., Cheek, T. R., and Norman, K. M.,** Identification of a secretory granule-binding protein as caldesmon, *Nature*, 319, 68, 1986.

60. **Sontag, J. M., Aunis, D., and Bader, M. F.,** Peripheral actin filaments control calcium-mediated catecholamine release from streptolysin-O-permeabilized chromaffin cells, *Eur. J. Cell Biol.*, 46, 316, 1988.

61. **Südhof, T. C. and Jahn, R.,** Proteins of synaptic vesicles involved in exocytosis and membrane recycling, *Neuron*, 6, 665, 1991.

62. **Burgoyne, R. D., Morgan, A., and O'Sullivan A. J.,** The control of cytoskeletal actin and exocytosis in intact and permeabilized adrenal chromaffin cells: role of calcium and protein kinase C, *Cell Signal.*, 1, 323, 1989.

63. **Vitale, M.-L., Rodriguez del Castillo, A., Tchakarov, L., and Trifaro, J.-M.,** Cortical filamentous actin disassembly and scinderin redistribution during chromaffin cell stimulation precede exocytosis, a phenomenon not exhibited by gelsolin, *J. Cell Biol.*, 113, 1057, 1991.

64. **Tchakarov, L., Vitale, M.-L., Jeyapragasan, A., Rodriguez del Castillo, A., and Trifaro, J.-M.,** Expression of scinderin, an actin filament-severing protein, in different tissues, *FEBS Lett.*, 268, 209, 1990.

65. **Maekawa, S. and Sakai, H.,** Inhibition of actin regulatory activity of the 74-kDa protein from bovine adrenal medulla (adseverin) by some phospholipids, *J. Biol. Chem.*, 265, 10940, 1990.

66. **Sakurai, T., Kurokawa, H., and Nonomura, Y.,** The calcium-dependent actin filament-severing activity of a 74-kDa protein (adseverin) resides in its NH_2-terminal half, *J. Biol. Chem.*, 266, 4581, 1991.

67. **Urrutia, R., McNiven, M. A., Albanesi, J. P., Murphy, D. B., and Kachar, B.,** Purified kinesin promotes vesicle motility and induces active sliding between microtubules *in vitro*, *Proc. Natl. Acad. Sci. U.S.A.*, 88, 6701, 1991.

68. **Fujimoto, T. and Ogawa, K.,** Retrieving vesicles in secretion-induced rat chromaffin cells contain fodrin, *J. Histochem. Cytochem.*, 37, 1589, 1989.

69. **Trifaró, J.-M., Fournier, S., and Novas, M. L.,** The p65 protein is a calmodulin-binding protein present in several types of secretory vesicles, *Neuroscience*, 29, 1, 1989.

70. **Schmidle, T. R., Weiler, R., Desnos, C., Scherman, D., Fischer-Colbrie, R., Floor, E., and Winkler, H.,** Synaptic/synaptophysin, p65 and SV2: their presence in adrenal chromaffin granules and sympathetic large dense core vesicles, *Biochim. Biophys. Acta*, 1060, 251, 1991.

71. **Trifaró, J.-M. and Fournier, S.,** Calmodulin and chromaffin cell secretion, in *Progress in Catecholamine Research, Part A: Basic Aspects and Peripheral Mechanisms*, Dahlström, A, Belmaker, R. H., and Sandler, M., Eds., Alan R. Liss, New York, 1988, 257.

72. **Burgoyne, R. D. and Geisow, M. J.,** The annexin family of calcium-binding proteins, *Cell Calcium*, 10, 1, 1989.

73. **Burgoyne, R. D. and Morgan, A.,** Evidence for a role of calpactin in calcium-dependent exocytosis, *Biochem. Soc. Trans.*, 18, 1101, 1990.

74. **Drust, D. S. and Creutz, C. E.,** Differential subcellular distribution of p36 (the heavy chain of calpactin I) and other annexins in the adrenal medulla, *J. Neurochem.*, 56, 469, 1991.

75. **Zaks, W. J. and Creutz, C. E.,** Annexin-chromaffin granule membrane interactions: a comparative study of synexin, p32 and p67, *Biochim. Biophys. Acta*, 1029, 149, 1990.

76. **Jones, P. G., Damni, A., and Waisman, D. M.,** Inability of annexin-II tetramer to stimulate exocytosis in detergent permeabilized adrenal-medullary cells, *FASEB J.*, 8, A1315, 1994.

77. **Terakawa, S., Fan, J. H., Kumakura, K., and Ohara-Imaizumi, M.,** Quantitative analysis of exocytosis directly visualized in living chromaffin cells, *Neurosci. Lett.*, 123, 82, 1991.

78. **Nakata, T., Sobue, K., and Hirokawa, N.,** Conformational change and localization of calpactin I complex involved in exocytosis as revaled by quick-freeze, deep-etch electron microscopy and immunocytochemistry, *J. Cell Biol.*, 110, 13, 1990.

79. **Leszczyszyn, D. J., Jankowski, J. A., Viveros, O. H., Diliberto, E. J., Near, J. A., and Wightman, R. M.,** Secretion of catecholamines from individual adrenal medullary chromaffin cells, *J. Neurochem.*, 56, 1855, 1991.

80. **von Grafenstein, H. and Knight, D. E.,** Triggered exocytosis and endocytosis have different requirements for calcium and nucleotides in bovine chromaffin cells, *J. Membr. Biol.*, 134, 1, 1993.

81. **Cheek, T. R. and Burgoyne, R. D.,** Cyclic AMP inhibits both nicotine-induced actin disassembly and catecholamine secretion from bovine adrenal chromaffin cells, *J. Biol. Chem.*, 262, 11663, 1987.

82. **Oset-Gasque, M. J., Parramon, M., and Gonzalez, M. P.,** GABAB receptors modulate catecholamine secretion in chromaffin cells by a mechanism involving cyclic AMP formation, *Br. J. Pharmacol.*, 110, 1586, 1993.

83. **Alburquerque, E. X., Deshpande, S. S., Aravaca, Y., Alkondon, M., and Daly, J. M.,** A possible involvement of cyclic AMP in the expression of desensitization of the nicotinic acetylcholine receptor, *FEBS Lett.*, 199, 113, 1986.

84. **Terbush, D. R. and Holz, R. W.,** Activation of protein kinase C is not required for exocytosis from bovine adrenal chromaffin cells: the effects of protein kinase C(19-31), Ca/CaM kinase II(291-317), and staurosporine, *J. Biol. Chem.*, 265, 21179, 1990.

85. **Tachikawa, E., Takahashi, S., and Kashimoto, T.,** p-Chloromercuribenzoate causes Ca2+-dependent exocytotic catecholamine secretion from cultured bovine adrenal medullary cells, *J. Neurochem.*, 53, 19, 1989.

86. **Messing, R. O., Stevens, A. M., Kiyasu, E., and Sneade, A. B.,** Nicotinic and muscarinic agonists stimulate rapid protein kinase C translocation in PC12 cells, *J. Neurosci.*, 9, 507, 1989.

87. **Wilson, S. P.,** Regulation of chromaffin cell secretion and protein kinase C activity by chronic phorbol ester treatment, *J. Biol. Chem.*, 265, 648, 1990.

88. **Ito, S., Mochizuki-Oda, N., Hori, K., Ozaki, K., Miyakawa, A., and Negishi, M.,** *J. Neurochem.*, 56, 531, 1991.

89. **Schneider, A. S., Cline, H. T., and Lemaire, S.,** Rapid rise in cGMP accompanies catecholamine secretion in suspension of isolated adrenal chromaffin cells, *Life Sci.*, 24, 1389, 1979.

90. **Waldman, S. A., Rapoport, R. M., Fiscus, R. R., and Murad, F.,** Effects of atriopeptin on particulate guanylate cyclase from rat adrenal, *Biochim. Biophys. Acta*, 845, 298, 1985.

91. **Warashina, A. and Fujiwara, N.,** Differential effects of protein kinase C activation on catecholamine secretions evoked by stimulations of various receptors in the rat adrenal medulla, *Neurosci. Lett.*, 129, 181, 1991.

92. **Keogh, R. and Marley, P. D.,** Regulation of cyclic AMP levels by calcium in bovine adrenal medullary cells, *J. Neurochem.*, 57, 1721, 1991.

93. **Moro, M. A., Michelena, P., Sánchez-García, P., Palmer, R., Moncada, S., and García, A. G.,** Activation of adrenal medullary L-arginine: nitric oxide pathway by stimuli which induce the release of catecholamines, *Eur. J. Pharmacol.*, 246, 213, 1993.

94. **Chritton, S. L., Dousa, M. K., Yaksh, T. L., and Tyce, G. M.,** Nicotinic- and muscarinic-evoked release of canine adrenal catecholamines and peptides, *Am. J. Physiol.*, 260, R589, 1991.

95. **Bjorklund, A. and Stenevi, U.,** Reconstruction of the nigrostriatal dopamine pathway by intracerebral nigral transplants, *Brain Res.*, 177, 555, 1979.

96. **Freed, W. J., Morihisa, J. M., Karoum, F., Seiger, A., Olson, L., Hoffer, L., and Wyatt, R. J.,** Transplanted adrenal chromaffin cells in rat brain reduce lesion-induced rotational behaviour, *Nature*, 292, 351, 1981.

97. **Sortwell, C. E. and Sagen, J.,** Induction of antidepressive activity by monoaminergic transplants in rat neocortex, *Pharmacol. Biochem. Behav.*, 46, 225, 1993.

98. **Winnie, A. P., Pappas, G. D., Gupta, T. K., Wang, H., Ortega, J. D., and Sagen, J.,** Subarachnoid adrenal medullary transplants for terminal cancer pain, *Anesthesiology*, 79, 644, 1993.

99. **García-Hernández, F., Pacheco-Cano, M. T., and Drucker-Colín, R.,** Reduction of motor impairment by adrenal medulla transplants in aged rats, *Physiol. Behav.*, 54, 589, 1993.

100. **Nishino, H.,** Intracerebral grafting of catecholamine producing cells and reconstruction of disturbed brain function, *Neurosci. Res.*, 16, 157, 1993.

101. **Hurtig, H., Joyce, J. N., Sladek, J. R., and Trojanowski, J. Q.,** Postmortem analysis of adrenal-medulla-to-caudate autograft in a patient with Parkinson's disease, *Ann. Neurol.*, 25, 607, 1989.

102. **Peterson, D. I., Price, M. L., and Small, C. S.,** Autopsy findings in a patient who had an adrenal-to-brain transplant for Parkinson's disease, *Neurology* 39, 235, 1989.

103. **Waters, C. H., Itabashi, H. H., Apuzzo, M. L. J., and Weiner, L. P.,** Adrenal to caudate transplantation: postmortem study, *Movement Disorders*, 5, 248, 1990.

104. **Kordower, J. H., Cochran, E., Penn, R. D., and Goetz, C. G.,** Putative chromaffin cell survival and enhanced host-derived TH-fiber innervation following a functional adrenal medulla autograft for Parkinson's disease, *Ann. Neurol.*, 29, 405, 1991.

105. **Hirsch, E. C., Duyckaerts, C., Javoy-Agid, F., Hauw, J.-J., and Agid, Y.,** Does adrenal graft enhance recovery of dopaminergic neurons in Parkinson's disease? *Ann. Neurol.*, 27, 676, 1990.

106. **Bohn, M. C., Cupit, L. C., Marciano, F., and Gash, D. M.,** Adrenal medulla grafts enhance recovery of striatal dopaminergic fibers, *Science*, 237, 913, 1987.

107. **Silani, V., Pizzuti, A., Falini, A., Borsani, G., Rugarli, E. I., Melo, C. A., Sidoli, A., Fillani, F., Baralle, F., and Scarlato, G.,** Beta-nerve growth factor mRNA expression in the parkinsonian adrenal gland, *Exp. Neurol.*, 113, 166, 1991.

108. **Sagen, J., Wang, H., Tresco, P. A., and Aebischer, P.,** Transplants of immunologically isolated xenogeneic chromaffin cells provide a long-term source of pain-reducing neuroactive substances, *J. Neurosci.*, 13, 2415, 1993.

109. **Schueler, S. B., Ortega, J. D., Sagen, J., and Kordower, J. H.,** Robust survival of isolated bovine adrenal chromaffin cells following intrastriatal transplantation: a novel hypothesis of adrenal graft viability, *J. Neurosci.*, 13, 4496, 1993.

110. **Date, I., Yoshimoto, Y., Gohda, Y., Furuta, T., Asari, S., and Ohmoto, T.,** Long-term effects of cografts of pretransected peripheral nerve with adrenal medulla in animal models of Parkinson's disease, *Neurosurgery*, 33, 685, 1993.

111. **Watts, R. L., Goetz, C., Graham, S., Zakers, G. O., Bakay, R. A., Stebbins, G. T., and Penn, R. D.,** Autologous intrastriatal adrenal medulla/nerve cografts in Parkinson's disease: early results, *Neurology*, 43, A222, 1993.

112. **Jousselin-Hosaja, M.,** A descriptive and quantitative morphometric study of long-term mouse adrenal medulla grafts implanted into the putamen: effect of nerve growth factor injected at grafting, *Brain Res.*, 627, 275, 1993.

113. **Pezzoli, G., Motti, E. D. F., Zecchinelli, A., Ferrante, C., Silani, V., Falini, A., Pizzuti, A., Mulazzi, D., Baratta, P., Vegeto, A., Villani, R., and Scarlato, G.,** Adrenal medulla autograft in 3 parkinsonian patients: results using 2 different approaches, *Prog. Brain Res.*, 82, 677, 1990.

114. **Mendelowitsch, A., Zhang, T.-M., Vereczkey, C., Gratzl, M., and Gratzl, O.,** Long-term survival of autologous adrenal medulla grafts in the great omentum of the rat, *Neurol. Res.*, 15, 269, 1993.

115. **López-Lozano, J. J., Bravo, G., Abascal, J., and CPH Neural Transplantation Group,** A long-term study of Parkinson's patients subjected to autoimplants of perfused adrenal medulla into the caudate nucleus, *Transplant. Proc.*, 22, 2243, 1990.

Chapter 2

CONGENITAL ADRENAL HYPERPLASIA

Perrin C. White and Phyllis W. Speiser

CONTENTS

INTRODUCTION

Congenital adrenal hyperplasia (CAH) is caused by defects in the genes encoding any of the five enzymes that contribute to the synthesis of cortisol from cholesterol in the adrenal cortex (Figure 1). Adrenal hyperplasia refers to glandular enlargement caused by excessive secretion of adrenocorticotropin compensating for inadequate cortisol synthesis. Another name for the syndrome is "adrenogenital syndrome," referring to the commonly associated ambiguity of female external genitalia due to altered adrenal androgen production. Particular enzyme deficiencies can be differentiated from one another by the manner in which the ratio of precursor/product hormones is perturbed, and by distinct phenotypic abnormalities including pseudohermaphroditism, disturbances in sodium and potassium homeostasis, blood pressure dysregulation, and abnormal somatic growth (Table 1).[1,2] The molecular genetic basis of CAH has been well described for each enzymatic deficiency, except for that of cholesterol desmolase (side chain cleavage enzyme).

CAH is most often caused by deficiency of 21-hydroxylase (~>90% of cases), followed in frequency by deficiencies of 11β-hydroxylase, 17α-hydroxylase/17,20-lyase, and 3β-hydroxysteroid dehydrogenase; deficiency of the side chain cleavage enzyme is rare. Classic forms of these enzymatic deficiencies are apparent at birth, whereas nonclassic variants are manifested in childhood or young adult life. This chapter will review clinical aspects of CAH, including diagnosis and treatment, as well as genetics.

EMBRYOLOGY

In order to better comprehend the pathophysiology of CAH, some background information about adrenal and gonadal development is helpful. The fetal gonads are undifferentiated until about the seventh week of gestation. At that time, 46XY fetuses undergo differentiation of testicular Leydig cells under the influence of the gene encoding the sex-determining factor of the Y chromosome (SRY), and perhaps other genes. Testosterone secretion begins about a week later. In normal 46XX fetuses, ovarian differentiation occurs by about 10 weeks' gestation in the presence of a dose-dependent feminizing gene and the absence of high local concentrations of a Sertoli cell product, anti-Mullerian hormone (AMH).

The internal genital duct structures are also recognizable by 7 weeks. Mullerian ducts will form the upper third of the vagina, the uterus, and the Fallopian tubes in the absence of high local concentrations of AMH. Wolffian ducts will form the epididymis, vas deferens, seminal vesicles, and ejaculatory ducts only if adequate local androgen concentrations are recognized by specific receptors.

Female external genital development is currently thought to be a default pathway in the absence of androgen action. The urogenital sinus is destined to separate into urethral and vaginal orifices in normal females, and the labioscrotal folds remain unfused. The labia minora hood the clitoris. In males the urethral and genital orifices fuse to form an elongated penile urethra, while the labioscrotal folds fuse to form the scrotum into which the testes descend. Labioscrotal fusion may also occur in 46XX fetuses exposed to high androgen levels from fetal adrenal or maternal sources. Conversely, male external genitals may be hypoplastic if a defect exists in testosterone metabolism or action.

The adrenal cortex differentiates from mesodermal tissues at about 7 weeks' gestation, the same time as gonadal differentiation occurs. Within a short interval, two adrenal zones form: a small peripheral adult cortex and a large inner fetal cortex. The fetal cortex begins to produce steroids by the latter half of the first trimester. Adrenal mass peaks at 15 weeks.[3] Early adrenal growth is thought to be only partly attributable to adrenocorticotropic hormone (ACTH). Other adrenal trophic hormones include TGF-β, bFGF, and IGF-II.[4] After 20 weeks' gestation, adrenal growth and steroidogenesis are almost exclusively responsive to ACTH. Thus, *in utero* administration of glucocorticoids can suppress fetal ACTH and thereby inhibit adrenal steroid production.

BIOCHEMISTRY OF ADRENAL STEROID BIOSYNTHESIS

The adrenal zona fasciculata synthesizes cortisol starting with cholesterol as substrate. This five-step process (Figure 1) is under the control of ACTH (corticotropin). The first step is cleavage of the cholesterol side chain to yield pregnenolone. This is followed by 3β-dehydrogenation to progesterone and successive hydroxylations at the 17α, 21, and 11β positions mediated by three separate cytochrome P450 enzymes. A "17-deoxy" pathway is also present, in which 17α-hydroxylation does *not* occur, and the final product is normally corticosterone.

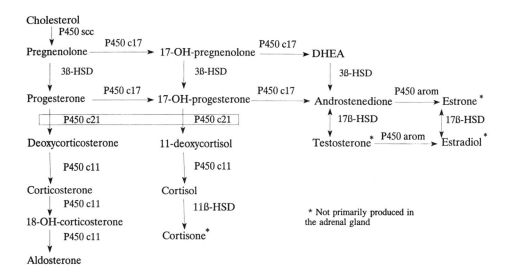

FIGURE 1. The pathways of steroid synthesis are diagrammed. Cholesterol is converted in several steps to aldosterone, cortisol, or sex steroids. Hormones marked by an asterisk are produced largely outside the adrenal cortex. Deficiency of a given enzyme causes accumulation of hormonal precursors and a deficiency of products. A box is drawn around P450c21, 21-hydroxylase, the most common enzyme deficiency causing congenital adrenal hyperplasia. HSD, hydroxysteroid dehydrogenase; DHEA, dehydroepiandrosterone.

In the adrenal zona glomerulosa, which does not possess 17α-hydroxylase activity, corticosterone is not the final product. Instead, corticosterone is successively hydroxylated and oxidized at the 18 position to yield aldosterone. The 18-hydroxylase and 18-oxidase activities are termed corticosterone methyloxidase I and II, respectively. Aldosterone synthesis is regulated mainly by angiotensin II and serum potassium levels. In normal individuals, aldosterone secretion is about 1000-fold lower than cortisol secretion.

CLINICAL FEATURES

21-HYDROXYLASE (P450c21/*CYP21*) DEFICIENCY

The fundamental problem in patients affected with this common enzyme deficiency is that they cannot adequately synthesize cortisol. Consequently, precursors such as 17-hydroxyprogesterone and 17-hydroxypregnenolone are overproduced. These precursors are converted into androgens in the adrenal gland, causing inappropriately rapid advancement of linear growth, early epiphyseal fusion, and short stature. Other clinical features of androgen excess include precocious development of sexual hair, apocrine body odor, and penile or clitoral enlargement. Reduced fertility may be observed in both sexes. Clinical features distinguishing 21-hydroxylase deficiency from other forms of CAH are outlined in Table 1.

The diagnosis of 21-hydroxylase deficiency is made by measuring blood levels of 17-hydroxyprogesterone in response to administration of intravenous ACTH.[5] A more extensive panel of adrenal hormones assayed before and after ACTH administration will aid in differentiating 21-hydroxylase deficiency from other enzymatic defects. Cortisol stimulation is almost always suboptimal following ACTH infusion in patients with severe defects in

TABLE 1

Clinical, Biochemical, and Genetic Characteristics of Various Forms of Congenital Adrenal Hyperplasia

	P450c21		P450c11	P450c17	3β-HSD		p450scc
Deficient phenotype	Classic	Nonclassic	Classic	Classic	Classic	Nonclassic	Classic
Ambiguous genitalia	+ in 46XX	—	+ in 46XX	+ in 46XY – puberty in ♀	+ in 46XY – mild in 46XX	—	+
Addisonian crisis	+ in SW	—	Rare	—	+	?	++ (lethal)
Incidence (general population)	1:14,000	1:100	1:100,000	~120 cases	?	? common	rare
Hormones							
Glucocorticoids	↓	nl	↓	↓	↓ often	NL	↓
Mineralocorticoids	↓ in SW	nl	↑	↑	↓ often	NL	↓
Androgens	↑↑ prenatally	↑ postnatally	↑↑ prenatally	↓	↓ in ♂ weak androgens	↑ in ♀	↓
Estrogens		Relative deficiency in ♀		↓	↓	↓	↓
Physiology							
Blood pressure	↓ untreated	nl	↑ often	↑ often	↓	NL	↓
Na balance	↓ in SW	nl	↑	↑	↓ often	NL	↓
K balance	↑ in SW	nl	↓	↓	↑ often	NL	↑
Acidosis	in SW	—	± alkalosis	± alkalosis	if SW	—	+
Diagnosis							
Metabolite increase	+++ 17-OHP	+ 17-OHP	DOC, S	DOC, B	DHEA, 17δ5Preg		none
Common mutations	SW:del; nt656 A→G; SV: I172N	V281L	R448H, frameshifts	term, frameshifts	term, frameshifts		StAR

↑ and ↓ signify increased and decreased levels, respectively. ♂ and ♀ denote male and female, respectively. + and − indicate present and absent, respectively. NL, normal. Hormonal abbreviations: DHEA, dehydroepiandrosterone; Preg, pregnenolone; 17-OHP, 17-hydroxyprogesterone; DOC, deoxycorticosterone. SW, salt-wasting; SV, simple virilizing; StAR, steroidogenic acute regulatory protein.

adrenal steroid synthesis. If blood testing cannot be employed, or radioimmunoassays for 17-hydroxyprogesterone are unavailable, one can measure 17-ketosteroids and/or pregnane-triol in a 24-h urine collection. The latter steroid is the principal direct metabolite of 17-hydroxyprogesterone in urine. These tests were standard prior to the advent of radio-immunoassays.

In the severe classic form of 21-hydroxylase deficiency, female fetuses are exposed to excess androgens *in utero* and are born with masculinized external genitalia. Postnatally clitoromegaly is exacerbated if treatment is not instituted promptly. Some genetic females are mistaken for males with hypospadias and cryptorchidism. Adjunctive tests commonly employed in the evaluation of infants with ambiguous genitalia include karyotype, pelvic and abdominal ultrasound, and sinugram of the urogenital orifice(s) using radiopaque dyes. The latter tests can identify internal genitourinary malformations potentially requiring surgical correction.

About 75% of classic patients have a defect beyond suboptimal cortisol synthesis and excess androgen secretion. They produce inadequate amounts of aldosterone due to inefficient 21-hydroxylation of progesterone. Such patients fail to conserve sodium normally and usually come to medical attention in the neonatal period with hyponatremia, hyperkalemia, and hypovolemic shock. Such salt-wasting "adrenal crises" can be lethal if medical care is not expeditiously administered. Patients without problems of sodium balance who show signs of prenatal virilization and markedly elevated hormonal precursors of 21-hydroxylase (e.g., 17-hydroxyprogesterone) are referred to as simple virilizers.

The milder nonclassic form of 21-hydroxylase deficiency is marked by signs of postnatal androgen excess.[6] Females with the nonclassic disorder are born with normal external genitalia, except for rare cases with mild clitoromegaly. The most common presentation is in young women with hirsutism and oligomenorrhea. A subset of women with the syndrome of polycystic ovaries has nonclassic 21-hydroxylase deficiency; some of these patients present with diminished fertility. It is more difficult to precisely delineate between the classic simple virilizing disease and nonclassic disease among males because hormonal reference standards for the diagnosis are on a continuum, with some overlap between the classic and nonclassic categories, and also because affected males do not manifest ambiguous genitalia as a sign of *in utero* androgen excess.

Phenotypic severity in nonclassic 21-hydroxylase deficiency varies greatly, and some individuals have been detected solely on the basis of hormonal or genetic testing in the course of family studies. Patients with nonclassic disease have 17-hydroxyprogesterone levels that exceed those seen in heterozygous carriers of an affected gene, but are lower than those of patients with the classic form of the disorder. In the nonstimulated state, the nonclassic individual may have nearly normal serum hormone levels. In some newborn screening programs these infants are detected with mildly elevated 17-hydroxyprogesterone levels. Aldosterone synthesis is normal in patients with nonclassic 21-hydroxylase deficiency. Table 2 describes features distinguishing salt-wasting, simple virilizing, and nonclassic forms of 21-hydroxylase deficiency.

The various 21-hydroxylase deficiency phenotypes have arisen by allelic variation in the active gene (*CYP21*). Some phenotypic variation is, however, not solely accounted for by this explanation, exemplified by siblings carrying the same *CYP21* who differ in their ability to conserve sodium. Other genetic factors obviously influence clinical outcome.

Neonatal screening for 21-hydroxylase deficiency measuring heel-prick 17-hydroxy-progesterone levels by radioimmunoassay[7-9] can be effective in reducing neonatal morbidity and mortality. It is particularly useful in males with salt-wasting disease in whom there is no obvious phenotypic clue to the diagnosis. The worldwide incidence of 21-hydroxylase deficiency CAH based on newborn screening is 1:14,554 live births; approximately 75% of infants detected in these programs manifest the salt-wasting phenotype.[9] There are genetically isolated populations with yet higher disease frequencies. According to the Hardy-Weinberg Law

TABLE 2
Phenotype in 21-Hydroxylase Deficiency

	Salt Wasting	Simple Virilizing	Nonclassic
Age at diagnosis	Infancy	Infancy (females) Childhood (males)	Childhood Adulthood
Aldosterone	Low	NL	NL
Virilization	Severe-moderate	Moderate-severe	None-mild
Mutation	Severe/severe	Severe/moderate or moderate/moderate	Severe/mild or moderate/mild or mild/mild

NL, normal.

for populations at equilibrium, the heterozygote frequency for all classic 21-hydroxylase gene defects is 1:61 persons.

A high frequency of nonclassic 21-hydroxylase deficiency has also been described among Ashkenazic Jews (~1:27), but it is also common among other ethnic groups such as Hispanics, Yugoslavs, and Italians.[10] In a mixed group of Caucasians, the disease occurred in ~1:100 individuals. Estimates of disease frequency were derived indirectly based on response to ACTH stimulation combined with HLA (human leukocyte antigen) typing.[11] Nonclassic 21-hydroxylase deficiency is thus among the most frequent autosomal recessive disorders in man. Clinical investigation to diagnose nonclassic 21-hydroxylase deficiency is warranted in any patient showing the various signs of androgen excess described above; particularly high-risk groups include Ashkenazic Jews, children with precocious pubarche, and girls or women with hirsutism and oligomenorrhea. Variations in disease frequency obtained by different investigators may be ascribed to different ethnic populations studied. It is assumed that many mildly affected individuals never seek medical attention.

11β-HYDROXYLASE (P450c11) DEFICIENCY

As with 21-hydroxylase deficiency, patients with 11-hydroxylase deficiency shunt accumulating precursor hormones into androgen pathways beginning in prenatal life, causing genital ambiguity in affected newborn females. Males have no abnormality of external genitalia. Signs of androgen excess become more prominent in 11β-hydroxylase deficiency if the disease is not promptly recognized and treated.[12] Patients with 11β-hydroxylase deficiency account for approximately 5% of all CAH cases, or about 1:100,000 live births. The disease frequency is considerably higher, ~1:5,000–7,000, among Jews of Moroccan descent.[13] There have been no systematic newborn screening programs to detect forms of CAH other than 21-hydroxylase deficiency. Nonclassic forms of 11-hydroxylase deficiency have also been described.[12]

Deficiency of 21- or 11β-hydroxylase may be distinguished on the basis of the hormonal profile. In the majority of cases, classic 21-hydroxylase deficiency is accompanied by deficient aldosterone synthesis and sodium wasting. In patients with 11-hydroxylase deficiency, however, excessive secretion of mineralocorticoid agonists (deoxycorticosterone or its metabolites) results in sodium retention, hypokalemia, volume expansion, suppressed plasma renin activity (PRA), and hypertension. The diagnosis of 11β-hydroxylase deficiency is made by the measurement of elevated basal or ACTH-stimulated deoxycorticosterone (DOC) and/or 11-deoxycortisol (compound S) in the serum, or elevated levels of the tetrahydro- compounds, -DOC or -S, in a 24-h urine collection.[14] Another useful marker in pediatric diagnosis is 6α-hydroxytetrahydro-11-deoxycortisol, which can be measured by gas chromatography/mass spectrometry of urine.[15] As in 21-hydroxylase deficiency, 17-ketosteroids are elevated in urine, reflecting adrenal androgen production. Low levels of aldosterone fail to induce a rise in PRA, because DOC is effectively suppressing PRA production. Hypertension may be absent in young children and is not the *sine qua non* for diagnosis of 11β-hydroxylase deficiency. In nonclassic cases DOC and 11-deoxycortisol (compound S) are variably elevated, and PRA may be normal.

17α-HYDROXYLASE/17,20-LYASE (P450c17) DEFICIENCY

In contrast to 21- and 11β-hydroxylase deficiencies, this defect is notable for a paucity of sex steroid hormones. The diagnosis of 17α-hydroxylase/17,20-lyase is made by measuring marked elevations of serum DOC and corticosterone (compound B) and the metabolites of these two steroids.[16] Aldosterone is often low secondary to suppression of renin by excess DOC, as in 11β-hydroxylase deficiency. Interestingly, 17α-hydroxylase-deficient patients do not suffer from adrenal crisis despite inadequate cortisol synthesis, because corticosterone, when present in sufficient quantities, apparently serves as a glucocorticoid agonist. Plasma ACTH levels are thus less elevated in 17α-hydroxylase deficiency than in other conditions of impaired cortisol production. Gonadotropin production is markedly elevated in both sexes because of absence of any sex steroid feedback; gonads are atrophic. Impaired production of glucocorticoids and sex steroids (C_{19}/C_{18} compounds) prevents 46XX individuals from developing female secondary sexual characteristics at puberty.[16] External genitals in 46XY individuals are also incompletely developed.[17] Precursor steroids are metabolized in the 17-deoxy pathway, producing mineralocorticoid agonists which cause hypokalemic alkalosis and hypertension as in 11-hydroxylase deficiency. In rare cases, selective 17,20-lyase deficiency is diagnosed. In such patients, cortisol levels are normal, but C_{21} to C_{19} steroid conversion is impaired, preventing normal sex steroid production.

Genetic and clinical features of complete 17-hydroxylase/17,20-lyase deficiency have been reviewed.[18] There have been reports of patients from Canadian-Dutch Mennonite kindreds in geographically distant locales who share the same genotype.[19] Relatively few genetic females have been detected; this diagnosis should be considered in adolescent girls with delayed puberty. Partial 17α-hydroxylase/17,20-lyase deficiency may be found in males with ambiguous genitalia.[20]

3β-HYDROXYSTEROID DEHYDROGENASE (3β-HSD) DEFICIENCY

3β-Hydroxysteroid dehydrogenase converts Δ^5 to Δ^4 steroids. A high ratio of Δ^5 to Δ^4 steroids characterizes the 3β-HSD deficiency.[21] Specifically, there are elevated serum levels of 17-hydroxypregnenolone and dehydroepiandrosterone (DHEA) (a weak androgen) before and after ACTH stimulation. Increased excretion of the Δ^5 metabolites pregnenetriol and 16-pregnenetriol in the urine is also diagnostic for this enzyme disorder. Affected individuals typically have cortisol insufficiency, salt wasting, and genital ambiguity. Whereas lack of potent androgens produces hypospadias in males, high levels of DHEA may cause mild virilization in females (clitoromegaly without urogenital sinus formation).[22] Males with either 3β-HSD or 17α-hydroxylase/17,20-lyase are predisposed to gynecomastia during adolescence due to deficient androgens in prenatal life. The precise frequency of severe defects in the adrenal 3β-HSD gene is unknown.

Nonclassic 3β-HSD deficiency is diagnosed with variable frequency in children with precocious pubarche and females with hirsutism and oligomenorrhea (reviewed in Refs. 23 and 24), but the hormonal profile with ACTH stimulation is less reliable compared with that described for 21-hydroxylase deficiency. Ovarian hyperandrogenism may also be confused with 3β-HSD deficiency.[25] Molecular genetic investigation has uncovered cases of mild 3β-HSD deficiency; preliminary data suggest that the established hormonal diagnostic criteria need to be revised such that the precursor/product ratios are far greater than 3 SD above the mean.[26]

Because normal fetuses are relatively deficient in 3β-HSD, apparent enzyme defects based on precursor/product ratios must be cautiously interpreted in neonates and infants. To date no marked variations in the ethnic incidence of this defect are known, although several classic cases have been identified in consanguineous families.

20,22-DESMOLASE (P450scc) DEFICIENCY

Also known as lipoid adrenal hyperplasia or cholesterol desmolase deficiency, this enzyme defect prevents any steroid production beyond cholesterol. Complete 20,22-desmolase deficiency produces complete adrenocortical insufficiency and is lethal due to marked cortisol deficiency and severe salt wasting. There are only about 30 cases reported in the world literature.[27,28] Partial defects result in pseudohermaphroditism in genetic males, and a lack of secondary sexual characteristics would be expected in genetic females. One case report describes a patient diagnosed in the newborn period and successfully treated for 18 years.[29] Cholesterol desmolase deficiency seems to occur with some frequency with moderate severity among Japanese.

OTHER STEROIDOGENIC DISORDERS

There are a number of disorders not included among the adrenal hyperplasias because they do not affect cortisol synthesis or disturb the hypothalamic-pituitary-adrenal axis. They are worthy of discussion here because the clinical manifestations are similar to those of the various forms of CAH.

AROMATASE DEFICIENCY

Defects in *CYP19* encoding cytochrome P450 aromatase (P450 arom) prevent normal synthesis of estrogens and create a relative abudance of androgens. Such defects have recently been identified as a novel cause of ambiguous genitalia in 46XX neonates[30] and of virilism in the setting of polycystic ovaries in young women.[31] Hormonal diagnosis rests on low levels of all estrogen metabolites in serum and urine and relatively high levels of testosterone, dihydrotestosterone, and androstenedione.

17-KETOSTEROID REDUCTASE DEFICIENCY

This enzyme is responsible for the conversion of androstenedione to testosterone, and estrone to estradiol. Classic deficiency of 17-ketosteroid reductase (a non-P450 enzyme, also termed 17β-hydroxysteroid dehydrogenase) is a cause of ambiguous genitalia and cryptorchidism in 46XY neonates, who have a tendency to virilize at puberty,[32] probably by means of extragonadal 17β-HSD activity and enhanced 5α-reductase activity.[33] Mild forms of this enzyme deficiency exist in young men with gynecomastia,[34] as well as in females with hirsutism and polycystic ovaries.[35] Specific defects in the gene encoding the type 3 isozyme of 17β-HSD have been identified and proven to reduce enzyme activity.[36] The most distinctive hormonal abnormality is elevation of androstenedione alone; serum testosterone may be within the normal range.

5α-REDUCTASE DEFICIENCY

The conversion of testosterone to its more potent form, dihydrotestosterone, requires enzymatic action by 5α-reductase. In many cases, 46XY patients with this enzyme deficiency are assigned to the female sex at birth. Anatomy in such patients consists of a perineoscrotal hypospadius with a blind-ending vagina. The phenotype may vary widely, and it has been suggested that *formes fruste* may account for some cases of familial hypospadius. At puberty affected males virilize, as do those with 17β-HSD deficiency. The phallus enlarges and testicular descent may occur. Internal anatomy described at surgery includes seminal vesicles and epididymis, vas deferens, and ejaculatory ducts, but no prostate and no Mullerian remnants. Hormonal diagnosis is made based on the extent of conversion of testosterone to dihydrotestosterone in genital skin, or on ratios of these hormones or their metabolites in blood or urine before and after stimulation with human chorionic gonadotropin.[37,38]

CORTICOSTERONE METHYLOXIDASE (CMO, ALDOSTERONE SYNTHASE) DEFICIENCY

A distal block in aldosterone synthesis results from defects in *CYP11B2* encoding 18-hydroxylase and 18-oxidase (CMO I and II, respectively). Deficiencies of either CMO I or II are rare autosomal recessive disorders of aldosterone biosynthesis that do not cause hypertension. Instead, patients with this disorder are subject to potentially lethal electrolyte abnormalities and failure to thrive in infancy and childhood, but they may have no symptoms as adults.[34,38] In CMO I deficiency, 18-hydroxycorticosterone levels are normal or decreased, whereas levels of this precursor are elevated in CMO II deficiency.

GLUCOCORTICOID-SUPPRESSIBLE HYPERALDOSTERONISM

This type of hypertension is inherited as an autosomal dominant disorder. It is distinguished from primary aldosteronism by suppression of (usually moderate) aldosterone hypersecretion within 48 h of dexamethasone administration[25] and by a high urinary concentration of 18-oxocortisol,[37] a 17α-hydroxylated analog of aldosterone that cannot be produced in the zona glomerulosa due to the zone's lack of 17α-hydroxylase activity. These features suggest that aldosterone is being synthesized in the zona fasciculata under the control of ACTH, implying that *CYP11B2* must be inappropriately regulated in a manner similar to the normal regulation of *CYP11B1*.

TREATMENT

Patients with either classic 21-hydroxylase deficiency, 11β-hydroxylase, 17α-hydroxylase/17,20-desmolase, or 3β-HSD deficiencies, as well as selected symptomatic patients with nonclassic forms of these diseases are treated with daily oral hydrocortisone or similar drugs. Treatment with glucocorticoids suppresses excessive secretion of ACTH, thereby correcting the adrenal hormone imbalance. Patients with salt-wasting CAH require supplementation with mineralocorticoids (e.g., fludrocortisone, [Florinef], 50–200 µg/day) and sodium supplements (1 g per 10 kg body weight). Many endocrinologists will empirically treat all CAH patients with Florinef and sodium chloride despite the lack of signs of salt wasting. Older children and adults with simple virilizing disease who are treated adequately with glucocorticoids usually do not have a clinically apparent deficiency of aldosterone. It is prudent to follow PRA in all patients as an index of the need for mineralocorticoid and salt supplements. Hypertension may arise as a complication of excessive or unnecessary treatment with fludrocortisone.

Glucocorticoid treatment also leads to reduction of endogenous mineralocorticoids in 11- and 17-hydroxylase deficiency, with amelioration of hypertension. In cases of long-standing hypertension, additional antihypertensive drugs may be required to completely normalize blood pressure.

The usual mode of treatment for CAH in childhood is 2–3 divided daily doses of hydrocortisone totalling ~15 mg/m^2/day. Even this relatively low dose may be supraphysiologic; healthy children and adolescents secrete an average of approximately 7 mg/m^2 of cortisol daily.[39,40] A single daily dose of hydrocortisone, due to its relatively rapid metabolism, is therapeutically suboptimal for the long term.

Treatment efficacy should be monitored in growing children with frequent measurements of serum 17-hydroxyprogesterone (good control <1000 ng/dL), androstenedione, testosterone, and PRA,[41] as well as assessment of growth, skeletal maturation, and pubertal status. There is some suggestion that children who begin treatment late (e.g., male simple virilizers treated at 2–5 years of age rather than in infancy) may benefit from the addition of a long-acting GnRH (gonadotropin-releasing hormone) analog to suppress central puberty.[42]

If the response to maintenance hydrocortisone at the standard dose is poor despite good medical compliance, a 2–4-day trial of dexamethasone (in a dose of ~20–30 µg/kg/day to a maximum of 2 mg/day) may be more effective in suppressing adrenal secretion. Maintenance hydrocortisone may then be resumed and adrenal hormone levels monitored. If epiphyses are fused, the maintenance regimen may be changed to either of the longer acting glucocorticoids, prednisone or dexamethasone. The greater potency of these drugs means that slight dosing errors may result in iatrogenic Cushing's syndrome and growth retardation in children. Life-threatening stress, severe illness, or surgery all demand parenteral therapy with high doses of hydrocortisone in any patient undergoing chronic treatment with exogenous glucocorticoids.

Clinical trials are currently being initiated using androgen receptor blockers and inhibitors of steroid synthesis in conjunction with glucocorticoids to ameliorate virilization and to prevent iatrogenic glucocorticoid-induced growth retardation.[43] Another potentially useful adjunct to standard therapy are the GnRH analogs, which serve to delay the onset of gonadarche.

It has been suggested that androgen receptor blockade may be preferable to glucocorticoids as primary treatment of mild 21-hydroxylase deficiency.[44] The latter therapeutic trials have been prompted by the observation that whereas menses usually resume in regularity within 2–6 months of beginning glucocorticoids in young women with nonclassic 21-hydroxylase deficiency, hirsutism is quite refractory to this mode of treatment.

Surgical therapy is required in cases of ambiguous genitalia. Most often this involves clitoroplasty and vaginoplasty in virilized females. Improved surgical techniques now permit these procedures to be performed in a single-stage operation by experienced urologists.[45]

With the recognition of disturbed gender identity and role among young women with CAH,[46,47] it is extremely important to provide early and continuing psychological counseling for these families. It is expected that with improved medical, surgical, and psychological treatments an improved psychosexual outcome will be achieved.

GENETICS

21-HYDROXYLASE DEFICIENCY

The genes encoding 21-hydroxylase and a homologous pseudogene (*CYP21* and *CYP21P*, respectively) each span 3 kb and are located 30 kb apart in the HLA complex on chromosome 6p21.3.[48,49] Although the two genes are 98% identical in nucleotide sequence, *CYP21P* has accumulated a number of mutations that render the putative gene product completely inactive. These include an 8-bp deletion in exon 3, a frameshift in exon 7, and a nonsense mutation in exon 8.

The vast majority of mutations causing 21-hydroxylase deficiency are caused by two types of recombinations between *CYP21* and *CYP21P*. About 20% of these are the result of unequal crossing over during meiosis, producing deletions of a 30-kb DNA segment that includes the 3' end of the pseudogene and the adjacent *C4B* serum complement gene, as well as the greater portion of the active *CYP21* gene.[50] This deleted haplotype is incapable of producing any active enzyme. Alternatively, deleterious mutations found in the pseudogene are transferred to *CYP21* by a process known as apparent gene conversion. The most common mutation in the latter class found in ~25% of affected chromosomes is a point mutation in the second intron that results in an abnormally spliced gene product. In these cases there may be some residual activity of the protein possibly due to some normally spliced mRNA. Less commonly found are seven missense mutations that cause changes in the protein's amino acid sequence.

Several large studies have examined the prevalence of individual mutations in an attempt to correlate specific mutations with particular clinical manifestations of the disease.[51-54] These correlations are most reliably made in individuals who are homozygous or hemizygous (i.e., the other chromosome carries a deletion) for each mutation. Mutations commonly found in classic and nonclassic forms of 21-hydroxylase deficiency can be grouped into three categories according to predicted level of enzymatic activity based on *in vitro* mutagenesis and expression. [55-58] One group with total ablation of enzyme activity is most often associated with salt-wasting disease; a second with 2% normal activity consists predominantly of patients with simple virilizing disease; and the third with 20–60% of normal activity is most often associated with the nonclassic disorder. As in several other inherited disorders in man, there are exceptions in which the phenotype does not correspond precisely with what one might expect based on *in vitro* expression of genes carrying discrete mutations. Factors outside the *CYP21* locus may influence disease expression.

A further point of interest in phenotype-genotype analysis is the wide range of clinical manifestations in patients carrying mutations such as Val-281→Leu and Pro-30→Leu, typically associated with nonclassic disease. These mutations are expected to reduce enzyme activity to 20–60% of normal, with 17-hydroxyprogesterone being the preferred substrate. An individual heterozygous for a deletion of *CYP21* (i.e., ablation of all enzyme activity derived from one chromosome) is also expected to have about 50% of normal 21-hydroxylase activity, but such individuals have no signs of disease and have hormonal abnormalities detectable only with ACTH stimulation. This suggests that *in vivo* 21-hydroxylase activity in patients with nonclassic 21-hydroxylase deficiency is often much less than 50% of normal. One plausible explanation for such differences in clinical manifestations of disease is fluctuating intraadrenal concentrations of progesterone, which at physiologic levels (2–4 μM)[59] acts as a competitive inhibitor of the nonclassic mutant enzyme for its main substrate, 17-hydroxyprogesterone. Thus, individuals carrying two nonclassic alleles might have more severely compromised 21-hydroxylase activity as intraadrenal progesterone concentration increases. Other factors contributing to phenotypic variability might include pseudosubstrate inhibition of other steroidogenic enzymes by accumulated precursors of 21-hydroxylase.

11β-HYDROXYLASE DEFICIENCY

There are two human genes[60] on chromosome 8q22[61] that encode 11β-hydroxylase (*CYP11B*) isozymes with predicted amino acid sequences that are 93% identical. Each has 9 exons spaced over approximately 7 kb. *CYP11B1*, expressed at high levels in normal adrenal glands,[60] is regulated by ACTH.[62] *CYP11B2*, not readily detectable in Northern blots using normal adrenal RNA,[60] is regulated primarily by angiotensin-II, rather than by ACTH. Transcripts of *CYP11B2* have been detected by hybridization to RNA from an aldosterone-secreting tumor,[63] or in normal adrenal mRNA by the more sensitive technique of reverse transcription coupled with the polymerase chain reaction.[64]

Defects in *CYP11B1* result in virilizing, hypertensive CAH, whereas defects in *CYP11B2* cause the rare salt-wasting disease CMO II deficiency. A third disease, glucocorticoid suppressible hyperaldosteronism, ensues when the regulatory region of *CYP11B1* is transposed by unequal crossing over to a position where it controls synthesis of *CYP11B2*, thus promoting glucocorticoid-suppressible and ACTH-stimulable aldosterone synthesis and hypertension (reviewed in Ref. 65).

Mutations in the *CYP11B1* gene tend to cluster in exons 6, 7, and 8; [66-68] the most common genetic alteration in Moroccan Jews with 11β-hydroxylase deficiency is Arg-448→His.[69] When introduced into *CYP11B1* cDNA and expressed in cultured cells, this mutation abolishes normal enzymatic activity and is therefore consistent with the classic, severe virilizing phenotype observed in these patients. Blood pressure was not uniformly elevated in all patients carrying this mutation, and thus, as observed in 21-hydroxylase deficiency, there are apparently other factors that modify phenotype.

Both forms of CMO deficiency are caused by mutations in the *CYP11B2* gene (Figure 2). CMO I deficiency in one Amish kindred was attributed to a frameshift mutation,[20] and CMO II deficiency in several Iranian Jewish kindreds was due to double homozygosity for two missense mutations.[29] *In vitro* expression studies indicate that less than 1–2% of normal aldosterone synthase activity permits levels of aldosterone biosynthesis adequate for normal

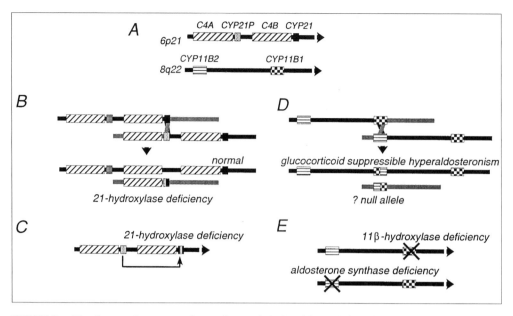

FIGURE 2.   Mutations causing common forms of congenital adrenal hyperplasia and related conditions. (**A**) The steroid 21-hydroxylase and 11β-hydroxylase genetic regions on chromosomes 6p and 8q, respectively. The gene encoding active 21-hydroxylase (CYP21) and a pseudogene (CYP21P) are adjacent to genes encoding the fourth component of serum complement (C4A, C4B). For simplicity, other genes in this region are not shown. CYP11B1 and CYP11B2 encode 11β-hydroxylase and aldosterone synthase, respectively. Arrows indicate direction of transcription of each gene. (**B**) Unequal meiotic crossovers between CYP21 and CYP21P cause 21-hydroxylase deficiency. (**C**) Gene conversions also cause 21-hydroxylase deficiency. (**D**) Unequal meiotic crossovers between CYP11B1 and CYP11B2 cause glucocorticoid suppressible hyperaldosteronism. (**E**) Point mutations in CYP11B1 and CYP11B2 cause 11β-hydroxylase and aldosterone synthase deficiencies, respectively.

sodium conservation. Thus major perturbations in enzyme activity are required for the salt-wasting phenotype to be clinically recognized.[29]

Affected glucocorticoid suppressible hyperaldosteronism (GRA) patients carry a chromosome 8 with three *CYP11B* genes that have presumably been generated by unequal crossing over.[18,19,30] The middle *CYP11B* gene on this chromosome is a chimera with 5′ and 3′ ends corresponding to *CYP11B1* and *CYP11B2*, respectively, so that transcriptional regulatory sequences are identical to *CYP11B1*. The encoded hybrid proteins (the amino terminal region is that of *CYP11B1*) retain the ability to synthesize aldosterone from deoxycorticosterone as long as the crossover point is before exon 5,[30] which is the case with all affected kindreds studied thus far.

17α-HYDROXYLASE/17,20-LYASE DEFICIENCY

The P450c17 structural gene (*CYP17*) spans 12.6 kb on chromosome 10q24.3,[70] with an intron-exon organization similar to that of *CYP21*. The same gene is expressed in both the adrenal and the testis.[71] Molecular characterization of specific mutations in *CYP17* has been reported in a number of patients (reviewed in Ref. 18). In patients with classic, severe 17α-hydroxylase and 17,20-lyase deficiencies, these have included a point mutation creating a stop codon in the first exon, a 7-bp duplication in exon 2 that produces a frameshift, and a 4-bp duplication in exon 8. Homozygous deletion of 3 bp in exon 1 was detected in a patient with apparent selective compromise of 17,20-lyase activity, a phenotypic female with sexual infantilism. A genetic male with ambiguous genitalia was found to be a compound heterozygote with a stop codon introduced by a single base substitution in exon 4 on one chromosome and a nonconservative proline→threonine substitution in exon 6 on the second chromosome.

3β-HYDROXYSTEROID DEHYDROGENASE DEFICIENCY

Two homologous genes encode 3β-HSD. The type I gene is expressed in placenta and skin, and the type II gene is expressed in adrenal and gonads.[72-74] Each gene occupies 8 kb, on chromosome 1p11-13.[75] This is the only enzyme discussed here that is not encoded by a gene in the cytochrome P450 superfamily. Mutations in the type II gene have been described in patients with classic 3β-HSD deficiency. These include two separate point mutations introducing termination codons[76,77] in exon 4, insertion of a single base causing a frame-shift,[76] and two separate amino acid substitutions in highly conserved portions of the protein.[78]

CHOLESTEROL DESMOLASE DEFICIENCY (LIPOID HYPERPLASIA)

The *CYP11A* gene encoding this enzyme encompasses 20 kb on chromosome 15q23-24.[79] Mutations in this gene have not yet been identified in patients with lipoid adrenal hyperplasia,[80] although *in vitro* studies suggest that the 20α-hydroxylase function is deficient in at least one patient with the syndrome. Lesions in the gene encoding steroidogenic acute regulatory protein (StAR) have been described in three patients with this disease.[80a] StAR is a cAMP inducible protein that facilitates cholesterol transport across the mitochondrial membrane, permitting cholesterol's conversion to pregnenolone by CYP11A.

PRENATAL DIAGNOSIS

Prenatal diagnosis of 21-hydroxylase deficiency has been practiced for some time[81,82] in pregnancies known to be at 25% risk by virtue of a previously diagnosed sibling. Hormonal diagnosis is performed by finding elevated levels of amniotic fluid 17-hydroxyprogesterone[83] or 21-deoxycortisol.[84] Genetic diagnosis was first accomplished by identifying the closely linked HLA markers on fetal cells cultured from the amniotic fluid.[85,86] Problems encountered with these diagnostic techniques included low 17-hydroxyprogesterone levels in non-salt-wasting cases and intra-HLA recombination[87] producing false negative results. To avoid these pitfalls, more direct genetic diagnosis has been attempted using allele-specific hybridization with oligonucleotide probes for the normal and mutant alleles of *CYP21* described below.[88,89] Early amniocentesis and chorionic villus sampling (CVS) have allowed such diagnostic studies to be done at the end of the first trimester.[90,91]

Pregnancies at high risk (1:4) for 21-hydroxylase deficiency may undergo prospective prenatal treatment of the fetus by administering dexamethasone to the mother beginning in the first trimester.[92-94] In light of the ontogeny of adrenal and gonadal development, deferral of therapy until fetal status is known could hamper the ability to prevent genital ambiguity.[95] Prenatal treatment has been efficacious in ameliorating genital ambiguity in a number of severely affected girls. Some treatment failures have been attributed to cessation of therapy in midgestation, noncompliance, or suboptimal dosing,[96,97] whereas others had no ready explanation.[98]

With respect to treatment safety, no fetus treated with low-dose dexamethasone has been born with a congenital malformation specifically attributable to dexamethasone therapy. The incidence of fetal deaths in treated pregnancies does not exceed that for the general population. This is in contrast to complications observed in a rodent model of *in utero* exposure to high-dose glucocorticoids,[99] which included cleft palate, placental degeneration, intrauterine growth retardation, or unexplained fetal death.

The incidence of maternal complications has varied among groups of investigators. Serious side effects such as overt Cushing's syndrome, massive weight gain, and hypertension have been reported in about 1% of all treated pregnancies.

Caution must be exercised in recommending prenatal therapy with dexamethasone, and women must be fully informed of these potential risks and nonuniformity of beneficial outcome to the affected female fetus. These caveats notwithstanding, many parents of affected girls still opt for prenatal medical treatment because of the severe psychological impact of ambiguous genitalia.

In principle, a similar diagnostic and therapeutic approach should be effective in 11-hydroxylase deficiency, in which affected female fetuses are also at risk for prenatal virilization.

SUMMARY AND CONCLUSIONS

The adrenal hyperplasias have been extensively studied from both the clinical and molecular genetic perspectives. The molecular basis of CAH resulting from deficiencies in all enzymes but cholesterol desmolase have been identified. From the foregoing discussion, it can be appreciated that severe mutations, such as deletions, frameshifts, and nonsense codons, in the genes encoding steroidogenic enzymes result in gene products with no enzymatic activity. In contrast, milder mutations, such as conservative or nonconservative substitutions, may cause a lesser degree of enzyme impairment. Indeed, the catalytic activity of such gene products may be differently affected for each of two different substrates.

One practical result of molecular genetic characterization is the ability to perform accurate and early prenatal diagnosis. Current research efforts are focused on the regulation of these genes, understanding more about gene and enzyme structure-function relationships, further clinical-genetic correlations, and optimizing treatment.

REFERENCES

1. **New, M. I., White P. C., Pang, S., Dupont, B., and Speiser P. W.,** The adrenal hyperplasias, in *The Metabolic Basis of Inherited Disease*, 6th ed., Scriver, C. R., Beaudet, A. L., Sly, W. S., and Valle, D., Eds., McGraw-Hill, New York, 1989, 1881.
2. **White, P. C., New, M. I., and Dupont, B.,** Congenital adrenal hyperplasia, *N. Engl. J. Med.*, 316, 1519, 1987.
3. **Branchaud, C. L. and Murphy, B. E. P.,** Physiopathology of the fetal adrenal, in *Hormones and Fetal Pathophysiology,* Pasqualini, J. R. and Scholler, R., Eds., Marcel Dekker, New York, 1992, 53.
4. **Estivariz, F. E., Lowry, P. J., and Jackson, S.,** Control of adrenal growth, in *The Adrenal Gland*, 2nd ed., James, V. H. T., Ed., Raven Press, New York, 1992, 43.
5. **New, M. I., Lorenzen, F., Lerner, A. J., et al.,** Genotyping steroid 21-hydroxylase deficiency: hormonal reference data, *J. Clin. Endocrinol. Metab.*, 57, 320, 1983.
6. **Kohn, B., Levine, L. S., Pollack, M. S., et al.,** Late-onset steroid 21-hydroxylase deficiency: a variant of classical congenital adrenal hyperplasia, *J. Clin. Endocrinol. Metab.*, 55, 817, 1982.
7. **Pang, S., Hotchkiss, J., Drash, A. L., Levine, L. S., and New, M. I.,** Microfilter paper method for 17α-progesterone radioimmunoassay: its application for rapid screening for congenital adrenal hyperplasia, *J. Clin. Endocrinol. Metab.*, 45, 1003, 1977.
8. **Pang, S., Murphey, W., Levine, L. S., et al.,** A pilot newborn screening for congenital adrenal hyperplasia (CAH) in Alaska, *Pediatr. Res.*, 15, 512, 1981.
9. **Pang, S. P., Wallace, M. A., Hofman, L., et al.,** Worldwide experience in newborn screening for classical congenital adrenal hyperplasia due to 21-hydroxylase deficiency, *Pediatrics*, 81, 866, 1988.
10. **Speiser, P. W., Dupont, B., Rubinstein, P., Piazza, A., Kastelan, A., and New, M. I.,** High frequency of nonclassical steroid 21-hydroxylase deficiency, *Am. J. Hum. Genet.*, 37, 650, 1985.
11. **Sherman, S. L., Aston, C. E., Morton, N. E., Speiser, P. W., and New, M. I.,** A segregation and linkage study of classical and nonclassical 21-hydroxylase deficiency, *Am. J. Hum. Genet.*, 42, 830, 1988.
12. **Zachmann, M., Tassinari, D., and Prader, A.,** Clinical and biochemical variability of congenital adrenal hyperplasia due to 11 beta-hydroxylase deficiency. A study of 25 patients, *J. Clin. Endocrinol. Metab.*, 56, 222, 1983.
13. **Rosler, A., Leiberman, E., and Cohen, T.,** High frequency of congenital adrenal hyperplasia (classic 11 beta-hydroxylase deficiency) among Jews from Morocco, *Am. J. Med. Genet.,* 42, 827, 1992.
14. **Eberlein, W. R. and Bongiovanni, A. M.,** Plasma and urinary corticosteroids in the hypertensive form of congenital adrenal hyperplasia, *J. Biol. Chem.*, 223, 85, 1956.

15. **Hughes, I. A., Arisaka, O., Perry, L. A., and Honour, J. W.,** Early diagnosis of 11 beta-hydroxylase deficiency in two siblings confirmed by analysis of a novel steroid metabolite in newborn urine, *Acta Endocrinol. (Copenhagen),* 111, 349, 1986.

16. **Biglieri, E. G., Herron, M. A., and Brust, M.,** 17-hydroxylation deficiency in man, *J. Clin. Invest.,* 45, 1946, 1966.

17. **New, M. I.,** Male pseudohermaphroditism due to 17α-hydroxylase deficiency, *J. Clin. Invest.,* 49, 1930, 1970.

18. **Yanase, T., Simpson, E. R., and Waterman, M. R.,** 17α-hydroxylase/17,20-lyase deficiency: from clinical investigation to molecular definition, *Endocr. Rev.,* 12, 91, 1991.

19. **Imai, T., Toshihiko, T., Waterman, M. R., Simpson, E. R., and Pratt, J. J.,** Canadian Mennonites and individuals residing in the Friesland region of the Netherlands share the same molecular basis of 17α-hydroxylase deficiency, *Hum. Genet.,* 89, 95, 1992.

20. **Ahlgren, R., Yanase, T., Simpson, E. R., Winter, J. S. D., and Waterman, M. R.,** Compound heterozygous mutations (Arg 239→stop, Pro 342→Thr) in the CYP17 (P45017α) gene lead to ambiguous external genitalia in a male patient with partial combined 17α-hydroxylase deficiency, *J. Clin. Endocrinol. Metab.,* 74, 667, 1992.

21. **Bongiovanni, A. M.,** Urinary excretion of pregnanetriol and pregnenetriol in two forms of congenital adrenal hyperplasia, *J. Clin. Invest.,* 60, 2751, 1971.

22. **Bongiovanni, A. M.,** The adrenogenital syndrome with deficiency of 3β-hydroxysteroid dehydrogenase, *J. Clin. Invest.,* 41, 2086, 1962.

23. **Bongiovanni, A. M.,** Acquired adrenal hyperplasia: with special reference to 3β-hydroxysteroid dehydrogenase, *Fertil. Steril.,* 35, 599, 1981.

24. **Zerah, M., Schram, P., and New, M. I.,** The diagnosis and treatment of nonclassical 3β-HSD deficiency, *The Endocrinologist,* 1, 75, 1991.

25. **Ehrmann, D. A. and Rosenfield, R. L.,** Hirsutism—beyond the steroidogenic block, *N. Engl. J. Med.,* 323, 909, 1990.

26. **Chang, Y. T., Zhang, L., Mason, J. I., et al.,** Redefining hormonal criteria for mild 3β-hydroxysteroid dehydrogenase deficiency congenital adrenal hyperplasia by molecular analysis of the type II 3β-HSD gene, *Pediatr. Res.,* 35, 96A, 1994.

27. **Prader, A. and Gurtner, H. P.,** Das Syndrom des Pseudohermaphroditismus masculinus bei kongenitaler Nebennierenrinden-Hyperplasia ohne Androgenüberproduktion (adrenaler Pseudoherm masc), *Helv. Paediatr. Acta,* 10, 397, 1955.

28. **Prader, A. and Siebenmann, R. E.,** Nebennereninsuffizienz bei kongenitaler Lipoid-hyperplasie der Nebennieren, *Helv. Paediatr. Acta,* 12, 569, 1957.

29. **Hauffa, B. P., Miller, W. L., Grumbach, M. M., Conte, F. A., and Kaplan, S. L.,** Congenital adrenal hyperplasia due to deficient cholesterol side-chain cleavage activity (20,22 desmolase) in a patient treated for 18 years, *Clin. Endocrinol.,* 23, 481, 1985.

30. **Harada, N., Ogawa, H., Shozu, M., and Yamada, K.,** Genetic studies to characterize the origin of the mutation in placental aromatase deficiency, *Am. J. Hum. Genet.,* 51, 666, 1992.

31. **Ito, Y., Fisher, C. R., Conte, F. A., Grumbach, M. M., and Simpson, E. R.,** Molecular basis of aromatase deficiency in an adult female with sexual infantilism and polycystic ovaries, *Proc. Natl. Acad. Sci. U.S.A.,* 90, 11673, 1993.

32. **Eckstein, B., Cohen, S., Farkas, A., and Rosler, A.,** The nature of the defect in familial male pseudohermaphroditism in Arabs of Gaza, *J. Clin. Endocrinol. Metab.,* 68, 477, 1989.

33. **Rosler, A., Belanger, A., and Labrie, F.,** Mechanisms of androgen production in male pseudohermaphroditism due to 17 beta-hydroxysteroid dehydrogenase deficiency, *J. Clin. Endocrinol. Metab.,* 75, 773, 1992.

34. **Castro-Magana, M., Angulo, M., and Uy, J.,** Male hypogonadism with gynecomastia caused by late-onset deficiency of testicular 17-ketosteroid reductase, *N. Engl. J. Med.,* 328, 1297, 1993.

35. **Pang, S., Softness, B., Sweeney, W. J., and New, M. I.,** Hirsutism, polycystic ovarian disease, and ovarian 17-ketosteroid reductase deficiency, *N. Engl. J. Med.,* 316, 1295, 1987.

36. **Geissler, W. M., Davis, D. L., Wu, L., Bradshaw, K. D., Patel, S., Mendonca, B. B., Elliston, K. O., Wilson, J. D., Russell, D. W., and Andersson, S.,** Male pseudohermaphroditism caused by mutations of testicular 17β-hydroxysteroid dehydrogenase 3, *Nat. Genet.,* 7, 34, 1994.

37. **Wilson, J. D., Griffin, J. E., and Russell, D. W.,** Steroid 5α-reductase deficiency, *Endocr. Rev.,* 14, 577, 1993.

38. **Imperato-McGinley, J., Guerrero, L., Gautier, T., and Peterson, R. E.,** Steroid 5α-reductase deficiency in man: an inherited form of male pseudohermaphroditism, *Science,* 186, 1213, 1974.

39. **New, M. I. and Seaman, M. P.,** Secretion rates of cortisol and aldosterone in various forms of congenital adrenal hyperplasia, *J. Clin. Endocrinol.,* 30, 361, 1970.

40. **Linder, B. L., Esteban, N. V., Yergey, A. L., Winterer, J. C., Loriaux, D. L., and Cassorla, F.,** Cortisol production rate in childhood and adolescence, *J. Pediatr.,* 117, 892, 1990.

41. **Golden, M. P., Lippe, B. M., Kaplan, S. A., Lavin, N., and Slavin, J.,** Management of congenital adrenal hyperplasia using serum dehydroepiandrosterone sulfate and 17-hydroxyprogesterone concentrations, *Pediatrics,* 61, 867, 1978.

42. **Dacou-Voutetakis, C. and Karidis, N.,** Congenital adrenal hyperplasia complicated by central precocious puberty: treatment with LHRH-agonist analogue, *Ann. N.Y. Acad. Sci.,* 687, 250, 1993.

43. **Cutler, G. B., Jr. and Laue. L.,** Seminars in medicine of the Beth Israel Hospital, Boston: congenital adrenal hyperplasia due to 21-hydroxylase deficiency, *N. Engl. J. Med.,* 323, 1806, 1990.

44. **Spritzer, P., Billaud, L., Thalabard, J.-C., et al.,** Cyproterone acetate versus hydrocortisone treatment in late-onset adrenal hyperplasia, *J. Clin. Endocrinol. Metab.,* 70, 642, 1990.

45. **Donahoe, P. K. and Gustafson, M. L.,** Early one-stage surgical reconstruction of the extremely high vagina in patients with congenital adrenal hyperplasia, *J. Pediatr. Surg.,* 29, 352, 1994.

46. **Mulaikal, R. M., Migeon, C. J., and Rock, J. A.,** Fertility rates in female patients with congenital adrenal hyperplasia due to 21-hydroxylase deficiency, *N. Engl. J. Med.,* 316, 178, 1987.

47. **Kuhnle, U., Bollinger, M., Schwarz, H. P., and Knorr, D.,** Partnership and sexuality in adult female patients with congenital adrenal hyperplasia. First results of a cross-sectional quality-of-life evaluation, *J. Steroid Biochem. Mol. Biol.,* 45, 123, 1993.

48. **White, P. C., Grossberger, D., Onufer, B. J., New, M. I., Dupont, B., and Strominger, J. L.,** Two genes encoding steroid 21-hydroxylase are located near the genes encoding the fourth component of complement in man, *Proc. Natl. Acad. Sci. U.S.A.,* 82, 1089, 1985.

49. **Carroll, M. C., Campbell, R. D., and Porter, R. R.,** The mapping of 21-hydroxylase genes adjacent to complement component C4 genes in HLA, the major histocompatibility complex in man, *Proc. Natl. Acad. Sci. U.S.A.,* 82, 521, 1985.

50. **White, P. C., Vitek, A., Dupont, B., and New, M. I.,** Characterization of frequent deletions causing steroid 21-hydroxylase deficiency, *Proc. Natl. Acad. Sci. U.S.A.,* 85, 4436, 1988.

51. **Owerbach, D., Crawford, Y. M., and Draznin, M. B.,** Direct analysis of CYP21B genes in 21-hydroxylase deficiency using polymerase chain reaction amplification, *Mol. Endocrinol.,* 4, 125, 1990.

52. **Mornet, E., Crete, P., Kuttenn, F., et al.,** Distribution of deletions and seven point mutations on CYP21B genes in three clinical forms of steroid 21-hydroxylase deficiency, *Am. J. Hum. Genet.,* 48, 79, 1991.

53. **Higashi, Y., Hiromasa, T., Tanae, A., et al.,** Effects of individual mutations in the P-450(C21) pseudogene on the P-450(C21) activity and their distribution in the patient genomes of congenital steroid 21-hydroxylase deficiency, *J. Biochem.,* 109, 638, 1991.

54. **Speiser, P. W., Dupont, J., Zhu, D., et al.,** Disease expression and molecular genotype in congenital adrenal hyperplasia due to 21-hydroxylase deficiency, *J. Clin. Invest.,* 90, 584, 1992.

55. **Higashi, Y., Tanae, A., Inoue, H., Hiromasa, T., and Fujii-Kuriyama, Y.,** Aberrant splicing and missense mutations cause steroid 21-hydroxylase [P-450(C21)] deficiency in humans: possible gene conversion products, *Proc. Natl. Acad. Sci. U.S.A.,* 85, 7486, 1988.

56. **Tusie-Luna, M. T., Traktman, P., and White, P. C.,** Determination of functional effects of mutations in the steroid 21-hydroxylase gene (CYP21) using recombinant vaccinia virus, *J. Biol. Chem.,* 265, 20916, 1990.

57. **Tusie-Luna, M. T., Speiser, P. W., Dumic, M., New, M. I., and White, P. C.,** A mutation (Pro-30 to Leu) in CYP21 represents a potential nonclassic steroid 21-hydroxylase deficiency allele, *Mol. Endocrinol.,* 5, 685, 1991.

58. **Higashi, Y., Hiromasa, T., Tanae, A., et al.,** Effects of individual mutations in the P-450(C21) pseudogene on the P-450(C21) activity and their distribution in the patient genomes of congenital steroid 21-hydroxylase deficiency, *J. Biochem.,* (Tokyo), 109, 638, 1991.

59. **Dickerman, Z., Grant, D. R., Faiman, C., and Winter, J. S. D.,** Intraadrenal steroid concentrations in man: zonal differences and developmental changes, *J. Clin. Endocrinol. Metab.,* 59, 1031, 1984.

60. **Mornet, E., Dupont, J., Vitek, A., and White, P. C.,** Characterization of two genes encoding human steroid 11β-hydroxylase (P-450 11β), *J. Biol. Chem.,* 264, 20961, 1989.

61. **Chua, S. C., Szabo, P., Vitek, A., Grzeschik, K. H., John, M., and White, P. C.,** Cloning of cDNA encoding steroid 11β-hydroxylase (P450c11), *Proc. Natl. Acad. Sci. U.S.A.,* 84, 7193, 1987.

62. **Kawamoto, T., Mitsuuchi, Y., Toda, K., Miyahara, K., Yokoyama, Y., Nakao, K., Hosoda, K., Yamamoto, Y., Imura, H., and Shizuta, Y.,** Cloning of cDNA and genomic DNA for human cytochrome P-450$_{11\beta}$, *FEBS Lett.,* 269, 345, 1990.

63. **Kawamoto, T., Mitsuuchi, Y., Ohnishi, T., et al.,** Cloning and expression of a cDNA for human cytochrome P-450aldos as related to primary aldosteronism, *Biochem. Biophys. Res. Commun.,* 173, 309, 1990.

64. **Curnow, K. M., Tusie-Luna, M. T., Pascoe, L., et al.,** The product of the CYP11B2 gene is required for aldosterone biosynthesis in the human adrenal cortex, *Mol. Endocrinol.,* 5, 1513, 1991.

65. **White, P. C., Pascoe, L., Curnow, K. M., Tannin, G., and Rosler, A.,** Molecular biology of 11β-hydroxylase and 11β-hydroxysteroid dehydrogenase enzymes, *J. Steroid Biochem. Mol. Biol.,* 43, 827, 1992.

66. **Curnow, K. M., Slutsker, L., Vitek, J., et al.,** Mutations in the CYP11B1 gene causing congenital adrenal hyperplasia and hypertension cluster in exons 6, 7, and 8, *Proc. Natl. Acad. Sci. U.S.A.,* 90, 4552, 1993.

67. **Naiki, Y., Kawamoto, T., Mitsuuchi, Y., et al.,** A nonsense mutation (TGG116TAG[Stop]) in CYP11B1 causes steroid 11β-hydroxylase deficiency, *J. Clin. Endocrinol. Metab.,* 77, 1677, 1993.

68. **Helmberg, A., Ausserer, B., and Kofler, R.,** Frame shift by insertion of 2 basepairs in codon 394 of CYP11B1 causes congenital adrenal hyperplasia due to steroid 11 beta-hydroxylase deficiency, *J. Clin. Endocrinol. Metab.,* 75, 1278, 1992.

69. **White, P. C., Dupont, J., New, M. I., Leiberman, E., Hochberg, Z., and Rösler, A.,** A mutation in CYP11B1 (Arg-448→His) associated with steroid 11β-hydroxylase deficiency in Jews of Moroccan origin, *J. Clin. Invest.,* 87, 1664, 1991.

70. **Matteson, K. J., Picado-Leonard, J., Chung, B.-C., Mohandas, T. K., and Miller, W. L.,** Assignment of the gene for adrenal P450c17 (steroid 17α-hydroxylase/17,20-lyase) to human chromosome 10, *J. Clin. Endocrinol. Metab.,* 63, 789, 1986.

71. **Chung, B-C., Picado-Leonard, J., Haniu, M., et al.,** Cytochrome P450c17 (steroid 17α-hydroxylase/17,20-lyase): cloning of human adrenal and testis cDNAs indicates the same gene is expressed in both tissues, *Proc. Natl. Acad. Sci. U.S.A.,* 84, 407, 1987.

72. **Lachance, Y., Luu-The, V., Labrie, C., et al.,** Characterization of human 3β-hydroxysteroid dehydrogenase/Δ^5-Δ^4 isomerase gene and its expression in mammalian cells, *J. Biol. Chem.,* 265, 20469, 1990.

73. **Lorence, M. C., Corbin, C. J., Kamimura, N., Mahendroo, M. S., and Mason, J. I.,** Structural analysis of the gene encoding human 3β-hydroxysteroid dehydrogenase/$\Delta^{5\text{-}4}$-isomerase, *Mol. Endocrinol.,* 4, 1850, 1990.

74. **Lachance, Y., Luu-The, V., Verreault, H., et al.,** Structure of the human type II 3β-hydroxysteroid dehydrogenase/Δ5-Δ4 isomerase (3β-HSD) gene: adrenal and gonadal specificity, *DNA Cell Biol.,* 10, 701, 1991.

75. **Berube, D., Luu-The, V., Lachance, Y., Gagne, R., and Labrie, F.,** Assignment of the human 3β-HSD gene to the p13 band of chromosome 1, *Cytogenet. Cell. Genet.,* 52, 199, 1989.

76. **Rheaume, E., Simard, J., Morel, Y., et al.,** Congenital adrenal hyperplasia due to point mutations in the type II 3β-hydroxysteroid dehydrogenase gene, *Nat. Genet.,* 1, 239, 1992.

77. **Chang, Y. T., Kappy, M. S., Iwamoto, K., Wang, J., Yang, X., and Pang, S.,** Mutations in the type II 3 beta-hydroxysteroid dehydrogenase (3 beta-HSD) gene in a patient with classic salt-wasting 3 beta-HSD deficiency congenital adrenal hyperplasia, *Pediatr. Res.,* 34, 698, 1993.

78. **Simard, J., Rheaume, E., Sanchez, R., et al.,** Molecular basis of congenital adrenal hyperplasia due to 3β-hydroxysteroid dehydrogenase deficiency, *Mol. Endocrinol.,* 7, 716, 1993.

79. **Chung, B. C., Matteson, K. J., Voutilainen, R., Mohandas, T. K., and Miller, W. M.,** Human cholesterol side-chain cleavage enzyme, P450scc: cDNA cloning, assignment of the gene to chromosome 15, and expression in the placenta, *Proc. Natl. Acad. Sci. U.S.A.,* 83, 8962, 1986.

80. **Lin, D., Gitelman, S. E., Saenger, P., and Miller, W. L.,** Normal genes for the cholesterol side chain cleavage enzyme, P450ssc, in congenital lipoid adrenal hyperplasia, *J. Clin. Invest.,* 88, 1955, 1991.

80a. **Lin, D., Sugawara, T., Strauss, J. F. I. Clark, B. J. Stocco, D. M., Saenger, P., Rogol, A., and Miller, W. L.,** Role of steroidogenic acute regulatory protein in adrenal and gonadal steroidogenesis, *Science,* 267, 1828, 1995.

81. **Merkatz, I. R., New, M. I., and Seaman, M. P.,** Prenatal diagnosis of adrenogenital syndrome by amniocentesis, *J. Pediatr.,* 75, 977, 1969.

82. **Jeffcoate, T. N. A., Fleigner, J. R. H., Russell, S. H., Davis, J. C., and Wade, A. P.,** Diagnosis of the adrenogenital syndrome before birth, *Lancet,* 2, 553, 1965.

83. **Frasier, S. D., Thorneycroft, I. H., Weiss, B. A., and Horton, R.,** Elevated amniotic fluid concentration of 17a-hydroxyprogesterone in congenital adrenal hyperplasia, *J. Pediatr.,* 86, 310, 1975.

84. **Gueux, B., Fiet, J., Couillin, P., et al.,** Prenatal diagnosis of 21-hydroxylase deficiency congenital adrenal hyperplasia by simultaneous radioimmunoassay of 21-deoxycortisol and 17-hydroxyprogesterone in amniotic fluid, *J. Clin. Endocrinol. Metab.,* 66, 534, 1988.

85. **Couillin, P., Nicolas, H., Boue, J., and Boue, A.,** HLA typing of amniotic-fluid cells applied to prenatal diagnosis of congenital adrenal hyperplasia, *Lancet,* 1, 1076, 1979.

86. **Pollack, M. S., Levine, L. S., Pang, S., et al.,** Prenatal diagnosis of congenital adrenal hyperplasia (21-hydroxylase deficiency) by HLA typing, *Lancet,* 1, 1107, 1979.

87. **Pang, S., Pollack, M. S., Loo, M., et al.,** Pitfalls of prenatal diagnosis of 21-hydroxylase deficiency congenital adrenal hyperplasia, *J. Clin. Endocrinol. Metab.,* 61, 89, 1985.

88. **Owerbach, D., Draznin, M. B., Carpenter, R. J., and Greenberg, F.,** Prenatal diagnosis of 21-hydroxylase deficiency congenital adrenal hyperplasia using the polymerase chain reaction, *Hum. Genet.,* 89, 109, 1992.

89. **Speiser, P. W., White, P. C., Dupont, J., Zhu, D., Mercado, A., and New, M. I.,** Prenatal diagnosis of congenital adrenal hyperplasia due to 21-hydroxylase deficiency by allele-specific hybridization and Southern blot, *Hum. Genet.,* 93, 424, 1994.

90. **Odink, R. J. H., Boue, A., and Jansen, M.,** The value of chorion villus sampling in early detection of 21-hydroxylase deficiency, *Pediatr. Res.,* 23, 131A/156, 1988.

91. **Shulman, D. I., Mueller, O. T., Gallardo, L. A., Stiff, D., and Ostrer, H.,** Treatment of congenital adrenal hyperplasia in utero, *Pediatr. Res.,* 25, 93A/543, 1989.

92. **David, M. and Forest, M. G.,** Prenatal treatment of congenital adrenal hyperplasia resulting from 21-hydroxylase deficiency, *J. Pediatr.,* 105, 799, 1984.

93. **Evans, M. I., Chrousos, G. P., Mann, D. W., et al.,** Pharmacologic suppression of the fetal adrenal gland in utero, *J. Am. Med. Assoc.,* 253, 1015, 1985.

94. **Forest, M. G., Betuel, H., and David, M.,** Traitement antenatal de l'hyperplasie congenitale des surrenales par deficit en 21-hydroxylase: etude multicentrique, *Ann. Endocrinol. (Paris),* 48, 31, 1987.

95. **Speiser, P. W., LaForgia, N., Kato, K., et al.,** First trimester prenatal treatment and molecular genetic diagnosis of congenital adrenal hyperplasia (21-hydroxylase deficiency), *J. Clin. Endocrinol. Metab.,* 70, 838, 1990.

96. **Migeon, C. J.,** Editorial: comments about the need for prenatal treatment of congenital adrenal hyperplasia due to 21-hydroxylase deficiency, *J. Clin. Endocrinol. Metab.,* 70, 836, 1990.

97. Editorial. Prenatal treatment of congenital adrenal hyperplasia, *Lancet,* i, 510, 1990.

98. **Pang, S., Pollack, M. S., Marshall, R. N., and Immken L.,** Prenatal treatment of congenital adrenal hyperplasia due to 21-hydroxylase deficiency, *N. Engl. J. Med.,* 322, 111, 1990.

99. **Goldman, A. S., Shapior, B. H., and Katsumata, M.,** Human foetal palatal corticoid receptors and teratogens for cleft palate, *Nature,* 272, 464, 1978.

Chapter 3

THE VITAMIN D ENDOCRINE SYSTEM

Reinhold Vieth and David E. C. Cole

CONTENTS

BASIC BIOLOGY

The term, *vitamin D*, strains the limits of its usual definitions as hormone, nutrient, and vitamin. In the strictest sense, vitamin D is none of these. If one defines a hormone as a molecule that is secreted in a regulated manner from one part of the body to signal other tissues via specific receptors, then vitamin D itself does not fit the definition. The vertebrate organism uses vitamin D to produce a true hormone, 1,25-dihydroxyvitamin D [1.25(OH)$_2$D], but the role of vitamin D itself is similar to that of cholesterol in the production of conventional steroid hormones. Vitamin D is not a prohormone, because, unlike a classic prohormone (e.g., proinsulin or proparathyroid hormone), the vitamin D precursor is not committed to the hormone synthetic pathway. Vitamin D is also not a prehormone in the classic sense of a peptide like angiotensinogen, because vitamin D itself is not secreted in a regulated manner and is not activated within the circulation. In many ways the vitamin D endocrine system is in a class by itself.*

The reader is advised that in the clinical literature, the term, *vitamin D*, is often used in a generic sense. The term is used carelessly to refer to 1,25(OH)$_2$D$_3$ or to any of its analogues. In recent years many experimental analogues have been developed that are based on the molecular structure of vitamin D. Unfortunately, in the jargon of the clinical setting, these potent drugs and hormone analogues are also then referred to as "vitamin D," and this practice may lead to dangerous misinterpretations. Recently, a more appropriate generic term, "deltanoid," has been proposed to indicate any vitamin D analogue.[1] The rationale for this new term is that it stems from *delta*, the letter D in the Greek alphabet, and the style of the word is similar to "retinoid," which is a generic term for molecules with a vitamin A (retinol) structure. An alternative and long-standing generic term for vitamin D-type molecules is "secosteroid," which stems from the Latin *seco*, to cut, and it means a fractured steroid molecule.

Authentic vitamin D comes in two forms, vitamin D$_2$ and D$_3$. In general, when vitamin D is discussed without a subscript, the point relates to either the D$_2$ or D$_3$ forms. What was once vitamin D$_1$ was found to be an impure mixture of materials and the term was dropped. Vitamin D$_2$ is ergocalciferol and is generated after ergosterol is exposed to ultraviolet (UV) light. Ergosterol is a plant steroid derived industrially from yeast.[2] Vitamin D$_3$ is cholecalciferol, the physiological form of vitamin D in mammals. Vitamin D$_2$ differs from vitamin D$_3$ by having a methyl group and double bond on the vitamin D side chain. In birds, vitamin D$_2$ is an ineffective agent. It was thought that vitamins D$_2$ and D$_3$ could be used interchangeably in primates, but clear differences have been demonstrated in monkeys.[3] The 1,25-dihydroxy D$_2$ and D$_3$ forms have different affinities for circulating binding protein (DBP), and for the intracellular receptor (VDR).[4] It is not yet settled whether there are differences in the biological efficacy of the D$_2$ and D$_3$ forms of the vitamin in humans.

If one thinks of steroid hormones as being derived from cholesterol (Figure 1), then vitamin D could have existed even before all the enzymatic machinery to synthesize steroid hormones was in place. It may be that the vitamin D system served to signal exposure to UV light. Essentially all fungi, plants, and animals produce photoactivatable, provitamin D.[5] Species of all mammalian classes require vitamin D, but this must be metabolized to 1,25(OH)$_2$D before it exhibits biological activity.[5,6]

SKIN AND VITAMIN D

Most mammals do not require vitamin D as a nutrient, because they are exposed to sufficient sunlight. For humans, the evolution of vitamin D into a nutrient stems from the

---

* An important aspect of vitamin D physiology is the complex interaction between the intracellular vitamin D receptor (VDR) for the activated form of vitamin D and the cellular genome. However, this area of active investigation is not extensively discussed here. The reader is referred to excellent reviews[61,95,122] and other chapters in this handbook.

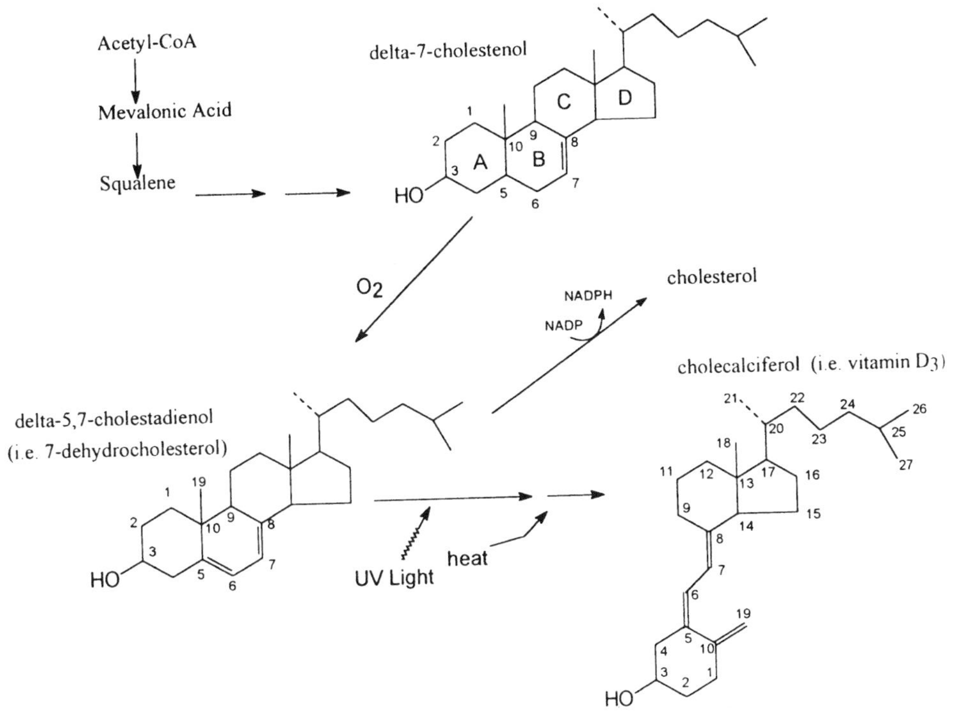

FIGURE 1. The dermal pathway toward cholesterol. This highlights how dermal cholesterol synthesis differs from that in other tissues. UV light disrupts 7-dehydrocholesterol to generate previtamin D_3, and this isomerizes with heat into vitamin D_3.

use of clothing, the migration of humans away from equatorial regions, and increased pollution. All of these lessen the exposure of skin to sunlight. The skin is an active and specialized site of sterol synthesis. The sequence of cholesterol-synthesizing reactions is different in the skin than the pathway that is typically shown for cholesterol synthesis in other tissues. In the skin, the removal of a double bond at C-24 during cholesterol synthesis occurs at an earlier step. Therefore, the last step in dermal cholesterol synthesis is from 7-dehydrocholesterol, an intermediate that is not present in other cholesterol-synthesizing tissues (Figure 1). In rat skin, 7-dehydrocholesterol comprises about 2% of the cholesterol content.[7] When 7-dehydrocholesterol is exposed to UV light of between 290 and 315 nm wavelength (UV-B), the B-ring of the steroid is cut between C-9 and C-10, to produce a secosteroid. With body heat, it takes about 24 h for the previtamin D_3 produced in this way to isomerize spontaneously into vitamin D_3. If there is sustained exposure to UV light, the previtamin D_3 and vitamin D_3 in skin deteriorate to tachysterol and other compounds.[8] This photodecomposition may explain why excess sun exposure does not cause vitamin D intoxication. It takes 1 to 4 days after sun exposure before increases in vitamin D are apparent in the circulation.[9]

In human aging, the skin loses its capacity for vitamin D production. In those over 70 years of age, a given amount of sun exposure produces only a fourth the vitamin D achieved in young adults.[10] Furthermore, the intensity of UV light from the sun diminishes during winter months. For example, at the latitude of Boston, Massachusetts (42°N), there is not enough outdoor UV intensity between November and February to generate any vitamin D in the skin, an effect that is accentuated by distance from the equator.[11]

Skin is comprised of an outer layer, the epidermis, with keratin protein at its surface, below which are aging keratinocytes, and reapidly reproducing, young keratinocytes deep in the epidermis. Vitamin D is thought to be generated from cholesterol precursor in the young keratinocytes. Skin blood vessels lie in the dermal tissue below the epidermis. The vitamin D_3 formed in this layer enters the circulation by mechanisms that have not been characterized. The skin blocks the absorption of most small molecules into the body because it is comprised of protective layers that are alternatively hydrophobic and aqueous. The absorption of vitamin D_3 from the skin into the circulation is unusual because this appears to be both specific and relatively efficient. It is thought that a remarkably high concentration of DBP in the circulation helps to draw vitamin D into the bloodstream.[12,13]

METABOLISM OF VITAMIN D BY LIVER AND KIDNEY

Natural vitamin D formed in the skin is taken into the circulation bound to DBP, from which it gains access to the liver slowly. In contrast, the vitamin D taken as part of the diet is absorbed from the gut in combination with cholesterol. Chylomicrons deliver fatty acids to adipose tissue, and chylomicron remnants are cleared by the liver, making both cholesterol and vitamin D available for metabolism.[9]

The liver readily converts vitamin D to 25-hydroxyvitamin D [25(OH)D]. The same liver mitochondrial enzyme carries out both the 25-hydroxylation of vitamin D and the 27-hydroxylation of cholesterol.[14] We do not know whether there is a biological consequence of this unusual situation of a shared liver enzyme.

The biological half-life of 25(OH)D in humans is several months, and its levels reflect vitamin D nutrition. Although 25(OH)D is unlikely to possess biological activity in itself,[15,16] its levels do affect serum $1,25(OH)_2D$ in an unexpected manner. Unless there is a near absolute lack of vitamin D, the serum $1,25(OH)_2D$ levels tend to be elevated in infants with rickets due to vitamin D deficiency.[17-19] Furthermore, dietary supplementation of rats with vitamin D, in amounts about ten times that normally added to commercial diets, results in lower serum $1,25(OH)_2D$ levels. There have been no studies aimed at explaining these inverse interactions between 25(OH)D and $1,25(OH)_2D$ levels. However, in rats, an increase in vitamin D nutritional status can increase VDR content.[20] Presumably, higher VDR levels increase tissue sensitivity to $1,25(OH)_2D$ so that lower serum $1,25(OH)_2D$ levels will have the same effect as the higher serum levels do when tissue VDR levels are lower.

The kidney functions as an endocrine gland synthesizing and secreting the $1,25(OH)_2D$ hormone. Production of $1,25(OH)_2D_3$ is stimulated by low calcium, low phosphate, and high circulating levels of parathyroid hormone (PTH). $1,25(OH)_2D_3$ stimulates the intestine to absorb calcium. Together with calcium, $1,25(OH)_2D_3$ suppresses the parathyroid gland. Together with PTH, $1,25(OH)_2D_3$ regulates both bone resorption and bone formation, thereby maintaining normal bone and mineral physiology. Figure 2 summarizes the way PTH and $1,25(OH)_2D$ interact to regulate calcium metabolism.

Kidney mitochondria can contain two enzymes to metabolize 25(OH)D, the 1α-hydroxylase to produce $1,25(OH)_2D$ and the 24-hydroxylase which produces $24,25(OH)_2D$.[21,22] The activities of these enzymes are inversely regulated in the kidney, because PTH will suppress 24-hydroxylase and stimulate 1α-hydroxylase.[23] In the absence of PTH or PTH receptors, $1,25(OH)_2D$ stimulates 24-hydroxylase, probably as a way of limiting the action of $1,25(OH)_2D$ by initiating its catabolism to $1,24,25(OH)_3D$—an inactive polar metabolite—both in the kidney and at target tissues.

CATABOLISM OF VITAMIN D METABOLITES AND ANALOGUES

Essentially all vitamin D that enters the body is metabolized to 25(OH)D, which is cleared from the circulation in several ways. The liver is a major site of clearance, through conjugation, oxidation, and biliary excretion of vitamin D metabolites. Some unaltered vitamin D metabolites are also secreted with bile, and they can be reabsorbed in what has been referred to as an enterohepatic cycle that probably comprises only a minor part of the body's vitamin D pool.[24] There is evidence that hepatic excretion vitamin D metabolites increase with calcium deprivation and hyperparathyroidism.[25] Normal human $1,25(OH)_2D$ production rates range between 0.3 and 1 µg/day,[26] but the adult recommended intake of vitamin D is only 5 µg/day.

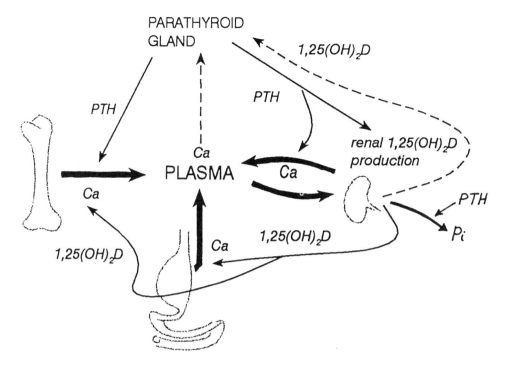

FIGURE 2. A schematic overview of calcium homeostasis. The heavy arrows represent the movement of calcium from bone, the intestine, and the kidney. The thinner arrows indicate actions that stimulate (solid arrows) and suppress (dashed arrows) what they point to. Note that $1,25(OH)_2D$ is one of two negative feedback signals to suppress the parathyroid gland. Also note the three classical target tissues of $1,25(OH)_2D$, the bone, the intestine, and the parathyroid gland.

From a pharmacological standpoint, the most important clearance route for vitamin D metabolites is 24-hydroxylation of the 25-hydroxyvitamin D side chain. Vitamin D itself and analogues without the 25-hydroxyl group are not metabolized by this pathway. Although 24-hydroxylase was originally demonstrated in the kidney, it has been demonstrated in all tissues with receptors for $1,25(OH)_2D$.[27] The vitamin D hormone brings about its own destruction in its target tissues. 24-Hydroxylase induction is classic evidence for tissue responsiveness to $1,25(OH)_2D$. After catabolism has been initiated by 24-hydroxylase, further metabolism results in the cleavage of the vitamin D side chain at carbon 23 to inactive calcitroic acid.[27,28]

TRANSPORT OF D METABOLITES VIA THE CIRCULATION

Vitamin D, its metabolites, and pharmaceutical analogues of vitamin D bind primarily to DBP in the circulation. DBP has a molecular weight of 58,000 Da and belongs to the same molecular family as albumin. DBP has been known to geneticists since the early 1960s as group-specific component (Gc), a circulating genetic marker detectable by electrophoresis or immunoassay. DBP is one of the most heterogeneous proteins in humans, with at least 120 allelic variants known, but only three of these account for the DBP found in most humans. For $1,25(OH)_2D$, DBP functions like a conventional hormone binding protein, such as thyroid hormone binding globulin, or sex-steroid binding globulin. However, DBP circulates at 5 μmol/L in humans, far in excess of the 100 nmol/L range that is the normal limit of the sum of all the vitamin D metabolites. Because of the high DBP concentration, the biologically available, free fraction of $1,25(OH)_2D$ is normally only 0.4% of the total $1,25(OH)_2D$.[29] At the cell level, this low free concentration makes $1,25(OH)_2D$ among the most potent of hormones, with free levels that are often in the femtomolar range. Direct measures of free

1,25(OH)$_2$D are difficult to perform and to reproduce. The classic approach to measuring free 1,25(OH)$_2$D uses dialysis,[29] but a far easier and valid method is based on quantitation of the specific binding capacity of DBP using an approach similar to that used for measuring the free thyroxine index.[30] Levels of DBP are lower when there is liver impairment, or in those suffering from anorexia nervosa, and they are higher during pregnancy.[29-31]

The forms of vitamin D differ in their relative affinities for DBP, and the metabolic clearance rates for analogues and metabolites is slower with greater DBP-binding affinity. In the human, the DBP affinity is greatest for 25(OH)D and relatively low for 1,25(OH)$_2$D and vitamin D.[4] The relative affinities of vitamin D metabolites for DBP are proportional to their circulating concentrations.[4]

DBP is cleared mainly by the liver but also by the kidney. The half-life of DBP in the circulation is normally about 72 h, much shorter than the half-lives of vitamin D metabolites. Recent studies have shown DBP to function as part of the actin scavenger system.[32,33] Actin is an intracellular, fibrous, structural protein that polymerizes spontaneously. When tissue is injured, actin is released from cells and can enter the circulation, where its polymerization would result in occlusion of microvasculature, particularly in the lung and brain. Once bound to actin, DBP complex is quickly cleared, with a half-life of about 30 min, and the components of DBP are recycled.[34] The body has another protein to remove actin from the circulation, gelsolin, which is an enzyme that binds and catabolizes actin.[33] For DBP, the actin-binding and vitamin D-binding functions are independent of each other, because neither ligand affects the interaction of DBP with the other.

A third role for DBP is as a circulating peptide that B cells metabolize to produce a proactivating factor further activated by T cells. With these activation steps, DBP becomes a signaling molecule that greatly enhances the phagocytic activity of macrophages.[32,35]

For other proteins in the circulation, such as albumin and other hormone-binding proteins, there exist rare individuals in whom one of those proteins is missing genetically. Affected individuals can adapt to the absence of the missing protein, with little obvious difficulty. However, there is no known case of DBP absence reported in humans or in animal models. It appears that DBP is essential for mammalian life. This may be due to its actions that do not involve the vitamin D system. The genetic heterogeneity of DBP, and the minimal variability in the functionality of DBP despite this heterogeneity, attest to the fundamentally important roles that DBP plays in mammalian physiology. It is equally remarkable that three so apparently disparate functions are combined in this one protein.

VITAMIN D NUTRITION
Definition of Vitamin D Deficiency

Calcium metabolism reflects only one aspect of vitamin D action. 1,25(OH)$_2$D, acts on many tissues that are *not* related to calcium metabolism, including the hematopoietic and lymphatic systems, skeletal muscle, vascular smooth muscle, skin, reproductive tissues, the brain, and the spinal cord.[36,37] More than 50 genes have been reported to be transcriptionally regulated by 1,25(OH)$_2$D.[37] It is not known which of the various other effects of the vitamin D endocrine system are important to health. Walters et al.[36] concluded that "vitamin D deficiency is a heterogeneous collection of physiologic conditions." *In the most general sense, vitamin D deficiency is a state in which the supply of vitamin D is not sufficient for the optimal operation of at least one of the various physiological functions that may depend on the vitamin D endocrine system.*

1,25(OH)$_2$D can be produced by several tissues in the body. These include the liver, keratinocytes, placenta, macrophages, aorta, skin, and bone cells.[38,39] This peripheral production of 1,25(OH)$_2$D$_3$ is thought to play a paracrine role to modulate cell proliferation and differentiation.[38] One thing that must certainly be a key aspect of paracrine 1,25(OH)$_2$D production is that 1α-hydroxylase activity *in vivo* is highly dependent on the availability of substrate.[15,40] That is, unlike other paracrine hormone systems, there is an unreliable and highly variable supply of substrate. Consequently, vitamin D nutritional status will affect potential paracrine roles of $1,25(OH)_2D$ that may not be related directly to mineral metabolism or even to serum $1,25(OH)_2D$.

In northern cities, vitamin D is by far the most common nutritional deficiency in elderly individuals.[41] There is now ample evidence that the combination of vitamin D supplements with calcium will reduce the risk of osteoporosis.[42] In light of this, there is a growing consensus that for the elderly, the recommended intake of vitamin D should be increased from the present adult level of 5 µg/day to 20 µg/day (800 IU/day).[42,43]

Table 1 summarizes the interpretations that can be applied to specific concentrations of serum 25(OH)D.

TABLE 1
Significance of Serum Levels of 25(OH)D in Animals and Humans

Serum 25(OH)D (nmol/L)	Significance
0	Target level in animal studies of vitamin D deficiency; the aim is to suppress 1,25(OH)2D, ideally to undetectable levels
<10	Distinctly osteomalacic or rachitic range in humans
20	Lower limit of reference range in Toronto[75]
25	"persistent 25(OH)D levels below 25nmol/L . . . should indicate vitamin D depletion"[76]
80	Upper limit of reference range in Toronto[75]
225	Upper limit of reference range in Puerto Rico[77]
>250	Pharmacologically achieved levels
731	Toxic levels in patients poisoned by erroneously excessive amounts of vitamin D_3 in milk from a U.S. dairy[78]

Vitamin D Nutrition during Reproduction and Infancy

The placenta actively transfers 25(OH)D from the mother to the fetus.[44] The placenta produces $1,25(OH)_2D$, thereby promoting maternal absorbtion of calcium from the diet. The fetus itself does not produce much $1,25(OH)_2D$.[45] Cord-blood levels of vitamin D metabolites are substantially lower than maternal values, and there is a substantial seasonal variation in fetal vitamin D metabolite levels.[46] At birth, serum 25(OH)D concentrations are about half those of children and adults.[47,48] Breast milk contains very little vitamin D, and breast-fed infants exhibit strikingly lower 25(OH)D concentrations than those given conventional vitamin supplements. In Finland, Markestad[48] reported median values of only 6 ng/ml in breast-fed infants, as compared to formula-fed infants (median 36 ng/ml, $p < .01$). Furthermore, the Pittard study[50] showed that infants in South Carolina had neonatal 25(OH)D concentrations essentially the same as the Finnish infants.[48] Therefore, it would be imprudent to assume that simply because individuals live at a more southern latitude, they are less in need of vitamin D supplementation—particularly if they have limited UV exposure.

A recent study from South America reports that in their winter at 55°S latitude, neonatal 25(OH)D levels average only 4 ng/ml, whereas at 34°S latitude they average 11 ng/ml.[49] For adults, 10 ng/ml is the decision level for clinically low 25(OH)D—below this, osteomalacia is anticipated. The published 25(OH)D levels in children with frank nutritional rickets range up to 20 nmol/L (8 ng/ml).[18,19] Clearly, the neonatal period is one in which there is a risk of vitamin D deficiency.

Even though the current recommendations for neonatal vitamin D intake were established 30 years ago (American Academy of Pediatrics, Committee on Nutrition, 1963) it was only in 1991 that an appropriate longitudinal study validated the 10 µg/day (400 IU/day) dose as the recommended intake for infants.[50] This dose is effective and safe.

USE OF 1,25(OH)$_2$D$_3$ ANALOGUES IN THE TREATMENT OF DISEASE

As kidney function deteriorates, there is a fall in its capacity to fulfill its endocrine role. This is partly due to the loss of functional kidney mass and partly due to the accumulation of uremic toxins that inhibit residual 1α-hydroxylase.[51] At the same time, the kidney loses its capacity to excrete phosphate. Together, the higher serum phosphate and low levels of 1,25(OH)$_2$D$_3$ result in hypocalcemia. Low calcium and low 1,25(OH)$_2$D$_3$ levels stimulate the parathyroid gland to secrete PTH. Renal osteodystrophy ensues because of the combination of high PTH secretion, low calcium, and low 1,25(OH)$_2$D. Uremic toxins not only impair the production of 1,25(OH)$_2$D$_3$, but blunt its peripheral action as well. The toxins lower VDR levels, impair VDR nuclear uptake, and alter the interaction of VDR with its hormone-responsive elements (HRE) in the genome.[52] For all these reasons, it is now generally accepted that treatment of uremic patients with 1,25(OH)$_2$D$_3$ is helpful in preventing secondary hyperparathyroidism and renal bone disease.

In addition to 1,25(OH)$_2$D$_3$, the agent, 1α-hydroxycholecalciferol (alfacalcidol) is commonly used in nephrology.[53] This is metabolized by the liver in an unregulated way to 1,25(OH)$_2$D$_3$. Of particular interest for renal patients is 1,25(OH)$_2$-22-oxa-D$_3$ (OCT), which is reported to have beneficial effects on bone[54] and suppresses parathyroid gland secretion without altering serum calcium.[55]

Other analogues have potential in cancer treatment. Treatment of postmenopausal osteoporosis with 1,25(OH)$_2$D$_3$ reduces fracture rate[56] and is reported to cause hypercalcemia only rarely. 1α-Hydroxyvitamin D$_3$ is also being evaluated and is thought to differ in its effects on serum and urine calcium, the only measures of toxicity used.[57] Lastly, 1,25(OH)$_2$D$_3$ and its analogues have become popular in the treatment of psoriasis. Treatment for psoriasis can involve dermal doses as large as 500 μg (cf. the usual oral dose of 1 μg/day). The approach has been called "safe and effective" as long as serum and urine calcium levels remain in the normal range.[58] Reports are appearing of hypercalcemia in psoriasis patients treated topically with 1,25(OH)$_2$D or its analogues.[59,60]

NONCALCEMIC ANALOGUES OF 1,25(OH)$_2$D$_3$

The only way to determine which analogues have selective actions is to empirically evaluate each of them *in vivo*. However, there is an interesting and unresolved question as to why equimolar doses of some analogues *do not* cause hypercalcemia. There are several aspects of vitamin D biology that could render an analogue "noncalcemic."

Affinity for DBP—The most common feature of noncalcemic analogues of 1,25(OH)$_2$D$_3$ is that they have lower affinity for DBP than 1,25(OH)$_2$D$_3$ itself.[4] With less adherence to DBP, an analogue will be cleared faster from the blood, but there is no logical reason why this feature should tend to minimize effects on serum calcium while selecting for other actions. Poor affinity for DBP might make the drug more selective if it is applied directly to the skin, as it may be in the treatment of psoriasis, and where poor affinity for DBP could impair absorption from the skin.

Metabolism by Target Tissues—Oxidation of 1,25(OH)$_2$D$_3$ at carbon 24 on its side chain initiates the deactivation of the hormone and its analogues.[27] If an analogue has a modified side chain, its catabolism will be altered and this may alter the spectrum of biological activity.

VDR Differences and Greater Affinity for Certain Ligand Structures—The classic VDR is present in many tissues, and it may be that there are tissue-specific differences in VDR, caused by posttranslational modifications, that could alter specificity for ligand structures. Whether such differences exist is not known.

Transcaltachia—This is a phenomenon whereby 1,25(OH)$_2$D$_3$ has been shown to increase calcium transport within minutes, through nongenomic means.[61] If this mechanism for 1,25(OH)$_2$D$_3$ were to function *in vivo*, this would be through cell-membrane receptors that probably bind 1,25(OH)$_2$D$_3$ differently from the classic VDR, and such a difference could be exploited to tailor vitamin D analogues with selective actions.

Intracellular Calcium Shift—One obvious way for $1,25(OH)_2D_3$ analogues to be non-calcemic would be to cause a shift of elemental calcium into the cellular compartment. This feature would make an analogue appear to be safer on the basis of a measured serum calcium, but it could render the drug more toxic to tissues.

TOXICITY OF VITAMIN D

Vitamin D can be toxic when taken in excess orally. This should not come as a surprise, in light of the way we naturally acquire vitamin D. Few foods that humans naturally eat contain vitamin D, and most of the vitamin D we acquire in the contemporary diet is an artificial additive to milk. The oil of certain fish, like salmon and cod, contains nutritionally useful amounts of vitamin D_3. Presumably the fish acquired the capacity to synthesize vitamin D as part of their evolutionary adaptation to deep ocean water, or they have acquired it nutritionally from plankton consumption. Even the leaves of certain species of plants contain vitamin D_3 and its metabolites. A pharmacological amount of $1,25(OH)_2D_3$, 1 µg, is present in 1 g of *Cestrum diurnum* leaf,[62] which has been shown to be responsible for toxic calcinosis in cattle. As a poison against pests, vitamin D—referred to as "calciferol" on the product label—is only exceeded in popularity by warfarin. Vitamin D is much less expensive, being required in only microgram amounts to be lethal to rodents.

Although the skin is normally the major source of vitamin D in humans, there has been no known case of vitamin D toxicity due to excessive dermal production. The explanation for this is that with increasing UV exposure, an equilibrium is established in the skin, where the amount of vitamin D remains constant. Vitamin D can be considered the intermediate between activated previtamin D and the degradation products of vitamin D. Although excess UV exposure may increase previtamin D and vitamin D production rates, the amount of vitamin D present at any time achieves equilibrium in the skin because the UV light also causes accelerated photodecomposition of these products.[58]

Vitamin D is unusual as a nutrient because there is very little vitamin D in most of the foods humans normally eat. Addition of vitamin D to dairy products was mandated in the mid-1960s, and this has virtually eliminated nutritional rickets in Canada.[92] Unfortunately, because of its potential toxicity, some have argued that the addition of vitamin D to foods may be doing more harm than good.[16,63] The arguments that nutritional amounts of vitamin D are harmful fail to consider the therapeutic index (ratio between effective and toxic doses) for the vitamin. To our knowledge, the lowest vitamin D dose causing a clinically reported case of vitamin D intoxication [validated by the presence of hypercalcemia and an elevated serum 25(OH)D] involved a cumulative dosage of 3.6 million units (90,000 µg) of vitamin D given over 12 weeks.[64] The highest recommended dietary intake for vitamin D is 10 µg/day, and this is less than the more than 300 µg vitamin D_3 attainable with a minimally erythemal UV exposure to 1 m² of skin.[65]

The large margin of safety for vitamin D is understandable in light of the probable biological mechanisms causing vitamin D toxicity.[16,66] Toxicity probably occurs because of saturation of DBP with 25(OH)D and other metabolites that displace $1,25(OH)_2D$ into the biologically active free form. Furthermore, unphysiologically high levels of 25(OH)D drive, by mass action, the production of $1,25(OH)_2D$ beyond the body's limited capacity to clear the hormone.[66] Although total serum $1,25(OH)_2D$ levels may not be particularly high in reported cases of vitamin D toxicity, even the normal levels are inappropriate in the face of hypercalcemia and the increased free hormone.

Vitamin D toxicity results in hypercalcemia, due to excessive absorption of calcium from the diet. In severe cases there may be a net resorption of calcium from bone, but it is very unlikely that this can go on long enough to lower bone mass. Vitamin D and its analogues will tend to raise bone mass, not lower it. Vitamin D excess causes accumulation of calcium in the aorta and in kidney mitochondria. In fact, a classic way to induce arteriosclerosis in rats is to give them extremely large doses of vitamin D along with nicotine.[67,68] This treatment substantially reduces the elasticity of aorta. A disconcerting feature of this arteriosclerotic model is that serum calcium rises only transiently with the initial "sensitizing" step with vitamin D. Serum calcium remains normal during the subsequent weeks when calcium continues to accumulate in the aortic wall.[69] Obviously, serum calcium is probably not an adequate reflection of the true toxicity of vitamin D excess. Likewise, serum calcium may not be a true index of safety for the noncalcemic analogues of vitamin D. In humans, calcium content of the aortic wall rises sixfold with age.[68] Although it is not established whether vitamin D, its metabolites, or its analogues play a contributory role, further clarification is warranted.

EFFECTS OF VITAMIN D ON BONE

Vitamin D has long been thought necessary for bone formation, because rickets and osteomalacia are the classic signs of vitamin D deficiency. However, this role has been hard to prove. The most striking acute effect of $1,25(OH)_2D$ is osteoclastic bone resorption through a complex mechanism that involves signaling from osteoblasts, the release by osteoclasts of lysosomal enzymes, and increases in osteoclast number, size, and nuclear area.[70]

Brommage and DeLuca[71] showed that vitamin D-deficient rats did not become rachitic if their circulating mineral levels were maintained at normal levels. They contended that the role of vitamin D in bone formation is to ensure that sufficient calcium and phosphorus is available by ensuring absorption of calcium from the gut. Osteoblasts respond to the hormone through changes in collagen, alkaline phosphatase (reflected clinically in increased circulating enzyme levels),[152] and 24-hydroxylase.[70] The effect of $1,25(OH)_2D$ on the calcium-binding protein, Calbindin-D9k, may be the best evidence for a mineralizing role of $1,25(OH)_2D$. Although it is present in the cytosol of most soft tissues, in bone it is localized to the matrix vesicles, particularly near the mineralizing front of trabecular bone. It also seems to remain in position over the crystallites formed from the matrix vesicles in heavily mineralized bone. The patterns of synthesis and distribution of calbindin-D9k in normal and rachitic bone and cartilage indicate that $1,25(OH)_2D$ has a direct effect on mineralizing tissues.[72] Osteocalcin or bone Gla-protein (BGP) is a vitamin K-dependent protein that is produced by osteoblasts as well as by other tissues in the body.[115] However, tissue accumulation of osteocalcin occurs only in bone and cartilage. In osteoblast and chondrocyte cultures, the osteocalcin synthesis is increased by $1,25(OH)_2D_3$. One way to assess osteoblast function *in vivo* is to measure the increase in osteocalcin after doses of $1,25(OH)_2D_3$ are given.[73] The selective accumulation of osteocalcin in bone and cartilage may be related to the maintenance or development of a collagenous matrix.[74] Although it remains difficult to prove that $1,25(OH)_2D_3$ is directly needed for bone growth and mineralization, it is clear that $1,25(OH)_2D_3$ is essential to normal mineralization of the human skeleton.

CLINICAL CORRELATES

EXCESS VITAMIN D
Extrinsic Causes

In humans, excess vitamin D intake produces a toxic state clinically referred to as hypervitaminosis D. It is associated with hypercalcemia and all the signs and symptoms associated with that. Some are apparent on examination—the clouded mental state and chronic fatigue—whereas those associated with calcium deposition in different internal organs, particularly the kidney, are subtle in the early stages but more permanent. Hypervitaminosis D was a more common occurrence in the first decades after the introduction of vitamin D supplements, until it was appreciated that toxicity is not immediately apparent to the patient or the physician. Nowadays, hypervitaminosis D is uncommon[79] but still occurs accidentally if vitamin D supplementation in the milk is excessive.[78] It has also been reported occasionally in infants,[81] but the problem is usually the opposite—too little or too late.[80]

Intrinsic Causes

In the disease hyperparathyroidism,[82] the primary cause of the hypercalcemia is a direct action of PTH to stimulate release of calcium from bone, but a secondary effect is to stimulate renal 1α-hydroxylase and generate $1,25(OH)_2D$. In longstanding hyperparathyroidism with hypercalcemia, though, serum $1,25(OH)_2D$ levels may be low.[83] Hypercalcemia of malignancy may be osteolytic (i.e., secondary to invasion of bone by tumor) but may also be mediated by humoral factors, including vitamin D.[84,85] This form of excess $1,25(OH)_2D$ is associated more frequently with leukemia, neuroblastoma, and renal tumors.[86,87] Patients with sarcoidosis (or other granulomatous diseases, such as histoplasmosis) and hypercalcemia have hypercalciuria and increased levels of $1,25(OH)_2D$ with appropriate suppression of immunoreactive PTH (iPTH).[88] The excess $1,25(OH)_2D$ is apparently not renal in origin[89,90] but rather is derived from constitutive synthesis by granulomatous macrophages. Both prednisone and chloroquine[91] act to normalize serum calcium by reducing circulating $1,25(OH)_2D$ concentrations.

INSUFFICIENT VITAMIN D

Insufficient vitamin D may result in either rickets or osteomalacia.[92] Rickets is a disorder that was first recognized as a distinct entity at the beginning of the industrial revolution when large numbers of marginally nourished children began working indoors where skin exposure to sunlight was minimal. As the effects of vitamin D deficiency began to affect bone metabolism, their growth was stunted, their lower limbs became bowed, and their energy capacity declined. When these conditions applied also to working pregnant women, the condition would be present from birth and the disturbance in mineral metabolism so severe that it was a cause of infant death. The different stages of what is a progressive process of vitamin D depletion are listed in Table 2.

In current scientific parlance, rickets is defined as a disorder of mineralization in the preosseous cartilage of epiphyseal growth plates and the matrix of growing bone.[92] Osteomalacia may be defined as a disorder confined to endosteal remodeling sites of the mature bone matrix. The stage of bone growth and development determines whether combined rickets and osteomalacia, or osteomalacia alone, will occur in a particular individual.[93] These mineral-deficient states may result primarily from either lack of calcium availability (calciopenia) or lack of phosphate availability (phosphopenia), but calciopenia is usually the result of defects in vitamin D metabolism or action. Phosphopenia usually results from excess phosphate loss or inadequate phosphate intake. The classification of rickets into these two classes has implications for treatment (see Figures 3 and 4). Whereas calciopenia usually responds to vitamin D, effective treatment of phosphopenia requires phosphate replacement as well.

Our understanding of the etiology and pathogenesis of rickets continues to change as more is discovered about vitamin D metabolism and the interaction of vitamin D with other mineral elements. The appearance of heritable rickets in modern societies has increased with the decrease in nutritional vitamin D deficiency. As noted before, however, there has been a corresponding increase in the size of vulnerable hospitalized populations,[94] requiring clinical sensitivity to the differing needs of infants,[95] adults with chronic disease, and the elderly.[96]

Intake and Absorption

Nutritional vitamin D deficiency is a continuing problem despite widespread addition of vitamin D to many foods.[93] If the maternal diet is vitamin D deficient, nutritional rickets may appear in the breast-fed infant.[97] Dietary regimens without fortified cows' milk (or formulas) and vitamin supplements may not provide sufficient vitamin D. Urban black infants from northern latitudes who are exclusively breast fed are at increased risk for nutritional rickets.[98,99] A careful dietary history will usually suggest the diagnosis. Earlier descriptions of severe

TABLE 2
Stages of Vitamin D Deficiency

	Stage I	Stage II	Stage III
Clinical features			
Age of onset in children	3–6 months	5–12 months	>6 months
Clinical presentation	Tetany (hypocalcemic muscle contractions)	Delayed growth Bowing (*genu varum*) Failure to thrive Incidental discovery on an X-ray	Tetany and hypocalcemic convulsions Growth failure Bowing or knock-knees (*genu valgum*) Bone tenderness Pneumonia due to chest collapse
Physical signs	Craniotabes (skull softening)	Enlarged tender bone ends (knees, wrists) Lethargy and decreased muscle tone	Delayed growth and irritability Bone pain Hoarse voice (*laryngeal stridor*) Spinal deformities
Radiologic features	Minimal changes, with decreased mineralization	Demineralization Widened and frayed epiphyses	As for stage II but more severe Signs of hyperparathyroidism Pathologic fractures
Biochemical features			
Serum calcium	$\leftrightarrow$	$\downarrow$	$\downarrow$
Serum phosphorus	Slight $\uparrow$	$\downarrow$	$\downarrow$
Alkaline phosphatase activity	Slight $\uparrow$	$\Uparrow$	$\downarrow$
Serum PTH	Slight $\uparrow$	$\uparrow$	$\uparrow\uparrow$
Urinary amino acid excretion	$\leftrightarrow$	$\uparrow$	$\uparrow\uparrow$

$\uparrow$, increased. $\uparrow\uparrow$, greatly increased. $\downarrow$, decreased. $\leftrightarrow$, unchanged.

disease emphasized hypocalcemia as a cardinal feature of nutritional rickets. However, serum calcium may be normal in less severe or partially treated states (stage I—see Table 2). Serum phosphate may be only slightly depressed, but alkaline phosphatase is almost always elevated. Normalization of serum calcium is believed to result from compensatory hyperparathyroidism. A consequence of this secondary hyperparathyroidism is the increased excretion of cAMP and the development of generalized aminoaciduria.[93] Secondary hyperparathyroidism also provides part of the stimulus for increased 1α-hydroxylation of 25(OH)D in nutritional rickets and is considered responsible for the finding (discussed earlier) of normal or elevated 1,25(OH)$_2$D concentrations when levels of 25(OH)$_2$D are low.[18,19,100-102] There may also be down-regulation of the renal phosphaturic response to endogenous circulating PTH, because phosphate excretion is normal in patients with elevated immunoreactive PTH and nephrogenous cAMP.

Malabsorption resulting from intestinal, pancreatic, or hepatic disease may impair vitamin D and mineral homeostasis. Although clinical history may suggest deficient dietary intake, occult malabsorptive disorders should be considered in children with active rickets or adults with osteomalacia that occurs while on a normal diet. In chronic malabsorption syndromes, attention must be paid to the adequacy of vitamin D intake. Decreased 25(OH)D levels in some patients with inadequate supplementation have been associated with decreases in serum calcium and reduced bone mass. With increased supplementation of 1000 IU/day, both 25(OH)D and 1,25(OH)$_2$D levels are reportedly normal.[103] Although bone mineralization may remain somewhat decreased, clinically significant complications of osteopenia are not reported.

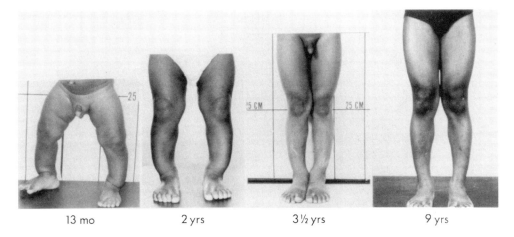

| 13 mo | 2 yrs | 3½ yrs | 9 yrs |

FIGURE 3. Photographs showing a child with leg bowing from nutritional rickets and the natural straightening that occurs with healing and normal growth if the treatment is started early enough.

Metabolic Defects
Altered Hepatic Metabolism

Osteopenia, rickets, and osteomalacia may complicate *chronic liver disease.*[104] Low serum levels of 25(OH)D and vitamin D may be found, but other defects arising from hepatic disease may include (1) decreased serum DBP (more significant in cirrhosis), (2) impaired 25-hydroxylation of vitamin D,[105] (3) impaired enterohepatic circulation of vitamin D and its metabolites,[106] and (4) deficient synthesis of other undefined vitamin D metabolites. Oral 1,25(OH)D$_3$ often does not correct the hepatic or malabsorptive osteomalacia of adults, but the ineffectiveness of 1,25(OH)$_2$D$_3$ may not be entirely explained by an altered intestinal response, because brisk increases in both calcium and phosphorus absorption have been noted.[107] In general, oral 1,25(OH)$_2$D is not recommended, and calcifidiol [25(OH)D$_3$] is used to treat hepatic osteodystrophy.[108]

Administration of anticonvulsants such as phenobarbital or diphenylhydantoin (phenytoin) may induce rachitic and osteomalacic changes in susceptible populations.[109] These changes are more likely to be of clinical significance when accompanied by decreased serum 25(OH)D levels usually brought on, in part, by associated risk factors, including decreased exposure to sunlight, poor nutritional status, and immobility. It has been stated that both agents induce hepatic metabolism of vitamin D to polyhydroxylated polar metabolites, thereby causing a depletion of active forms—25(OH)D and 1,25(OH)$_2$D—although *in vitro* studies show that phenobarbital increases conversion of D$_3$ to 25(OH)D$_3$.[110] Also, concentrations of 25(OH)D levels tend to be in the normal range in active, ambulatory patients on anticonvulsants. 1,25(OH)$_2$D levels may be normal or increased even in those with hypocalcemia and active bone disease. These findings suggest an anticonvulsant-induced end-organ resistance to vitamin D metabolites. In bone organ culture, diphenylhydantoin suppresses 1,25(OH)$_2$D- or PTH-induced bone resorption.[111] Use of diphenylhydantoin and sodium valproate, another anticonvulsant, is associated with secondary hyperparathyroidism in humans and animals.[112]

Altered Renal Metabolism

The progression of chronic renal failure is associated with growth retardation in children and bone disease in adults.[113-115] Because elements of osteitis fibrosa and osteomalacia are often mixed with frank rickets/osteomalacia and other histologic or radiographic abnormalities, this metabolic disorder has been collectively referred to as *renal osteodystrophy.* As noted above, replacement with vitamin D, or with one of its metabolites, is effective in promotion of growth and correction of secondary hyperparathyroidism.[116] 1,25(OH)D$_3$ and 1α(OH)D$_3$ do not require 1α-hydroxylation and are probably superior alternatives, but adverse

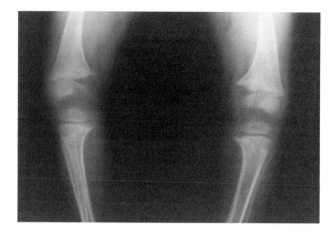

A

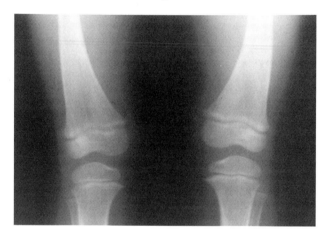

B

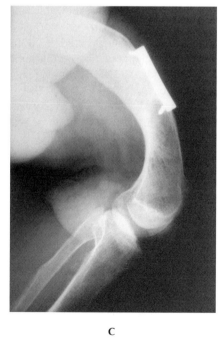

C

effects of these agents on the renal failure itself may occur if hypercalcemia intervenes.[117] Despite these measures, some degree of renal osteodystrophy often remains, and hormone resistance due to uremic factors undoubtedly contributes to the pathogenesis of this complex bone disorder.[118] As well as the analogues mentioned earlier, the concomitant use of $24,25(OH)_2D_3$ or $25(OH)D_3$ along with $1,25(OH)_2D_3$ may be beneficial.[119,120]

25-Hydroxylase Deficiency

An inherited defect of the 25-hydroxylase enzyme has seemed a likely possibility, but only recently has sufficient evidence been amassed to suggest that it may be a clinical entity. This has been reported in two siblings with severe rickets that was unresponsive to adequate vitamin D intake and low serum 25-hydroxylase levels that responded to pharmacological doses of vitamin D and physiological doses of calcifidiol.[121] The condition is probably uncommon and needs to be validated as a distinct disorder by molecular studies demonstrating inactivating mutations of the gene or absence of the enzymatic activity in tissue.[120]

1α-Hydroxylase Deficiency

Type 1 autosomal recessive vitamin D dependency (ARVDD-l) arising from a deficiency of renal 25(OH)D-lα-hydroxylase enzyme is a disorder that usually presents with hypocalcemia or rickets early in the newborn period.[122] It is accompanied by depressed serum calcium and phosphorus, marked secondary hyperparathyroidism, and elevated nephrogenic cAMP excretion.[123] Serum 25(OH)D levels are either normal or high due to previous vitamin D therapy, but $1,25(OH)_2D$ concentrations are universally low. Although the condition has been treated with pharmacologic doses (often 50,000 to 100,000 U/day) of vitamin D, it is very effectively treated with either alfacalcidol or calcitriol. Careful monitoring is required if optimum treatment is to be maintained.

RESISTANCE TO VITAMIN D ACTION
Vitamin D Receptor Deficiency

Also known as type II vitamin-D-dependency rickets, this rare syndrome of autosomal recessive inheritance presents with clinical and radiological features similar to severe vitamin D deficiency rickets.[122] A distinctive feature in most affected kindreds is alopecia totalis, which may be present from birth.[124] Other clinical features of rickets, such as widened wrists and ankles, may be apparent at birth, unlike other forms of inherited rickets. Adolescent- or adult-onset syndromes have also been reported. These patients present with hypocalcemia, modest hypophosphatemia, secondary hyperparathyroidism, and increased alkaline phosphatase activity. Circulating 25(OH)D is normal, but $1,25(OH)_2D$ levels are elevated in the untreated state. Patients with alopecia have generally been refractory to pharmacologic administration of $1,25(OH)_2D$, 25(OH)D, or lα(OH)D. Early death has been reported in affected kindreds.[122] A more effective therapy for those with alopecia has been suggested by Balsan et al.,[125] who used nocturnal parenteral calcium infusions. A striking correction of skeletal deformities and biochemical parameters occurred after 7 months of therapy in one affected

---

FIGURE 4. X-rays showing the lower limbs (femur, knee, and tibia-fibula). In the first X-ray (**A**), the lower leg bowing in this 2½-year-old girl can be recognized. She has an inherited disorder of phosphate transport—X-linked hypophosphatemic rickets. The gap between the shaft of the femur and the end (epiphysis) is the growth zone and does not show on X-ray because it is nonmineralized cartilage. Note how frayed and ragged the end of the femoral shaft is. In the next X-ray (**B**), taken at 5½ years after proper treatment with vitamin D and phosphate, her legs have straightened considerably and the growth plate is much more even. A zone of calcification (increased whiteness on the X-ray) can be see on both sides of the growth plate. The last figure (**C**) shows the patient's father at 32 years of age who was never properly treated as a child. His femur is so shortened and twisted that it is hardly recognizable. The radiodense area in the middle is a metallic plate inserted by the orthopedic surgeon in an effort to strengthen and straighten the bone surgically. This man has been partially crippled since he was a child and will have severe arthritis in the joints when he is older. This problem is now entirely avoidable with proper diagnosis and treatment.

girl. She had been resistant to oral calcium therapy and pharmacologic 25(OH)D therapy producing circulating 1,25(OH)$_2$D levels as high as 11,000 pg/ml.

Molecular studies have shown that the various defects in the vitamin D receptor lead to failure of intracellular binding of the ligand—1,25(OH)$_2$D—to the receptor, failure of the ligand/receptor complex to translocate to the nucleus, failure of the complex to bind essential cofactors, and failure of the complex to bind to its cognate hormone-responsive element(s) of the target genes.[122]

Hypomagnesemia

Calcium homeostasis is often severely affected in the condition of hypomagnesemia.[126-128] Numerous factors can predispose one to hypomagnesemia, and several inborn errors of magnesium homeostasis are known.[129] Primary hypomagnesemia usually refers to an isolated defect in intestinal magnesium transport.[130,131] Inherited defects in renal tubular reabsorption of magnesium and potassium, and of magnesium alone, also occur.[132] The most frequently encountered cases of magnesium deficiency in childhood are probably related to generalized malabsorptive disorders and excess renal losses related to the use of aminoglycoside antibiotics and cisplatin.[133] Patients receiving digoxin are at risk for developing hypomagnesemia, and newborns can present with hypomagnesemia secondary to maternal hypomagnesemia.[134] Hypomagnesemia is also seen in cases of pancreatitis, diabetes, and in both hyper- and hypoparathyroidism.[129] Dysregulation of calcium homeostasis in magnesium deficiency may occur for several reasons. Impaired secretion and activity of both PTH and vitamin D in hypomagnesemia has been reported by several investigators.[135-138] Synthesis of the active hormone is impaired, because the enzyme activity is magnesium dependent, and activity *in vitro* normalizes when magnesium is added.[139,140] There is also a failure to respond to exogenously administered 1,25(OH)$_2$D.[139,141]

The Neonate

Preterm and small-for-gestational-age (SGA) neonates, particularly when they fall in the very-low-birth-weight (VLBW) category (<1500 g),[142] are at risk for developing metabolic bone disease. Mild bone disease in these infants may be evident only as minimal osteopenia on radiographs or bone mineral densitometry.[143] In moderate disease, osteopenia is more pronounced, and zones of provisional calcification in the long bones may be narrowed. With severe osteopenia, the zone of provisional calcification may disappear altogether. Radiolucent bands in the metaphyses, as well as frank rachitic changes, may also be apparent. In addition to increased risks for fractures and bony deformities,[144] cardiorespiratory function may be compromised by the impairment of myocardial and diaphragmatic contractility. Ventilation requirements may increase, and preexisting cardiac failure may be exacerbated. Although milder disease is not usually associated with clinical problems, the disorder is progressive if not treated and is often slow to correct.

The pathogenesis of this disorder is complex, and more than one predisposing or causative factor is often implicated.[142,145,146] However, there is little doubt that inadequate mineral intake is a major cause of disease in these infants.[143] Maternal vitamin D deficiency,[147] preeclampsia, and perinatal asphyxia have also been described as significant prenatal risk factors. Postnatal risk factors include many indicators of neonatal morbidity such as assisted ventilation, late metabolic acidosis, sepsis, and recurrent apnea. Coincident cardiac anomalies, hepatobiliary dysfunction, or intestinal disease have also been associated with metabolic bone disease.[148] Aluminum loading, which is associated with intravenous therapy, may also be a contributing factor.[145,149,150] A contributory role for disordered regulation of calciotropic hormones in this disease has been more difficult to define.[147] Levels of 25(OH)D may be normal or low, but increased concentrations brought on by vitamin D supplementation may not be sufficient to stimulate mineralization, particularly if mineral substrates are limited.[151] Similarly, serum 1,25(OH)$_2$D concentrations may be increased by treatment,[19] but VLBW infants can be extremely resistant to the calcemic effect of the hormone.[50,153] Correction of early hypocalce-mia and a skeletal response may not be evident until doses of more than 3000 ng/kg/day are used.[154] The use of vitamin D metabolites should probably be restricted to specific indications, but up to 2000 IU/day of vitamin D can be safely used.[155] In infants with hepatic or renal failure, for instance, parenteral administration of $1,25(OH)D_3$ may be the only means of ensuring an adequate supply of active hormone.

DYSREGULATION OF VITAMIN D METABOLISM
Williams Syndrome and Idiopathic Hypercalcemia of Infancy

Williams syndrome has been considered synonymous with infantile idiopathic hypercal-cemia.[156] Fanconi and Girardet[157] initially noted that severe hypercalcemia accompanied a syndrome of mental deficiency, growth retardation, cardiovascular anomalies, and distinctive facial appearance. The increased incidence in Europe subsequent to the introduction of vitamin D supplements during pregnancy pointed to a role for prenatal vitamin D toxicity in the etiology of this disorder.[156,158,159] Clinical evidence for abnormal sensitivity to vitamin D was soon forthcoming[160] and was followed later by studies in the rabbit showing induction of cardiovascular anomalies and bony changes in the offspring by large intakes of vitamin D during pregnancy.[61,162] However, further efforts to confirm a primary defect in vitamin D metabolism have been unsuccessful.[163-166] A different experience in the United States led to the report of a syndrome by Williams et al.[167] that included the characteristic "elfin" facies, supravalvular aortic stenosis, and, less frequently, evidence of hypercalcemia with hypercal-ciuria. Beuren et al.[168] delineated the somatic phenotype further, while Jones and Smith[169] have emphasized the rarity of hypercalcemic signs or symptoms in their series of patients with Williams' elfin facies syndrome.

Martin et al.,[170] in a comprehensive study of 117 affected individuals, found that most of the patients could be classified as having either the Fanconi-type idiopathic hypercalcemia or the Williams-Beuren syndrome with developmental delay, facial features, and cardiovas-cular signs but without evidence for hypercalcemia. The groups show distinctive differences in clinical presentation and natural history, but the facial features, cardiovascular findings, and neurological deficits are the same.

Definition of a single metabolic abnormality has proven more difficult.[171] Early observers noted that the hypercalcemia arises, in part, from increased gastrointestinal absorption.[172] Vitamin D appears to have a permissive role, as evidenced by the efficacy of reduced vitamin D intake in the treatment of the disorder.[170] Moreover, asymptomatic patients given an oral or intravenous calcium load may demonstrate a more rapid rise in serum calcium than normal and a delay in calcium clearance.[173,174]

There are conflicting reports regarding serum concentrations of $25(OH)D$ and $1,25(OH)_2D$, but these metabolites do not appear to be consistently altered in either normo-calcemic or hypercalcemic individuals.[163,166,175-177] Suppression of iPTH release by high cal-cium concentrations may be less than expected, but the responses to PTH stimulation tests are normal.

Although case reports of familial recurrence have appeared, the syndrome is usually sporadic.[156,170,178-180] More recently, evidence has emerged to indicate that the dysmorphic features are associated with a *de novo* submicroscopic deletion on chromosome 7 that includes deletion of the elastin gene.[181,182] The challenge now is to relate this important molecular finding to the biochemical defect in mineral metabolism.

Hypoparathyroidism

Classic laboratory findings of hypoparathyroidism include hyperphosphatemia and hypo-calcemia. In the absence of PTH action, circulating levels of $1,25(OH)_2D$ are generally decreased.[183] Indeed, both rickets[184] and osteomalacia[185] have been reported in longstanding untreated disease; both appear to respond to treatment.[186] However, some $1,25(OH)_2D$ is detectable in the circulation of hypoparathyroid patients, and some may have levels in the normal range.

Long-term treatment of the hypocalcemia can be achieved with vitamin D,[187-189] dihydrotachysterol,[189] $1\alpha(OH)D_3$,[187,189] or $1,25(OH)_2D_3$.[186,189-191] Both $1\alpha(OH)D_3$ and $1,25(OH)_2D_3$ have the theoretical advantage that their potency and short serum half-lives allow for rapid normalization of serum calcium and rapid readjustment thereafter. Although resistance has been reported,[192] most patients will respond to doses of up to 100 ng/kg/day of calcitriol or about twice that amount of $1\alpha(OH)D_3$.[189,191] There may also be a slower response to increases or decreases in dosage than the serum half-lives for these metabolites would suggest.[193] Symptomatic adults can be treated with 2 μg/day of $1\alpha(OH)D_3$ but may require only 1 μg daily when normocalcemia is achieved. Treatment should be individualized. In this regard, it is probably most helpful to monitor the therapeutic response by measuring urinary calcium excretion along with serum calcium.[194] Maintenance of a reasonable serum calcium (about 8 mg/dl) at the expense of optimal levels of 9.5 to 10.5 mg/dl (which may be associated with hypercalciuria) should be the therapeutic goal. Further adjustment can be based on the maintenance of urinary calcium levels at less than 300 to 400 mg/day per 1.73 m^2 body surface area or less than 4 mg/kg body weight per day in infants and children.[195] In this group, it may prove more practical to follow calcium/creatinine ratios on consecutive early morning random specimens, with the aim of maintaining an average ratio of less than 0.4 (mg/mg). The risks of renal complications from calcitriol therapy are still being debated, although the common experience has been that hypercalcemic episodes are transient and well controlled and that renal glomerular filtration is not markedly affected.[190,196] $1\alpha(OH)D_3$ appears equally effective if increased doses are used, the exception being patients with liver disease, such as those with polyglandular failure and hepatitis.[105] For the patients in which some degree of hypercalciuria is unavoidable, hypocalciuric diuretics may be useful adjunctive therapy.[197] Thiazides have been used in idiopathic hypoparathyroidism but may present some risk to those with polyglandular failure in whom latent adrenal insufficiency is a possibility. Nevertheless, supplemental hydrochlorthiazide therapy has been used to effectively treat the hypercalciuria of pediatric hypoparathyroid patients receiving optimal doses of calcitriol.[198] The long-term safety of this agent has not been established.

X-Linked Hypophosphatemia

A sex-linked dominantly inherited form of rickets that is characterized by (1) hypophosphatemia present from birth, (2) low to normal serum calcium, and (3) rachitic changes appearing in infancy is variously termed familial or X-linked hypophosphatemic rickets (XLH) and is attributed to a defect in renal conservation of phosphorus.[199-201] Studies of the homologous X-linked phenotype in mouse (*Hyp*) have suggested that phosphate reabsorption in the proximal tubule is decreased as a result of a defect in sodium-dependent uptake in the luminal brush-border membrane. The severity of the condition tends to be more variable in females, in part because of random X-chromosome inactivation. The gene has been localized to a small region of Xp22.1-22.2,[202] but the presence of a phosphate transporter on chromosome 5q35[203] extends the controversy about the function of the X-linked gene responsible for this condition.

In untreated XLH patients, serum phosphate is quite low and alkaline phosphatase is elevated. Levels of 25(OH)D are in the normal range, and levels of $1,25(OH)_2D$ are not elevated, despite the hypophosphatemia. Decreased $1,25(OH)_2D$ levels may be seen in patients on some form of phosphate and vitamin D supplementation.[204] Similarly, the *Hyp* mouse model suggests that renal 1α-hydroxylation of 25(OH)D may be abnormally insensitive to hypophosphatemia,[205-207] a defect that can be demonstrated indirectly in the XLH patient.[208]

Effective therapy is directed toward maintenance of both normal serum calcium and phosphorus by supplemental oral phosphate (1 g/day elemental phosphorus) and vitamin D.[209]

In maintaining optimum levels of both agents, renal calcium excretion can be used as an early indicator of excess vitamin D intake. Both the $l\alpha(OH)D_3$ and $1,25(OH)_2D_3$ metabolites may offer some therapeutic advantages over vitamin D, including improved linear growth rate and reduced requirement for supplemental phosphate.[148,199,210,211] This effect is probably attributable to an action of $1,25(OH)_2D$ on bone mineralization that is independent of calcium and phosphorus concentrations.[210]

Hypercalciuria leading to nephrocalcinosis (which may be detected ultrasonographically) remains a significant complication.[212-215] Alon and Chan[216] have reported on the use of thiazides (and spironolactone or amiloride if hypokalemia ensues) to reduce the calciuria and minimize the risk of renal calcium deposition. In the younger patient, hyperparathyroidism probably occurs in some untreated patients, although it is not the commonly reported finding, perhaps because it is more likely to occur at night.[217] It more frequently arises in older patients as a result of therapy and can be difficult to manage. In patients who develop hypercalcemia, reduction of the vitamin D supplement may be sufficient to correct the problem. In those with some degree of hyperparathyroidism, however, reduction of phosphate intake for a period of time may be required.[199] For situations where PTH secretion has become autonomous,[218] surgical extirpation and autotransplantation has been advocated.[219]

Now that adequately treated children are reaching adulthood, the long-term complications of this disorder are receiving more intense scrutiny.[201,220,221] Hearing deficits,[222] arthritis,[200] calcification of the entheses (joints, tendons, ligaments),[223] and spinal canal stenosis[224] are some of the recently reported findings.

Hypercalciuric Hypophosphatemic States

Another variant of absorptive hypercalciuria has been described in a large kindred with hypophosphatemic rickets.[225] A primary renal tubular defect in phosphate reabsorption occurs, but, unlike patients with classic XLH, these individuals maintain the ability to generate elevated circulating $1,25(OH)_2D$ levels in response to hypophosphatemia, resulting in marked intestinal hyperabsorption of calcium, hypercalciuria, and nephrolithiasis.

Phosphate supplementation has been shown to be particularly useful in hypercalciuric hypophosphatemic rickets.[225] The skeletal disease responds directly to increased phosphate availability, thereby increasing serum phosphate levels and resulting in a reduction of circulating $1,25(OH)_2D$, which, in turn, removes the stimulus for increased calcium absorption.

Idiopathic Hypercalciuria

The term idiopathic hypercalciuria has been reserved for excessive urinary calcium excretion in the absence of hyperresorption or other primary skeletal disorder.[226,227] In absorptive hypercalciuria, increased intestinal calcium absorption occurs and results in the subsequent delivery of excess filtered calcium to the renal tubule. Increased intestinal absorption has been described in the absence of elevated $1,25(OH)_2D$ levels. Others suggest a $1,25(OH)_2D$-dependent hyperabsorption of calcium.[228] A group of these latter individuals is speculated to have dysregulation of the $25(OH)D$-$l\alpha$-hydroxylase in the proximal renal tubular cell.[229] Bone demineralization is not thought to be a component of absorptive hypercalciuria, and calcium balance is maintained.

Other Conditions

Hypothyroidism and hyperthyroidism have been associated with hypercalcemia.[230] In hypothyroidism, excess iPTH and increased $1,25(OH)_2D$ are found, but the reversibility of the hypocalciuria suggests that this is another condition in which the parathyroid gland set-point for calcium has been altered.[231,232] In congenital hypothyroidism, hypercalcemia may be avoided by forgoing vitamin D supplementation for the first few months. Hypercalcemia in hyperthyroid infants and children is rare but does occur.[232] Multiple endocrine adenopathies should always be considered in this group.[110,233]

In *nephrotic syndrome* with normal renal function, low serum ionized calcium, elevated iPTH, and osteomalacia have been reported.[234,235] Although serum 25(OH)D levels are low, presumably due to renal loss of protein-bound 25(OH)D, total serum $1,25(OH)_2D$ may be normal. It has been suggested that these "normal" levels of $1,25(OH)_2D$ are insufficient to prevent the development of osteomalacia and lead to the exacerbation of accompanying osteodystrophy when renal failure is also present, probably as a result of impaired 1α-hydroxylation of 25(OH)D.[236]

ACKNOWLEDGMENTS

We thank Dr. S.W. Kooh for Figure 3 and Dr. Jovan Evrovski for expert assistance in preparing the manuscript. We acknowledge with gratitude the teaching of Drs. C. Scriver, D. Fraser, and S. Salisbury that provided us with such a rich field of knowledge about vitamin D, both clinical and applied. We also appreciate the frequent collegial contributions of Drs. D. Hanley, S. Atkinson, S.W. Kooh, J.W. Balfe, and T. Carpenter in our clinical endeavors.

REFERENCES

1. **Anzano, M.A., Smith, J.M., Uskokovic, M.R., et al.,** $1\alpha,25$-dihydroxy-16-ene-23-yne-26,27-hexafluoroc-holecalciferol (RO24-5531), a new deltanoid (vitamin D analogue) for prevention of breast cancer in the rat, *Cancer Res.*, 54, 1653, 1994.
2. **Feiser, L.F., Feiser, M., Feiser, L.F., and Feiser, M., Eds.,** Vitamin D, in *Steroids,* Reinhold, New York, 1959, 90.
3. **Marx, S.J., Jones, G., Weinstein, R.S., Chrousos, G.P., and Renquist, D.M.,** Differences in mineral metabolism among nonhuman primates receiving diets with only vitamin D_3 or only vitamin D_2, *J. Clin. Endocrinol. Metab.,* 69, 1282, 1989.
4. **Bishop, J.E., Collins, E.D., Okamura, W.H., and Norman, A.W.,** Profile of ligand specificity of the vitamin D binding protein for $1\alpha,25$-dihydroxyvitamin D_3 and its analogs, *J. Bone Miner. Res.,* 9, 1277, 1994.
5. **Holick, M.F.,** Evolutionary biology and pathology of vitamin D, *J. Nutr. Sci. Vitaminol.,* 79, 1992.
6. **Henry, H. and Norman, A.W.,** Presence of renal 25-hydroxyvitamin-D-1-hydroxylase in species of all vertebrate classes, *Comp. Biochem. Physiol.,* 50B, 431, 1975.
7. **Esvelt, R.P., DeLuca, H.F., Wichmann, J.K., Yoshizawa, S., Zurcher, J., Sar, M., and Stumpf, W.E.,** 1,25-Dihydroxyvitamin D_3 stimulated increase of 7,8-didehydrocholesterol levels in rat skin, *Biochemistry,* 19, 6158, 1980.
8. **Webb, A.R., DeCosta, B.R., and Holick, M.F.,** Sunlight regulates the cutaneous production of vitamin D_3 by causing its photodegradation, *J. Clin. Endocrinol. Metab.,* 68, 882, 1989.
9. **Haddad, J.G., Matsuoka, L.Y., Hollis, B.W., Hu, Y.Z., and Wortsman, J.,** Human plasma transport of vitamin D after its endogenous synthesis, *J. Clin. Invest.,* 91, 2552, 1993.
10. **MacLaughlin, J. and Holick, M.F.,** Aging decreases the capacity of human skin to produce vitamin D_3, *J. Clin. Invest.,* 76, 1536, 1985.
11. **Ladizesky, M., Lu, Z., Oliveri, B., San Roman, N., Diaz, S., Holick, M.F., and Mautalen, C.,** Solar UV B radiation and photoproduction of vitamin D_3 in central and south areas of Argentina, *J. Bone Miner. Res.,* 10, 545, 1995.
12. **Bikle, D.D. and Pillai, S.,** Vitamin D, calcium, and epidermal differentiation, *Endocr. Rev.,* 14, 3, 1993.
13. **Holick, M.F.,** The use and interpretation of assays for vitamin D and its metabolites, *J. Nutr.,* 120 (Suppl. 11), 1464, 1990.
14. **Okuda, K.I.,** Liver mitochondrial P450 involved in cholesterol catabolism and vitamin D activation, *J. Lipid Res.,* 35, 361, 1994.
15. **Vieth, R.,** The mechanisms of vitamin D toxicity, *Bone Miner.,* 11, 267, 1990.
16. **Fraser, D.R.,** Vitamin D, *Lancet,* 345, 104, 1995.
17. **Steichen, J.J., Tsang, R.C., Greer, F.R., Ho, M., and Hug, G.,** Elevated serum 1,25-dihydroxyvitamin D concentrations in rickets of very low birthweight infants, *J. Pediatr.,* 99, 293, 1981.

18. **Garabedian, M., Bainsel, M., Mallet, E., Guillozo, H., Toppet, M., Grimberg, R., Nguen, T.M., and Balsan, S.,** Circulating vitamin D metabolite concentrations in children with nutritional rickets, *J. Pediatr.,* 103, 381, 1983.

19. **Chesney, R.W., Hamstra, A.J., and DeLuca, H.F.,** Rickets of prematurity: supranormal levels of serum 1,25-dihydroxyvitamin D, *Am. J. Dis. Child.,* 135, 34, 1981.

20. **Sandgren, M.E. and DeLuca, H.F.,** Serum calcium and vitamin D regulate 1,25-dihydroxyvitamin D3 receptor concentration in rat kidney in vivo, *Proc. Natl. Acad. Sci. U.S.A.,* 87, 4312, 1990.

21. **Henry, H.L.,** Vitamin D hydroxylases, *J. Cell. Biochem.,* 49, 4, 1992.

22. **Arabian, A., Grover, J., Barre, M.G., and Delvin, E.E.,** Rat kidney 25-hydroxyvitamin D3 1 alpha- and 24-hydroxylases: evidence for two distinct gene products, *J. Steroid. Biochem. Mol. Biol.,* 45, 513, 1993.

23. **Shinki, T., Jin, C.H., Nishimura, A., Nagai, Y., Ohyama, Y., Moshiro, N., Okuda, K., and Suda, T.,** Parathyroid hormone inhibits 25-hydroxyvitamin D_3-24-hydroxylase mRNA expression stimulated by 1,25-dihydroxyvitamin D_3 in rat kidney but not in intestine, *J. Biol. Chem.,* 267, 13757, 1992.

24. **Fraser D.R.,** The physiological economy of vitamin D, *Lancet,* i, 969, 1983.

25. **Clements, M.R., Davies, M., Hayes, M.E., Mawer, E.B., and Adams, P.H.,** The role of 1,25-dihydroxyvitamin D in the mechanism of acquired vitamin D deficiency, *Clin. Endocrinol.,* 37, 17, 1992.

26. **Gray, R.W., Caldes, A.E., Wilz, A.E., Lemann, J., Smith, G., and DeLuca, H.F.,** Metabolism and excretion of ^{3}H-1,25-$(OH)_2D_3$ in healthy adults, *J. Clin. Endocrinol. Metab.,* 46, 756, 1978.

27. **Makin, G., Lohnes, D., Byford, V., Ray, R., and Jones, G.,** Target cell metabolism of 1,25-dihydroxyvitamin D_3 to calcitroic acid, *Biochem. J.,* 262, 173, 1989.

28. **Reddy, G.S., Tsering, K.Y., Thomas, B.R., Dayal, R., and Norman, A.W.,** Isolation and identification of 1,23-dihydroxy-24,25,26,27-tetranorvitamin D_3, a new metabolite of 1,25-dihydroxyvitamin D_3 produced in rat kidney, *Biochemistry,* 26, 324, 1987.

29. **Bikle, D.D., Gee, E., Halloran, B., and Haddad, J.G.,** Free 1,25-dihydroxyvitamin D levels in serum from normal subjects, pregnant subjects, and subjects with liver disease, *J. Clin. Invest.,* 74, 1966, 1984.

30. **Vieth, R.,** Simple method for determining specific binding capacity of vitamin D-binding protein and its use to calculate the concentration of "free" 1,25-dihydroxyvitamin D, *Clin. Chem.,* 40, 435, 1994.

31. **Olmos, J.M., Riancho, J.A., Amado, J.A., Freijanes, J., and Menendez-Arango, J.G.J.,** Vitamin D metabolism and serum binding proteins in anorexia nervosa, *Bone,* 12, 43, 1991.

32. **Constans, J.,** Group-specific component is not only a vitamin-D-binding protein, *Exp. Clin. Immunogenet.,* 9, 161, 1992.

33. **Lee, W.M. and Galbraith, R.M.,** The extracellular actin-scavenger system and actin toxicity, *N. Engl. J. Med.,* 326, 1335, 1992.

34. **Dueland, S., Blomhoff, R., and Pedersen, J.I.,** Uptake and degradation of vitamin D binding protein and vitamin D binding protein-actin complex *in vivo* in the rat, *Biochem. J.,* 267, 721, 1990.

35. **Yamamoto, N. and Kumashiro, R.,** Conversion of vitamin D_3 binding protein (group-specific component) to a macrophage activating factor by the stepwise action of β-galactosidase of B cells and sialidase of T cells, *J. Immunol.,* 151, 2794, 1993.

36. **Walters, M.R., Kollenkirchen, U., and Fox, J.,** What is vitamin D deficiency? *Proc. Soc. Exp. Biol. Med.,* 199, 385, 1992.

37. **Hannah, S.S. and Norman, A.W.,** 1,25$(OH)_2$Vitamin D_3 regulated expression of the eucaryotic genome, *Nutr. Rev.,* 52, 376, 1994.

38. **Dusso, A.S., Finch, J., Brown, A., Ritter, C., Delmez, J., Schreiner, G., and Slatopolsky, E.,** Extrarenal production of calcitriol in normal and uremic humans, *J. Clin. Endocrinol. Metab.,* 72, 157, 1991.

39. **Bikle, D.D., Halloran, B.P., and Riviere, J.E.,** Production of 1,25 dihydroxyvitamin D_3 by perfused pig skin, *J. Invest. Dermatol.,* 102, 796, 1994.

40. **Dusso, A., Lopez-Hilker, S., Lewis-Finch, J., Grooms, P., Brown, A., Martin, K., and Slatopolsky, E.,** Metabolic clearance rate and production rate of calcitriol in uremia, *Kidney Int.,* 35, 860, 1989.

41. **Cals, M.J., Bories, P.N., Devanlay, M., Desveaux, N., Luciani, L., Succari, M., Duche, J.C., de Jaeger, C., Blonde-Cynober, F., and Coudray-Lucas, C.,** Extensive laboratory assessment of nutritional status in fit, health-conscious, elderly people living in the Paris area, *J. Am. Coll. Nutr.,* 13, 646, 1994.

42. **Meunier, P.J.,** Prevention of hip fractures, *Am. J. Med.,* 95, 75S, 1993.

43. **Heaney, R.P.,** Bone mass, nutrition, and other lifestyle factors, *Am. J. Med.,* 95, 29S, 1993.

44. **Clements, M.R. and Fraser, D.R.,** Vitamin D supply to the rat fetus and neonate, *J. Clin. Invest.,* 81, 1768, 1988.

45. **Kooh, S.W. and Vieth, R.,** 25-Hydroxyvitamin D metabolism in the sheep fetus and lamb, *Pediatr. Res.,* 14, 360, 1980.

46. **Garel, J.M.,** Hormonal control of calcium metabolism during the reproductive cycle in mammals, *Physiol. Rev.,* 67, 1, 1987.

47. **Weisman, Y., Reiter, E., and Root, A.R.,** Measurement of 24,25-dihydroxyvitamin D in sera of neonates and children, *J. Pediatr.,* 91, 904, 1977.

48. **Markestad, T.,** Plasma concentrations of 1,25-dihydroxyvitamin D, 24,25-dihydroxyvitamin D, and 25,26-dihydroxyvitamin D in the first year of life, *J. Clin. Endocrinol. Metab., 57, 755, 1983.*

49. **Oliveri, M.B., Mautalen, C.A., Alonso, A., Velazquez, H., Trouchot, H.A., Porto, R.M.L., and Barata, A.D.,** Nutritional status of vitamin D in mothers and neonates of Ushuaia and Buenos Aires, *Medicina (Buenos Aires), 53, 315,1993 (in Spanish).*

50. **Pittard, W.B., Geddes, K.M., Hulsey, T.C., and Hollis, B.W.,** How much vitamin D for neonates? *Am. J. Dis. Child., 145, 1147, 1991.*

51. **Hsu, C.H. and Patel, S.,** Uremic plasma contains factors inhibiting 1-alpha-hydroxylase activity, *J. Am. Soc. Nephrol., 3, 947, 1992.*

52. **Hsu, C.H., Patel, S.R., and VanHolder, R.,** Mechanism of decreased intestinal calcitriol receptor concentration in renal failure, *Am. J. Physiol., 264, F662, 1993.*

53. **Watson, A.R., Kooh, S.W., Tam, C.S., Reilly, B.J., Balfe, J.W., and Vieth, R.W.,** Renal osteodystrophy in children on CAPD: a prospective trial of 1-alpha-hydroxycholecalciferol therapy, *Child. Nephrol. Urol., 9, 220, 1989.*

54. **Sato, K., Nishii, Y., Woodies, F.N., and Raisz, L.G.,** Effects of two new vitamin D_3 derivatives, 22-oxa-1a-25-dihydroxyvitamin D_3 (OCT) and 2β-(3-hydroxypropoxy)-1α,25-dihydroxyvitamin D_3 (ED-71), on bone metabolism in tissue culture, *Bone, 14, 47, 1993.*

55. **Brown, A.J. and Finch, J.L.,** New active analogues of vitamin D with low calcemic activity, *Kidney Int., Suppl. 38, S22, 1990.*

56. **Tilyard, M.W., Spears, G.F.S., Thomson, J., and Dovey, S.,** Treatment of postmenopausal osteoporosis with calcitriol or calcium, *N. Engl. J. Med., 326, 357, 1992.*

57. **Gallagher, J.C., Bishop, C.W., Knutson, J.C., Mazess, R.B., and DeLuca, H.F.,** Effects of increasing doses of 1α-hydroxyvitamin D_2 on calcium homeostasis in postmenopausal osteopenic women, *Bone Miner. Res., 9, 607, 1994.*

58. **Holick, M.F.,** Active vitamin D compounds and analogues: a new therapeutic era for dermatology in the 21st century [editorial; comment], *Mayo Clin. Proc., 68, 925, 1993.*

59. **Hoeck, H.C., Laurberg, G., and Laurberg, P.,** Hypercalcaemic crisis after excessive topical use of a vitamin D derivative, *J. Intern. Med., 235, 281, 1994.*

60. **Russell, J.A.,** Osteomalacic myopathy, *Muscle Nerve, 17, 578, 1994.*

61. **Norman, A.W.,** Vitamin D research frontiers, *J. Cell. Biochem., 49, 1, 1992.*

62. **Prema, T.P. and Raghuramulu, N.,** Free vitamin D_3 metabolites in *Cestrum Diurnum* leaves, *Phytochemistry, 37, 677, 1994.*

63. **Moon, J., Bandy, B., and Davison, A.J.,** Hypothesis: etiology of atherosclerosis and osteoporosis: Are imbalances in the calciferol endocrine system implicated? *J. Am. Coll. Nutr., 11, 567, 1992.*

64. **Rizzoli, R., Stoermann, C., Ammann, P., and Bonjour, J.-P.,** Hypercalcemia and hyperosteolysis in vitamin D intoxication: effects of clodronate therapy, *Bone, 15, 193, 1994.*

65. **Adams, J.S., Clemens, T.L., Parrish, J.A., and Holick, M.F.,** Vitamin D synthesis and metabolism after UV irradiation of normal and vitamin D-deficient subjects, *N. Engl. J. Med., 306, 722, 1982.*

66. **Vieth, R.,** Vitamin D metabolism in Mexican-Americans [letter; comment], *J. Bone Miner. Res., 5, 791, 1990.*

67. **Atkinson, J., Poitevin, P., Chillon, J.-M., Lartaud, I., and Levy, B.,** Vascular Ca overload produced by vitamin D_3 plus nicotine diminishes arterial distensibility in rats, *Am. J. Physiol., 266, H540, 1994.*

68. **Strates, B., Lian, J., Nimni, M.E., Nimni, I., Marcel, E., Eds.,** Calcification in cardiovascular tissues and bioprostheses, in *Collagen,* CRC Press, Boca Raton, FL, 1988, 273.

69. **Henrion, D., Chillon, J.-M., Capdevelle-Atkinson, C., and Atkinson, J.,** Effect of chronic treatment with the calcium entry blocker, isradipine, on vascular calcium overload produced by vitamin D_3 and nicotine in rats, *J. Pharmacol. Exp. Ther., 260, 1, 1992.*

70. **Stern, P.H.,** Vitamin D and bone, *Kidney Int., (Suppl. 29), S17, 1990.*

71. **Brommage, R. and DeLuca, H.F.,** Evidence that 1,25-dihydroxyvitamin D_3 is the physiologically active metabolite of vitamin D_3, *Endocr. Rev., 6, 491, 1985.*

72. **Balmain, N.,** Calbindin-D9k. A vitamin-D-dependent, calcium-binding protein in mineralized tissues, *Clin. Orthop. Relat. Res., 265, 265, 1991.*

73. **Saggese, G., Federico, G., Bertelloni, S., and Baroncelli, G.I.,** Mineral metabolism in Turner's syndrome: evidence for impaired renal vitamin D metabolism and normal osteoblast function, *J. Clin. Endocrinol. Metab., 75, 998, 1992.*

74. **Barone, L.M., Owen, T.A., Tassinari, M.S., Bortell, R., Stein, G.S., and Lian, J.B.,** Developmental expression and hormonal regulation of the rat matrix Gla protein (MGP) gene in chondrogenesis and osteogenesis, *J. Cell. Biochem., 46, 351, 1991.*

75. **Vieth, R., Chan, A., and Pollard, A.,** 125I-RIA kit cannot distinguish vitamin D deficiency as well as a more specific assay for 25-hydroxyvitamin D, *Clin. Biochem., 28, 175, 1995.*

76. **Marel, G.M., McKenna, M.J., Frame, B., and Peck, W.A., Eds.,** Osteomalacia, in *Bone and Mineral Research,* 4th ed., Elsevier Science Publishers, Amsterdam, 1986, 335.

77. **Haddock, L., Corcino, J., and Vazquez, M.D.,** 25(OH)D serum levels in the normal Puerto Rican population and in subjects with tropical sprue and parathyroid disease, *P.R. Health Sci. J.,* 1, 85, 1982.

78. **Jacobus, C.H., Holick, M.F., Shao, Q., Chen, T.C., Holm, I.A., Kolodny, J.M., Fuleihan, G.E., and Seely, E.W.,** Hypervitaminosis D associated with drinking milk, *N. Engl. J. Med.,* 326, 1173, 1992.

79. **Haddad, J.G.,** Vitamin D—Solar rays, the Milky Way, or both? *N. Engl. J. Med.,* 326, 1213, 1992.

80. **Holick, M., F., Shao, Q., Liu, W.W., and Chen, T.C.,** The vitamin D content of fortified milk and infant formula, *N. Engl. J. Med.,* 326, 1178, 1992.

81. **Nako, Y., Fukushima, N., Tomomasa, T., and Nagashima, K.,** Hypervitaminosis D after prolonged feeding with a premature formula, *Pediatrics,* 92, 862, 1993.

82. **Potts, J.T.J.,** Management of asymptomatic hyperparathyroidism, *J. Clin. Endocrinol. Metab.,* 70, 1489, 1990.

83. **Shaker, J.L., Krawczyk, K.W., and Findling, J.W.,** Primary hyperparathyroidism and severe hypercalcemia with low circulating 1,25-dihydroxyvitamin D, *J. Clin. Endocrinol. Metab.,* 71, 1305, 1990.

84. **Breslau, N.A., McGuire, J.L., Zerwekh, J.E., Frenkel, E.P., and Pak, C.Y.C.,** Hypercalcemia associated with increased calcitriol levels in three patients with lymphoma, *Ann. Intern. Med.,* 100, 1, 1984.

85. **Kelly, P.J. and Eisman, J.A.,** Hypercalcaemia of malignancy, *Cancer Metast. Rev.,* 8, 23, 1989.

86. **McKay, C. and Furman, W.L.,** Hypercalcemia complicating childhood malignancies, *Cancer,* 72, 256, 1993.

87. **Rosseau-Merck, M.F., Nogues, C., Nezelof, C., Marin-Cudraz, B., and Paulin, D.,** Infantile renal tumors associated with hypercalcemia, *Arch. Pathol. Lab. Med.,* 107, 311, 1983.

88. **Nocton, J.J., Stork, J.E., Jacobs, G., and Newman, A.J.,** Sarcoidosis associated with nephrocalcinosis in young children, *J. Pediatr.,* 121, 937, 1992.

89. **Barbour, G.L., Coburn, J.W., Slatopolsky, E., Norman, A.W., and Horst, R.L.,** Hypercalcemia in an anephric patient with sarcoidosis: evidence for extrarenal generation of 1,25-dihydroxyvitamin D, *N. Engl. J. Med.,* 305, 440, 1981.

90. **Steele, C.J. and Kleiman, M.B.,** Disseminated histoplasmosis, hypercalcemia and failure to thrive, *Pediatr. Infect. Dis. J.,* 13, 421, 1994.

91. **O'Leary, T.J., Jones, G., Yip, A., Lohnes, D., Cohanim, M., and Yendt, E.R.,** The effects of chloroquine on serum 1,25-dihydroxyvitamin D and calcium metabolism in sarcoidoisis, *N. Engl. J. Med.,* 315, 727, 1986.

92. **Cole, D.E.C., Carpenter, T.O., and Goltzman, D.,** Calcium homeostasis and disorders of bone and mineral metabolism, in *Pediatric Endocrinology,* 2nd ed., Collu, R., Ducharme, J.R., Guyda, H.J., Eds., Raven Press, New York, 1989, 509.

93. **Klein, G.L. and Simmons, D.J.,** Nutritional rickets: thoughts about pathogenesis, *Ann. Intern. Med.,* 25, 379, 1993.

94. **Anderson, J.J.B. and Toverud, S.U.,** Diet and vitamin D: a review with an emphasis on human function, *J. Nutr. Biochem.,* 5, 58, 1994.

95. **Pike, J.W.,** Vitamin D$_3$ receptors: structure and function in transcription, *Annu. Rev. Nutr.,* 11, 189, 1991.

96. **Gloth, F.M., Tobin, J.D., Sherman, S.S., and Hollis, B.W.,** Is the recommended daily allowance for vitamin D too low for the homebound elderly? *J. Am. Geriatr. Soc.,* 39, 137, 1991.

97. **Haworth, J.C. and Dilling, L.A.,** Vitamin-D-deficient rickets in Manitoba, 1972, *Can. Med. Assoc. J.,* 134, 237, 1986.

98. **Curtis, J.A., Kooh, S.W., Fraser, D., and Greenberg, M.L.,** Nutritional rickets in vegetarian children, *Can. Med. Assoc. J.,* 128, 150, 1983.

99. **Saal, H.M., Ratzan, S.K., and Carey, D.E.,** Yogurt: contributory factor in development of nutritional rickets, *Clin. Pediatr.,* 24, 452, 1985.

100. **Seino, Y., Shimotsuji, T., Yamaoka, K., Ishida, M., Ishii, T., Matsuda, S., Matsuda, S., Ikehara, C., Yabuuchi, H., and Dokoh, S.,** Plasma 1,25-dihydroxyvitamin D concentrations in cords, newborns, infants, and children, *Calcif. Tissue Int.,* 30, 1, 1980.

101. **Markestad, T., Halvorsen, S., Halvorsen, K.S., Aksnes, L., and Aarskog, D.,** Plasma concentrations of vitamin D metabolites before and during treatment of vitamin D deficiency rickets in children, *Acta Pediatr. Scand.,* 73, 225, 1984.

102. **Venkataraman, P.S., Tsang, R.C., Buckley, D.D., Ho, M., and Steichen, J.J.,** Elevation of serum 1,25-dihydroxyvitamin D in response to physiologic doses of vitamin D in vitamin D-deficient infants, *J. Pediatr.,* 103, 416, 1983.

103. **Reiter, E.O., Brugman, S.M., Pike, J.W., Pitt, M., Dokoh, S., Haussler, M.R., et al.,** Vitamin D metabolites in adolescents and young adults with cystic fibrosis: effects of sun and season, *J. Pediatr.,* 106, 21, 1985.

104. **Clark, J.H. and Hudson, S.D.,** Hypocalcemia as the initial manifestation of occult cholestatic liver disease, *Clin. Pediatr.,* 31, 428, 1992.

105. **Gustafsson, J., Holmberg, I., Hardell, L.I., and Foucard, T.,** Hypoparathyroidism and liver disease—evidence for a vitamin D hydroxylation defect. A case report, *Acta Endocrinol.,* 105, 211, 1984.

106. **Wiesner, R.H., Kumar, R., Seeman, E., and Go, V.L.W.,** Enterohepatic physiology of 1,25-dihydroxyvitamin D$_3$ metabolites in normal man, *J. Lab. Clin. Med.,* 96, 1094, 1980.

107. **Farrinton, K., Epstein, O., Varghese, Z., Newman, S.P., Moorhead, J.F., and Sherlock, S.,** Effect of oral 1,25-dihydroxycholecalciferol on calcium and phosphate malabsorption in primary biliary cirrhosis, *Gut,* 20, 616, 1979.

108. **Rao, D.S.,** Metabolic bone disease in gastrointestinal and biliary disorders, in *Primer on the Metabolic Bone Diseases and Disorders of Mineral Metabolism,* 2nd ed., Favus, M.J., Ed., Raven Press, New York, 1993, 268.

109. **Hahn, T.J., Hendin, B.A., Scharp, C.R., Boisseau, V.C., and Haddad, J.G.J.,** Serum 25-hydroxycalciferol levels and bone mass in children on chronic anticonvulsant therapy, *N. Engl. J. Med.,* 292, 550, 1975.

110. **Hahn, T.J.,** Steroid and drug-induced osteopenia, in *Primer on the Metabolic Bone Diseases and Disorders of Mineral Metabolism,* 2nd ed., Favus, M.J., Ed., Raven Press, New York, 1993, 250.

111. **Somerman, M.J., Rifkin, B.R., Pinton-Miska, S., and Au, W.Y.W.,** Effect of phenytoin on rat bone resorption *in vitro, Arch. Oral Biol.,* 31, 267, 1986.

112. **Kruse, K., Bartels, H., Ziegler, R., Dreller, E., and Kracht, U.,** Parathyroid function and serum calcitonin in children receiving anticonvulsant drugs, *Eur. J. Pediatr.,* 133, 151, 1980.

113. **Hodson, E.M., Shaw, P.F., Evans, R.A., Dunstan, C.R., Hills, E.E., Wong, S.Y.P., et al.,** Growth retardation and renal osteodystrophy in children with chronic renal failure, *J. Pediatr.,* 103, 735, 1983.

114. **Hsu, A.C., Kooh, S.W., Fraser, D., Cumming, W.A., and Fornasier, V.L.,** Renal osteodystrophy in children with chronic renal failure: an unexpectedly common and incapacitating complication, *Pediatrics,* 70, 742, 1982.

115. **Cole, D.E.C. and Hanley, D.A.,** Osteocalcin, in *Bone Matrix and Bone Specific Products,* Vol. 3 in *Bone* series, Hall, B.K., Ed., CRC Press, Boca Raton, FL, 1991, 239.

116. **Hodson, E.M., Evans, R.A., Dunstan, C.R., Hills, E., Wong, S.Y.P., Rosenberg, A.R., et al.,** Treatment of childhood renal osteodystrophy with calcitriol or ergocalciferol, *Clin. Nephrol.,* 24, 192, 1985.

117. **Trachtman, H. and Gauthier, B.,** Parenteral calcitriol for treatment of severe renal osteodystrophy in children with chronic renal insufficiency, *J. Pediatr.,* 110, 966, 1987.

118. **Reed, A.M., Haugen, M., Pachman, L.M., and Langman, C.B.,** Repair of osteopenia in children with juvenile rheumatoid arthritis, *J. Pediatr.,* 122, 693, 1994.

119. **Piraino, B.M., Rault, R., Greenberg, A., Dominguez, J.H., Wallia, R., Houck, P., et al.,** Spontaneous hypercalcemia in patients undergoing dialysis, *Am. J. Med.,* 80, 607, 1986.

120. **Buccianti, G., Bianchi, M.L., Valenti, G., Lorenz, M., Cresseri, D.,** Effects of calcifediol treatment on the progression of renal osteodystrophy during continuous ambulatory peritoneal dialysis, *Nephron,* 56, 353, 1990.

121. **Casella, S.J., Reiner, B.J., Chen, T.C., Holick, M.F., and Harrison, H.E.,** A possible genetic defect in 25-hydroxylation as a cause of rickets, *J. Pediatr.,* 124, 929, 1994.

122. **Marx, S.J.,** Vitamin D and other calciferols, in *The Metabolic and Molecular Bases of Inherited Disease,* 7th ed., Scriver, C.R., Beaudet, A.L., Sly, W.S., and Valle, D., Eds., McGraw-Hill, New York, 1995, 3091.

123. **Aarskog, D., Aksnes, L., and Markestad, T.,** Effect of parathyroid hormone on cAMP and 1,25-dihydroxyvitamin D formation and renal handling of phosphate in vitamin D-dependent rickets, *Pediatrics,* 71, 59, 1983.

124. **Rosen, J.F., Fleischman, A.R., Finberg, L., Hamstra, A., and Deluca, H.F.,** Rickets with alopecia, an inborn error of vitamin D metabolism, *J. Pediatr.,* 94, 729, 1979.

125. **Balsan, S., Garabedian, M., Larchet, M., Gorski, A., Cournot, G., Tau, C., et al.,** Long-term nocturnal calcium infusions can cure rickets and promote normal mineralization in hereditary resistance to 1,25-dihydroxyvitamin D, *J. Clin. Invest.,* 77, 1661, 1986.

126. **Pronicka, E. and Gruszczynska, B.,** Familial hypomagnesaemia with secondary hypocalcaemia—autosomal or X-linked inheritance? *J. Inherited Metab. Dis.,* 14, 397, 1991.

127. **Chery, M., Biancalana, V., Philippe, C., Malpuech, G., Carla, H., Gilgenkrantz, S., et al.,** Hypomagnesemia with secondary hypocalcemia in a female with balanced X;9 translocation, mapping of the Xp22 chromosome breakpoint, *Hum. Genet.,* 93, 587, 1994.

128. **Abbott, L.G. and Rude, R.K.,** Clinical manifestations of magnesium deficiency, *Miner. Electr. Metab.,* 19, 314, 1993.

129. **Anast, C.S. and Gardner, D.W.,** Magnesium metabolism, in *Disorders of Mineral Metabolism,* Anonymous Academic Press, New York, 1981, 423.

130. **Dudin, K.I. and Teebi, A.S.,** Primary hypomagnesaemia, a case report and literature review, *Eur. J. Pediatr.,* 146, 303, 1987.

131. **Nutbeam, H.M., Sinclair, L., and Oberholzer, V.G.,** Magnesium transport defect with hypercalcaemia, *J. R. Soc. Med.,* 72, 932, 1979.

132. **Sutton, R.A.L. and Domrongkitchaiporn, S.,** Abnormal renal magnesium handling, *Miner. Electr. Metab.,* 19, 232, 1993.

133. **Green, C.G., Doershuk, C.F., and Stern, R.C.,** Symptomatic hypomagnesemia in cystic fibrosis, *J. Pediatr.,* 107, 425, 1985.

134. **Schindler, A.M.,** Isolated neonatal hypomagnesaemia associated with maternal overuse of stool softener, *Lancet,* 2, 822, 1984.

135. **Fatemi, S., Ryzen, E., Flores, J., Endres, D.B., and Rude, R.K.,** Effect of experimental human magnesium depletion on parathyroid hormone secretion and 1,25-dihydroxyvitamin D metabolism, *J. Clin. Endocrinol. Metab.,* 73, 1067, 1991.

136. **Fuss, M., Cogan, E., Gillet, C., Karmali, R., Geurts, J., Bergans, A., et al.,** Magnesium administration reverses the hypocalcemia secondary to hypomagnesemia despite low circulating levels of 25-hydroxyvitamin D and 1,25-dihydroxyvitamin D, *Clin. Endocrinol.,* 22, 807, 1985.

137. **Rude, R.K., Oldham, S.B., and Singer, F.R.,** Functional hypoparathyroidism and parathyroid hormone end-organ resistance in human magnesium deficiency, *Clin. Endocrinol.,* 5, 209, 1976.

138. **Leicht, E., Schmidt-Gayk, H., Langer, H.-J., Sneige, N., and Biro, G.,** Hypomagnesaemia-induced hypocalcaemia, concentrations of parathyroid hormone, prolactin and 1,25-dihydroxyvitamin D during magnesium replenishment, *Magnesium Res.,* 5, 33, 1992.

139. **Leicht, E. and Biro, G.,** Mechanisms of hypocalcaemia in the clinical form of severe magnesium deficit in the human, *Magnesium Res.,* 5, 37, 1992.

140. **Rude, R.K., Adams, J.S., Ryzen, E., Endres, D.B., Niimi, H., Horst, R.L., et al.,** Low serum concentrations of 1,25-dihydroxyvitamin D in human magnesium deficiency, *J. Clin. Endocrinol. Metab.,* 61, 933, 1985.

141. **Graber, M.L. and Schulman, G.,** Hypomagnesemic hypocalcemia independent of parathyroid hormone, *Ann. Intern. Med.,* 104, 804, 1986.

142. **Brooke, O.G. and Lucas, A.,** Metabolic bone disease in preterm infants, *Arch. Dis. Child.,* 60, 682, 1985.

143. **Bishop, N.,** Bone disease in preterm infants, *Arch. Dis. Child.,* 64, 1403, 1989.

144. **Gefter, W.B., Epstein, D.M., Anday, E.K., and Dalinka, M.K.,** Rickets presenting as multiple fractures in premature infants on hyperalimentation, *Radiology,* 142, 371, 1982.

145. **Koo, W.W.K., Oestreich, A.E., Sherman, R., Buckley, D., Tsang, R.C., and Steichen, J.J.,** Failure of high calcium and phosphorus supplementation in the prevention of rickets of prematurity, *Am. J. Dis. Child.,* 14, 857, 1986.

146. **McIntosh, N., DeCurtis, M., and Williams, J.,** Failure of mineral supplementation to reduce incidence of rickets in very-low-birthweight infants, *Lancet,* 2, 981, 1986.

147. **Delvin, E.E., Salle, B.L., Glorieux, F.H., Adeleine, P., and David, L.S.,** Vitamin D supplementation during pregnancy, effect on neonatal calcium homeostasis, *J. Pediatr.,* 109, 328, 1986.

148. **Toomey, F., Hoag, R., Batton, D., and Vain, N.,** Rickets associated with cholestasis and parenteral nutrition in premature infants, *Radiology,* 142, 85, 1982.

149. **Sedman, A.B., Miller, N.L., Warady, B.A., Lum, G.M., and Alfrey, A.C.,** Aluminum loading in children with chronic renal failure, *Kidney Int.,* 26, 201, 1984.

150. **Koo, W.W.K., Krug-Wispe, S.K., Succop, P., Bendon, R., and Kaplan, L.A.,** Sequential serum aluminum and urine aluminum, creatinine ratio and tissue aluminum loading in infants with fractures/rickets, *Pediatrics,* 89, 877, 1992.

151. **Hillman, L.S., Hoff, N., Salmons, S., Martin, L., McAlister, W., and Haddad, J.,** Mineral homeostasis in very premature infants, serial evaluation of serum 25-hydroxyvitamin D, serum minerals, and bone mineralization, *J. Pediatr.,* 106, 970, 1985.

152. **Chesney, R.W., Hamstra, A.J., and Deluca, H.F.,** Rickets of prematurity, supranormal levels of serum 1,25-dihydroxyvitamin D, *Am. J. Dis. Child.,* 135, 34, 1981.

153. **Venkataraman, P.S., Tsang, R.C., Steichen, J.J., Grey, I., Neylan, M., and Fleishman, A.R.,** Early neonatal hypocalcemia in extremely preterm infants, *Am. J. Dis. Child.,* 140, 1004, 1986.

154. **Koo, W.W.K., Tsang, R.C., Poser, J.W., Laskarzewski, P., Buckley, D., Johnson, R., et al.,** Elevated serum calcium and osteocalcin levels from calcitriol in preterm infants, *Am. J. Dis. Child.,* 140, 1152, 1986.

155. **Evans, J.R., Allen, A.C., Stinson, D.A., Hamilton, D.C., Brown, B.S.J., Vincer, M.J., et al.,** Effect of high-dose vitamin D supplementation on radiographically detectable bone disease of very low birth weight infants, *J. Pediatr.,* 115, 779, 1989.

156. **Fraser, D., Langford Kidd, B.S., Kooh, S.W., and Paunier, L.,** A new look at infantile hypercalcemia, *Pediatr. Clin. North Am.,* 13, 506, 1966.

157. **Fanconi, G. and Girardet, P.,** Chronische Hypercalcamie, kombiniert mit Osteosklerose, Hyperazotamie, Minderwuchs und kongenitalen Missbildungen, *Helv. Paediatr. Acta,* 7, 314, 1952.

158. **Forfar, J.O., Balf, C.L., Maxwell, G.M., and Tompsett, S.L.,** Idiopathic hypercalcemia of infancy, *Lancet,* i, 981, 1956.

159. **Lightwood, R.,** Idiopathic hypercalcemia with failure to thrive, *Arch. Dis. Child.,* 27, 302, 1952.

160. **Fellers, F.X. and Schwartz, R.,** Etiology of the severe form of idiopathic hypercalcemia of infancy, a defect in vitamin D metabolism, *N. Engl. J. Med.,* 259, 1050, 1958.

161. **Chan, G.M., Buchino, J.J., Mehlhorn, D., Bove, K.E., Steichen, J.J., and Tsang, R.C.,** Effect of vitamin D on pregnant rabbits and their offspring, *Pediatr. Res.,* 13, 121, 1979.

162. **Friedman, W.F. and Mills, L.F.,** The relationship between vitamin D and the craniofacial and dental anomalies of the supravalvular aortic stenosis syndrome, *Pediatrics,* 43, 12, 1969.

163. **Chesney, R.W., Deluca, H.F., Gertner, J.M., and Genel, M.,** Increased plasma 1,25-dihydroxyvitamin D in infants with hypercalcemia and elfin facies, *N. Engl. J. Med.,* 313, 889, 1985.

164. **Forbes, G.B.,** Vitamin D in pregnancy and the infantile hypercalcemic syndrome, *Pediatr. Res.,* 13, 1382, 1979.
165. **Martin, N.D.T., Snodgrass, G.J.A.I., Cohen, R.D., Porteous, C.E., Coldwell, R.D., Trafford, D.J.H., et al.,** Vitamin D metabolites in idiopathic infantile hypercalcemia, *Arch. Dis. Child.,* 60, 1140, 1985.
166. **Kruse, K., Pankau, R., Gosch, A., and Wohlfahrt, K.,** Calcium metabolism in Williams-Beuren syndrome, *J. Pediatr.,* 121, 902, 1992.
167. **Williams, J.C.P., Barratt-Boyes, B.G., and Lowe, J.B.,** Supravalvular aortic stenosis, *Circulation,* 24, 1311, 1961.
168. **Beuren, A.J., Schulze, C., Eberle, P., Harmijanz, D., and Apitz, J.,** The syndrome of supravalvular aortic stenosis, peripheral pulmonary stenosis, mental retardation and similar facial appearance, *Am. J. Cardiol.,* 13, 471, 1964.
169. **Jones, K.L. and Smith, D.W.,** The Williams elfin facies syndrome, *J. Pediatr.,* 86, 718, 1975.
170. **Martin, N.D.T., Snodgrass, G.H.A.I., and Cohen, R.D.,** Idiopathic infantile hypercalcemia—a continued enigma, *Arch. Dis. Child.,* 59, 605, 1984.
171. **Jones, K.L.,** Williams syndrome, an historical perspective of its evolution, natural history, and etiology, *Am. J. Med. Genet.,* (Suppl. 6), 89, 1990.
172. **Morgan, H.G., Mitchell, R.G., Stowers, J.M., and Thomson, J.,** Metabolic studies on two infants with idiopathic hypercalcemia, *Lancet,* 1, 925, 1956.
173. **Barr, D.G.D. and Forfar, J.O.,** Oral calcium-loading test in infancy, with particular reference to idiopathic hypercalcemia, *Br. Med. J.,* 1, 477, 1969.
174. **Culler, F.L., Jones, K.L., and Deftos, L.J.,** Impaired calcitonin secretion in patients with Williams syndrome, *J. Pediatr.,* 107, 720, 1985.
175. **Aarskog, D., Aksnes, L., and Markestad, T.,** Vitamin D metabolism in idiopathic infantile hypercalcemia, *Am. J. Dis. Child.,* 135, 1021, 1981.
176. **Garabedian, M., Jacqz, E., Gillozo, H., Grimberg, R., Guillot, M., Gagnadoux, M.F., et al.,** Elevated plasma 1,25-dihydroxyvitamin D concentrations in infants with hypercalcemia and an elfin facies, *N. Engl. J. Med.,* 312, 948, 1985.
177. **Taylor, A.B., Stern, P.B., and Bell, N.H.,** Abnormal regulation of circulating 25-hydroxyvitamin D in the Williams syndrome, *N. Engl. J. Med.,* 306, 972, 1982.
178. **White, R.A., Preus, M., Watters, G.V., and Fraser, F.C.,** Familial occurrence of the Williams syndrome, *J. Pediatr.,* 91, 614, 1977.
179. **Wiltse, H.E., Goldbloom, R.B., Anita, A.U., Ottesen, O.E., Rowe, R.D., and Cooke, R.E.,** Infantile hypercalcemia syndrome in twins, *N. Engl. J. Med.,* 275, 1157, 1966.
180. **Morris, C.A., Thomas, I.T., and Greenberg, F.,** Williams syndrome, autosomal dominant inheritance, *Am. J. Med. Genet.,* 47, 478, 1993.
181. **Ewart, A.K., Morris, C.A., Ensing, G.J., Loker, J., Moore, C., Leppert, M., et al.,** A human vascular disorder, supravalvular aortic stenosis, maps to chromosome 7, *Proc. Natl. Acad. Sci. U.S.A.,* 90, 3226, 1993.
182. **Ewart, A.K., Morris, C.A., Atkinson, D., Jin, W., Sternes, K., Spallone, P., et al.,** Hemizygosity at the elastin locus in a developmental disorder, Williams syndrome, *Nat. Genet.,* 5, 11, 1993.
183. **Chesney, R.W., Rosen, J.F., Hamstra, A.J., and Deluca, H.F.,** Serum 1,25-dihydroxyvitamin D levels in normal children and in vitamin D disorders, *Am. J. Dis. Child.,* 134, 135, 1980.
184. **Schutt-Aine, J.C., Young, M.A., Pescovitz, O.H., Chrousos, G.P., and Marx, S.J.,** Hypoparathyroidism, a possible cause of rickets, *J. Pediatr.,* 106, 255, 1984.
185. **Drezner, M.K., Neelson, F.A., Jowsey, J., and Lebovitz, H.E.,** Hypoparathyroidism, a possible cause of osteomalacia, *J. Clin. Endocrinol. Metab.,* 45, 114, 1977.
186. **Epstein, S., Meunier, P.J., Lambert, P.W., Stern, P.H., and Bell, N.H.,** 1,25-Dihydroxyvitamin D_3 corrects osteomalacia in hypoparathyroidism and pseudohypoparathyroidism, *Acta Endocrinol.,* 103, 241, 1983.
187. **Aksnes, L. and Aarskog, D.,** Vitamin D metabolites in serum from hypoparathyroid patients treated with vitamin D_2 and 1-hydroxyvitamin D_3, *J. Clin. Endocrinol. Metab.,* 51, 1223, 1980.
188. **Kind, H.P., Handysides, A., Kooh, S.W., and Fraser, D.,** Vitamin D therapy in hypoparathyroidism and pseudohypoparathyroidism, weight-related dosages for initiation of therapy and maintenance therapy, *J. Pediatr.,* 91, 1006, 1977.
189. **Okano, K., Furukawa, Y., Morii, H., and Fujita, T.,** Comparative efficacy of various vitamin D metabolites in the treatment of various types of hypoparathyroidism, *J. Clin. Endocrinol. Metab.,* 55, 238, 1982.
190. **Chan, J.C.M., Young, R.B., Hartenberg, M.A., and Chinchilli, V.M.,** Calcium and phosphate metabolism in children with idiopathic hypoparathyroidism or pseudohypoparathyroidism, effects of 1,25-dihydroxyvitamin D_3, *J. Pediatr.,* 106, 421, 1985.
191. **Markowitz, M.E., Rosen, J.F., Smith, C., and Deluca, H.F.,** 1,25-Dihydroxyvitamin D_3-treated hypoparathyroidism, 35 patient years in 10 children, *J. Clin. Endocrinol. Metab.,* 55, 727, 1982.
192. **Chesney, R.W., Horowitz, S.D., Kream, B.E., Eisman, J.A., Hong, R., and Deluca, H.F.,** Failure of conventional doses of 1,25-dihydroxycholocalciferol to correct hypocalcemia in a girl with idiopathic hypoparathyroidism, *N. Engl. J. Med.,* 297, 1272, 1977.

193. **Miller, J.D., Bowker, B.M., Cole, D.E.C., and Guyda, H.J.,** DiGeorge's syndrome in monozygotic twins, *Am. J. Dis. Child.,* 137, 438, 1983.
194. **Smothers, R.L., Levine, B.S., Singer, F.R., Bryce, G.F., Malloon, J.P., Miller, O.N., et al.,** Relationship between urinary calcium and calcium intake during calcitriol administration, *Kidney Int.,* 29, 578, 1986.
195. **Stapleton, F.B., Noe, H.N., Jerkins, G., and Roy, S.,** Urinary excretion of calcium following an oral calcium loading test in healthy children, *Pediatrics,* 60, 594, 1982.
196. **Levine, M.A., Jap, T.S., and Hung, W.,** Infantile hypothyroidism in two sibs, an unusual presentation of pseudohypoparathyroidism type Ia, *J. Pediatr.,* 107, 919, 1985.
197. **Li, X.Q., Tembe, V., Horwitz, G.M., Bushinsky, D.A., and Favus, M.J.,** Increased intestinal vitamin D receptor in genetic hypercalciuric rats. A cause of intestinal calcium hyperabsorption, *J. Clin. Invest.,* 91, 661, 1993.
198. **Sadeghi-Nejad, A. and Senior, B.,** Hypercalcemia, an unusual complication of hyperthyroidism in a child, *Acta Pediatr. Scand.,* 75, 504, 1986.
199. **Glorieux, F.H., Marie, P.J., Pettifor, J.M., and Delvin, E.E.,** Bone response to phosphate salts, ergo-calciferol, and calcitriol in hypophosphatemic vitamin D-resistant rickets, *N. Engl. J. Med.,* 303, 1023, 1980.
200. **Rasmussen, H. and Tenenhouse, H.S.,** Mendelian hypophosphatemias., in *The Metabolic and Molecular Bases of Inherited Disease,* 7th ed., Scriver, C.R., Beaudet, A.L., Sly, W.S., and Valle, D., Eds, McGraw-Hill, New York, 1995, 3717.
201. **Cole, D.E.C.,** Rickets, osteomalacia, and pediatric bone disease, *Curr. Opin. Orthop.,* 3, 93, 1992.
202. **Rowe, P.S.N., Goulding, J., Read, A., Lehrach, H., Francis, F., Hanauer, A., et al.,** Refining the genetic map for the region flanking the X-linked hypophosphataemic rickets locus (Xp22.1-22.2), *Hum. Genet.,* 93, 291, 1994.
203. **Ghishan, F.K., Knobel, S., Dasuki, M., Butler, M., and Phillips, J.,** Chromosomal localization of the human renal sodium phosphate transporter to chromosome 5, implications for X-linked hypophosphatemia, *Pediatr. Res.,* 35, 510, 1994.
204. **Mason, R.S., Rohl, P.G., Lissner, D., and Posen, S.,** Vitamin D metabolism in hypophosphatemic rickets, *Am. J. Dis. Child.,* 136, 909, 1982.
205. **Cunningham, J., Gomes, H., Seino, Y., and Chase, L.R.,** Abnormal 24-hydroxylation of 25-hydroxyvitamin D in the X-linked hypophosphatemic mouse, *Endocrinology,* 112, 633, 1983.
206. **Lobaugh, B. and Drezner, M.K.,** Abnormal regulation of renal 25-hydroxyvitamin D-1α-hydroxylase activity in the X-linked hypophosphatemic mouse, *J. Clin. Invest.,* 71, 400, 1983.
207. **Nesbitt, T., Drezner, M.K., and Lobaugh, B.,** Abnormal parathyroid hormone stimulation of 25-hydroxyvitamin D-1α-hydroxylase activity in the hypophosphatemic mouse, *J. Clin. Invest.,* 77, 181, 1986.
208. **Lyles, K.W. and Drezner, M.K.,** Parathyroid hormone effects on serum 1,25-dihydroxyvitamin D levels in patients with X-linked hypophosphatemic rickets, evidence for abnormal 25-hydroxyvitamin D-1α-hydroxylase activity, *J. Clin. Endocrinol. Metab.,* 54, 638, 1982.
209. **Latta, K., Hisano, S., and Chan, J.C.M.,** Therapeutics of X-linked hypophosphatemic rickets, *Pediatr. Nephrol.,* 7, 744, 1993.
210. **Harrell, R.M., Lyles, K.W., Harrelson, J.M., Friedman, N.E., and Drezner, M.K.,** Healing of bone disease in X-linked hypophosphatemic rickets/osteomalacia, *J. Clin. Invest.,* 75, 1858, 1985.
211. **Tsuru, N., Chan, J.C.M., and Chinchilli, V.M.,** Renal hypophosphatemic rickets, growth and mineral metabolism after treatment with calcitriol (1,25-dihydroxyvitamin D_3) and phosphate supplementation, *Am. J. Dis. Child.,* 141, 108, 1987.
212. **Goodyer, P.R., Kronick, J.B., Jequier, S., Reade, T.M., and Scriver, C.R.,** Nephrocalcinosis and its relationship to treatment of hereditary rickets, *J. Pediatr.,* 111, 700, 1987.
213. **Verge, C.F., Lam, A., Simpson, J.M., Cowell, C.T., Howard, N.J., and Silink, M.,** Effects of therapy in X-linked hypophosphatemic rickets, *N. Engl. J. Med.,* 325, 1843, 1991.
214. **Cole, D.E.C.,** Nephrocalcinosis in X-linked hypophosphataemic rickets, just how serious is the problem?, *Clin. Invest. Med.,* 17, 131, 1994.
215. **Kooh, S.W., Binet, A., and Daneman, A.,** Nephrocalcinosis in X-linked hypophosphataemic rickets, its relationship to treatment, kidney function, and growth, *Clin. Invest. Med.,* 17, 123, 1994.
216. **Alon, U. and Chan, J.C.M.,** Effects of hydrochlorothiazide and amiloride in renal hypophosphatemic rickets, *Pediatrics,* 75, 754, 1985.
217. **Carpenter, T.O., Mitnick, M.A., Ellison, A., Smith, C., and Insogna, K.L.,** Nocturnal hyperparathyroidism: afrequent feature of X-linked hypophosphatemia., *J. Clin. Endocrinol. Metab.,* 78, 1378, 1994.
218. **Alon, U., Newsome, H., and Chan, J.C.M.,** Hyperparathyroidism in patients with X-linked dominant hypophosphatemic rickets—application of the calcium infusion test as an indicator for parathyroidectomy, *Int. J. Pediatr. Nephrol.,* 5, 39, 1984.
219. **Kinder, B.K. and Rasmussen, H.,** New applications of total parathyroidectomy and autotransplantation: use in proximal renal tubular dysfunction, *World J. Surg.,* 9, 156, 1985.

220. **Reid, I.R., Hardy, D.C., Murphy, W.A., Teitelbaum, S.L., Bergfeld, M.A., and Whyte, M.P.,** X-linked hypophosphatemia: a clinical, biochemical, and histopathologic assessment of morbidity in adults, *Medicine,* 68, 336, 1989.

221. **Hardy, D.C., Murphy, W.A., Siegel, B.A., Reid, I.R., and Whyte, M.P.,** X-linked hypophosphatemia in adults: prevalence of skeletal radiographic and scintigraphic features, *Radiology,* 171, 403, 1989.

222. **Davies, M., Kane, R., and Valentine, J.,** Impaired hearing in X-linked hypophosphataemic (vitamin-D-resistant) osteomalacia, *Ann. Intern. Med.,* 100, 230, 1984.

223. **Polisson, R.P., Martinez, S., Khoury, M., Harrell, R.M., Lyles, K.W., Friedman, N., et al.,** Calcification of enthesis associated with X-linked hypophosphatemic osteomalacia, *N. Engl. J. Med.,* 313, 1, 1985.

224. **Cartwright, D.W., Masel, J.P., and Latham, S.C.,** The lumbar spinal canal in hypophosphataemic vitamin D-resistant rickets, *Aust. N.Z.J. Med.,* 11, 154, 1981.

225. **Tieder, M., Modai, D., Samuel, R., Arie, R., Halabe, A., Bab, I., et al.,** Hereditary hypophosphatemic rickets with hypercalciuria, *N. Engl. J. Med.,* 312, 611, 1985.

226. **Coe, F.L., Parks, J.H., and Asplin, J.R.,** The pathogenesis and treatment of kidney stones, *N. Engl. J. Med.,* 326, 1141, 1992.

227. **Harangi, F. and Mehes, K.,** Family investigations in idiopathic hypercalciuria, *Eur. J. Pediatr.,* 152, 64, 1993.

228. **Misselwitz, J., Hesse, V., and Markestad, T.,** Nephrocalcinosis, hypercalciuria and elevated serum levels of 1,25-dihydroxyvitamin D in children, *Acta Paediatr. Scand.,* 79, 637, 1990.

229. **Insogna, K.L., Broadus, A.E., Dreyer, B.E., Ellison, A.F., and Gertner, J.M.,** Elevated production rate of 1,25-dihydroxyvitamin D in patients with absorptive hypercalciuria, *J. Clin. Endocrinol. Metab.,* 61, 490, 1984.

230. **Auwerx, J. and Bouillon, R.,** Mineral and bone metabolism in thyroid disease: a review, *Q.J. Med.,* 60, 737, 1986.

231. **Zaloga, G.P., Eil, C., and O'Brian, J.T.,** Reversible hypocalciuric hypercalcemia associated with hypothyroidism., *Am. J. Med.,* 77, 1101, 1984.

232. **Tau, C., Garabedian, M., Farriaux, J.P., Czernichow, P., Pomarede, R., and Balsan, S.,** Hypercalcemia in infants with congenital hypothyroidism and its relation to vitamin D and thyroid hormone, *J. Pediatr.,* 109, 808, 1986.

233. **Estelle, M., Lamothe, F., Narod, S.A., Miller, S., Goodfellow, P.J., Cole, D.E.C., et al.,** Screening for multiple endocrine neoplasia type 2A with DNA-polymorphism analysis, *Henry Ford Hosp. Med. J.,* 40, 224, 1992.

234. **Freudlich, M., Bourgoignie, J.J., Zillerueleo, G., Abitbol, C., Canterbury, J.M., and Strauss, J.,** Calcium and vitamin D metabolism in children with nephrotic syndrome, *J. Pediatr.,* 108, 383, 1986.

235. **Freundlich, M., Bourgoignie, J.J., Zilleruelo, G., Jacob, A.I., Canterbury, J.M., and Strauss, J.,** Bone, modulating factors in nephrotic children with normal glomerular filtration rate, *Pediatrics,* 76, 280, 1986.

236. **Mizokuchi, M., Kubota, M., Tomino, Y., and Koide, H.,** Possible mechanism of impaired calcium and vitamin D metabolism in nephrotic rats, *Kidney Int.,* 42, 335, 1992.

Chapter 4

CLINICAL MANIFESTATIONS
OF GASTROINTESTINAL HORMONES

Leon J. Yoder

CONTENTS

"Hormones," named by Starling and Bayliss in 1905, were a new class of chemical substances, peptides, that became increasingly important in explaining the complex function of multicellular organisms. Peptides are chemical compounds that can be hydrolyzed by various enzymatic processes to amino acids. Gastrointestinal hormones may consist of as many as 40 such amino acids.[1] Organ function becomes increasingly more specialized the higher the class of vertebrae. This function can be achieved only by the interaction of the nervous and endocrine systems, where both play roles in transmitting signals through specialized pathways. The endocrine system uses its messengers, called hormones, to transmit these signals through the circulatory system. When a target organ or cell is reached, the hormone binds itself to a specific binding site called a receptor, and then the physiologic action occurs.[2]

The family of hormones is increasing and includes neuropeptides, paracrine agents, growth factors, and cytokines.[3] Gastrointestinal hormones will be discussed in this chapter. Most of these hormones are localized in specific areas of the intestinal tract corresponding to their function. Gastrin is found in the stomach; insulin, glucagon, and pancreatic polypeptide in the pancreas; secretin, cholecystokinin (CCK), motilin, and gastrointestinal polypeptide in the duodenum and jejunum; enteroglucagon, peptide YY, and neurotensin in the ileum and colon; and somatostatin in all areas from stomach through colon.[4]

Yalow and Berson have developed a method where antibodies are directed against peptide hormones and are measured quantitatively.[5] This test, the radioimmunoassay (RIA), is the best for measuring gastrointestinal hormones. Caution must be exercised in obtaining serum and plasma samples properly because sampling error can be very high. Treating the blood samples by immediate freezing after centrifugation minimizes degradation by plasma enzymes. Gastrin radioimmunoassay should be performed fasting because physiologic increases of gastrin follow a meal. Gastric distension will also affect gastrin levels positively. With the additions of fluorescent labeling and immunohistochemical testing more peptide hormones have been uncovered.

Gastrointestinal hormones have been divided into families according to their amino acid sequences. The sequences for some families are very similar structurally because their evolution originates from common precursor cells.

Gastrin-Cholecystokinin Family
Secretin-Glucagon-Vasoactive Intestinal Polypeptide-Gastrointestinal Polypeptide Family
Pancreatic Polypeptide Family

Some families are not structurally related.

Somatostatin
Motilin
Neurotensin

The physiologic responses of gastrointestinal hormones are dependent on specific receptor sites on target organs. This interaction causes a cellular response for a specific physiologic function. An example is gastrin, which has receptor sites located in antral and duodenal mucosa. The physiologic response is acid secretion. Another example is CCK, with receptor sites in duodenal and jejunal mucosa. Cell response results in pancreatic enzyme secretion and gallbladder contraction. Table 1 lists the principal gastrointestinal hormones, locations, and main physiologic effects.

TABLE 1
Gastrointestinal Hormones and Effects

Hormone	Location	Effect
Gastrin	Gastric antral, duodenal	HCl acid secretion
Cholecystokinin	Duodenal, jejunal mucosa	Pancreatic enzyme secretion; gallbladder contraction
Secretin	Duodenal, jejunal mucosa	Pancreatic secretion of water and bicarbonate
Glucagon	Small intestinal mucosa	Glucose metabolism
Vasoactive intestinal polypeptide	Gastrointestinal tract	Smooth muscle relaxation
Gastrointestinal polypeptide	Duodenal, jejunal mucosa	Insulin release
Pancreatic polypeptide	Pancreatic islet cells	Pancreatic secretion inhibition
Somatostatin	Gastrointestinal tract	GI motility and.gastric release inhibition
Motilin	Duodenal mucosa	Gastric acid stimulation
Neurotensin	Ileal, colonic mucosa	Gastric emptying inhibition

GASTROINTESTINAL HORMONAL DISEASES[6-9]

GASTRINOMA (ZOLLINGER-ELLISON SYNDROME)

Uncontrolled release of gastrin by a pancreatic endocrine tumor results in severe hyperacidity and ulcer disease. Although rare as a cause of peptic ulcer disease, less than 1%, it is suspected under the following conditions:

1. Multiple ulcers refractory to usual ulcer therapy
2. Ulcers recurring after ulcer surgery

3. Ulcers with associated diarrhea
4. Ulcers associated with multiple endocrine neoplasias (MEN-1)
5. Ulcers found in usual places but also in unusual areas such as third and fourth parts of duodenum and jejunum.

The Zollinger-Ellison syndrome is characterized by very high serum gastrin levels. Fasting serum gastrin levels are usually less than 200 pg/ml. Between 200 and 1000 pg/ml gastrinoma is only one of the conditions to be considered. Others include antral G-cell hyperplasia, retained gastric antrum after ulcer surgery, gastric outlet obstruction, atrophic gastritis, pernicious anemia, and chronic renal failure. Above 1000 pg/ml only gastrinoma, pernicious anemia, and atrophic gastritis are considered. In equivocal cases provocative testing can help differentiate other hypergastrinemic-hyperacidic conditions. The secretin test is the best and most reliable. After secretin is given intravenously for 30–60 seconds (2 U/kg) serum gastrins are drawn at 5-min intervals for 30 min. In normal patients there is little, if any, increase in serum gastrin levels. In gastrinoma patients the gastrin levels significantly increase within 10 min (usually more than 50% of baseline level). Meal stimulation is another provocative test but is less sensitive than secretin stimulation. The meal may consist of 2 eggs, one piece of toast, and 2 bouillon cubes dissolved in 4 oz of hot water. Serum gastrin levels are then checked fasting and then at 15-min intervals to 90 min following the meal. In gastrinoma patients no significant increase (less than 50% of fasting level) is observed. A third provocative test is the calcium stimulation infusion. Calcium gluconate (5 mg/kg/h) is infused intravenously over 3 h. Serum gastrins are drawn at fasting and at 30-min intervals for 4 h following the infusion. In gastrinoma patients there is a significant rise (greater than 50% of baseline level) in serum gastrins. This test is limited because it does not differentiate gastrinoma patients from patients with hypergastrinemia from other causes such as achlorhydric states. Of the three provocative tests the secretin stimulation is positive in greater than 95% of gastrinoma patients, which makes it the most sensitive. It remains the test of choice in equivocal hypergastrinemic states. A summary of serum gastrin responses is shown in Table 2.

TABLE 2
Serum Gastrin Responses to Provocative Tests

Disorder	Secretin	Test Meal	Calcium
Gastrinoma	Greater than 50% of baseline level	Less than 50% of baseline level	Greater than 50% of baseline level
Duodenal ulcer	Little, if any increase	Very mild increase	Very mild increase
Pernicious anemia	No response	No response	No response
G-cell hyperplasia	No response	Greater than 50% of baseline level	No response or exaggerated

The treatment for gastrinoma depends on whether the tumor can be localized by radiographic methods and removed surgically, or treated medically. Usually less than 50% of the tumors are found radiographically and are either localized and resectable or metastatic and unresectable. If resectable then complete cure is anticipated, but this is only about 20%. If not resectable then treatment with omeprazole has become the medical treatment of choice. Omeprazole is a powerful proton pump inhibitor that has a profound effect on decreasing gastric acid secretion. Hypergastrinemia results as a normal physiologic response to acid suppression. Omeprazole, being a more potent acid suppressor than H_2 receptor antagonists, raises serum gastrin levels to much higher values. In sustained hypergastrinemia, gastric enterochromaffin-like (ECL) cell hyperplasia has developed in rats in which some have progressed to gastric carcinoid tumors. This phenomenon has occurred in patients with pernicious anemia and gastrinomas. Omeprazole has no effect on serum gastrins that are already increased in gastrinomas, so the ECL hyperplasia and the possible progression to carcinoid tumors are not an issue. Total gastrectomy was once the treatment of choice before H_2 receptor antagonists and omeprazole. It is still considered when medical treatment fails with maximum doses of acid suppression or when undesirable side effects prohibit continued use.

CARCINOID

Carcinoid tumors are the most common gastrointestinal (GI) endocrine tumors, even though their occurrence is only 1.5% of all GI neoplasms. Most carcinoids occur in the appendix, terminal ileum, and rectum. Lesser sites are the stomach, duodenum, and colon. Rarely have they been found in the pancreas, biliary tract, esophagus, and lung.

Carcinoids are slow-growing neoplasms arising from enterochromaffin (EC) or ECL cells. If found primarily in the appendix they usually do not have metastatic potential, but in other sites metastasis may occur to the liver. Bone, heart, lung, spleen, pancreas, ovaries, and adrenals are not as common metastatic sites.

Once metastasis occurs a variety of vasoactive substances are secreted systemically and the carcinoid syndrome is now described. Vasomotor symptoms such as flushing, perspiring, palpitations, borborygmus, diarrhea, and bronchospasm are early manifestations of the syndrome. Hepatomegaly, ascites, and edema are late manifestations and signify a poor prognosis. The substances responsible for the vasomotor symptoms include serotonin, somatostatin, histamine, tachykinins, substance P, kallikreins, and peptide YY.

The diagnosis of carcinoid tumor is made by biopsy, and oftentimes this is done coincidentally at the time of abdominal exploratory for another condition. The carcinoid syndrome is diagnosed by the clinical presentation and the measurement of a urine metabolite of serotonin, 5-hydroxyindoleacetic acid (5-HIAA). A 24-h urine collection will show increases above normal levels of 2–8 mg per 24 h. Provocative testing can be used in equivocal cases with epinephrine or pentagastrin. Both stimulate serotonin. Serotonin-rich foods such as tomatoes, eggplants, pineapples, bananas, avocados, and kiwi need to be avoided while testing because they will cause false-positive values. Medications such as mandelamine and phenathiazines may cause false-negative values and so also need to be avoided. Radiographic studies such as computed tomographic scanning, magnetic resonance imaging, ultrasound, and angiography may suggest carcinoids when suspected.

Treatment consists of surgical removal if no metastasis is found, and pharmacologic antagonists, if metastatic, to control the carcinoid symptoms. These antagonists have only limited success. Death usually results from extensive hepatic or pulmonary metastasis.

INSULINOMAS

Insulinomas are mostly benign neoplasms of the pancreas that secrete excessive insulin and thereby cause significant hypoglycemia; 90% are benign and resectable and the others can be treated by chemotherapy. The classic Whipple's triad of insulinoma includes hypoglycemia symptoms after a 24-h fast, documented hypoglycemia during symptoms, and relief of these symptoms by glucose administration. Plasma insulin levels drawn simultaneously with serum glucoses show inappropriately high insulin levels during these hypoglycemic episodes.

Most symptomatic hypoglycemia is related to diabetic treatment, alcoholic liver disease, and less likely to adrenal insufficiency and panhypopituitarism. The simultaneous plasma insulin-serum glucose determinations will help differentiate these conditions from insulinomas because appropriate responses are seen in the former.

Surgical resection is the treatment of choice because most of these tumors are benign. Unfortunately, radiographic methods are not very helpful because the tumors are usually smaller than 1 cm. Various chemotherapeutic regimens for metastatic disease have had limited success.

VIPOMAS

A syndrome of watery diarrhea, hypokalemia, and achlorhydria was initially described by Verner and Morrison in 1958. This syndrome is caused by a non-B-cell islet pancreatic tumor which secretes VIP.

Diagnosis is suggested by an unexplained secretory diarrhea, where the diarrhea continues despite fasting. A high-serum VIP level is virtually diagnostic in this setting. Unfortunately, nearly 50% of vipomas are malignant and successful resection is not possible in most.

Treatment is surgical resection after the metabolic abnormalities are corrected. Diarrhea is controlled symptomatically with prednisone, but this does not always work. Octreotide, a congener of somatostatin, has now become the preferred treatment in controlling secretory diarrhea in this syndrome. It has been effective in other secretory diarrheas such as carcinoid syndrome and enteropathies.

GLUCAGONOMAS

Unexplained migratory necrolytic skin lesions, glossitis, stomatitis, and catabolism may suggest a glucagon-secreting tumor. The majority of these tumors are malignant and resectable in 30% of cases. Diagnosis is confirmed by increased plasma glucagon levels.

SOMATOSTATINOMA

A very rare tumor of pancreatic or small intestinal origin that secretes excessive somatostatin inhibits GI motility and insulin release. This gives rise to a myriad of clinical findings including diabetes, gallstones, and diarrhea. Most of these tumors are found coincidentally at the time of surgical exploratory surgery. If clinical findings are considered, an elevated plasma somatostatin level will be confirmatory. Unfortunately, delay in diagnosis is common because of the insidious nature of this tumor. By the time the diagnosis is made the tumor is usually no longer resectable.

CLINICAL APPLICATIONS OF GI HORMONES[10,11]

GI hormones have become increasingly valuable in diagnosing and treating various clinical conditions.

Secretin, as previously mentioned, has become invaluable in provocative testing for suspected gastrinoma. The secretin test for suspected pancreatic insufficiency remains the most sensitive method in detecting malabsorption secondary to pancreatic diseases. Secretin is given intravenously at a dose of 1 U/kg. Duodenal aspirates are then taken at 20-min intervals for 80 min. Total volume and bicarbonate levels are measured in each aliquot. In chronic pancreatitis, volume is decreased (less than 2 ml/kg per 80 min), and bicarbonate concentration also is decreased (less than 90 mEq/L). When volume remains normal and the bicarbonate concentration is decreased, pancreatic carcinoma is considered, although not reliable. Secretin stimulation also has been used in collecting pancreatic secretions for cytology.

CCK has not been as helpful in evaluating pancreatic-biliary disorders. CCK stimulates gallbladder contraction and has been used in various imaging techniques to diagnose acalculous gallbladder disease. Opacification of the gallbladder normally occurs after ingestion of an oral contrast agent taken 12 h previously. After intravenous injection of CCK, gallbladder emptying is normally expected. If emptying is poor and right upper quadrant is produced the test is considered abnormal and supports a diagnosis of acalculous cholecystitis. Similar interpretation with isotope scanning was thought to be more sensitive than oral cholecystography initially. Both tests, however, are influenced by such things as age, drugs, diabetes, weight, and diet, and therefore caution is necessary for interpretation.

Glucagon has been helpful in radiographic studies where smooth muscle relaxation of the gut is necessary at times for performing adequate examinations. These studies include endoscopic retrograde cholangio-pancreatography (ERCP), hypotonic duodenography, colonoscopy, and barium enema. Parenteral glucagon has also been used in treating symptomatic hypoglycemia, along with intravenous dextrose, because it increases glucose by glycogenolysis.

Somatostatin analogues have become increasingly important in the symptomatic treatment of various hormonal tumors. These include vipomas, metastatic carcinoids, insulinomas, glucagonomas, and gastrinomas. Octreotide, an analogue of somatostatin, has a much longer half-life (90–120 min) than somatostatin and can be used with fewer doses. Somatostatin is ubiquitous in the GI tract and it has effects, from inhibiting salivary, gastric, pancreatic, and biliary secretions to inhibiting the release of various GI hormones. Its beneficial effects have been seen notably in decreasing secretory diarrhea in vipomas and decreasing diarrhea and flushing in metastatic carcinoids. Somatostatin has also been used to control diarrheas secondary to enteropathies, short bowel syndromes, postvagotomy states, and pseudointestinal obstructions, with varied responses.

I-(Tyr)-octreotide scintigraphy is becoming a valuable test in attempts to localize primary endocrine pancreatic tumors. This test has also been useful in diagnosing some lymphomas, whether Hodgkin's or non-Hodgkin's.

Since hormones were first described at the start of this century, more than 50 different biologically active hormones have been isolated, as well as many of their receptor sites. An understanding of their physiologic responses has contributed greatly to our knowledge of various homonal conditions and their syndromes. With the development of stable analogues of peptide hormones many disease states formerly untreatable may now be effectively managed.

REFERENCES

1. **Gitnick, G.,** Gastrointestinal hormones and other chemical messengers, in *Gastroenterology and Hepatology,* Elsevier, New York, 1988, 1526.
2. **Despopoulos, A.,** *Color Atlas of Physiology,* Thieme Medical Publishers, New York, 1991, 234.
3. **Walsh, J. H.,** Gastrointestinal hormones: past, present, and future, *Gastroenterology,* 104, 653, 1993.
4. **Walsh, J. H.,** Gastrointestinal peptide hormones, in *Gastrointestinal Disease,* 4th ed., Sleisenger, M. H. and Fordtran, J. S., Eds., W. B. Saunders, Philadelphia, 1989, 78.
5. **Vinik, A.,** A personal historical perspective of the development of the gastrointestinal endocrine system, *Endocrinol. Metab. Clin. North Am.,* 22, 709, 1993.
6. **Modlin, I. M. and Basson, M. D.,** Clinical applications of gastrointestinal hormones, *Endocrinol. Metab. Clin. North Am.,* 22, 829, 1993.
7. **Lloyd, K.,** Gut hormones in gastric function, *Bailliere's Clin. Endocrinol. Metab. (England),* 8, 111, 1994.
8. **Klinkenberg-Knol, E. C.,** Long term treatment with omeprazole for refractory reflux esophagitis: efficacy and safety, *Ann. Intern. Med.,* 121, 161, 1994.
9. **McGuigan, J. C.,** Peptic ulcer, in *Principles of Internal Medicine,* 11th ed., McGraw-Hill, New York, 1988, 1250.
10. **Jensen, R. T. and Coy, D. H.,** Peptide receptor agonists/antagonists: discovery, present and possible future uses, *Regulat. Peptide Lett.,* 5, 45, 1994.
11. **Redfern, J. S. and O'Dorisio, T. M.,** Therapeutic uses of gastrointestinal hormones, *Endocrinol. Metab. Clin. North Am.,* 22, 845, 1993.

Chapter 5

HORMONAL EFFECTS ON URINARY ACIDIFICATION

Alexander J. Rouch

CONTENTS

INTRODUCTION: ACID-BASE BALANCE

In general terms, whole-body acid-base balance can be defined as the maintenance of a normal plasma pH, or $[H^+]$ (pH = $-\log [H^+]$). The two organ systems that play major roles in acid-base balance are the respiratory system and the renal system. Normally, dietary metabolism produces volatile and nonvolatile acid. The respiratory system controls the excretion of the volatile acid, or CO_2, and the renal system controls the excretion of the nonvolatile acid that originates from amino acid metabolism, organic acids, and phosphate.

To understand the key principles of acid-base homeostasis, one should first look at the CO_2/HCO_3^- buffering system.

$$CO_2 + H_2O \overset{CA}{\Leftrightarrow} H_2CO_3 \Leftrightarrow H^+ + HCO_3^- \qquad [5.1]$$

The reaction of CO_2 with water is catalyzed by the enzyme carbonic anhydrase (CA) and forms H_2CO_3, which ionizes into H^+ and HCO_3^- instantaneously. Using fundamental laws of mass action and dissociation of a weak acid, one can determine the $[H^+]$ (or pH) from this reaction. This yields the well-known Henderson-Hasselbalch equation:

$$pH = pK' + \log \frac{\left[HCO_3^-\right]}{\alpha \cdot P_{CO_2}} \qquad [5.2]$$

where pK' is the apparent dissociation constant (for plasma at 37°C, pK' = 6.1), P_{CO_2} is the partial pressure of CO_2 gas, and α is the CO_2 solubility coefficient (α = 0.03). Substituting the normal values for plasma $[HCO_3^-]$ and P_{CO_2} (24 mEq/L and 40 mmHg, respectively) yields a normal pH = 7.4 or $[H^+] = 4.0 \times 10^{-8}\ M$.

The physiological significance of the CO_2/HCO_3^- buffering system is that it is under the dual control of the lungs and kidneys. To illustrate the functions of the respiratory and renal systems in acid-base balance, the Henderson-Hasselbalch equation is often expressed as:

$$pH = pK' + \log \frac{\text{kidneys}}{\text{lungs}} \qquad [5.3]$$

This shows that the basic responsibility of the lungs is to control P_{CO_2} and the responsibility of the kidneys is to control plasma [HCO_3^-]. The lungs perform their function by altering ventilation and kidneys perform theirs by urinary acidification.

The purpose of this chapter is to review evidence of the hormonal effects on urinary acidification. Two subjects have been studied extensively in this respect. One involves corticosteroids and the other parathyroid hormone (PTH). After a brief description of the basic mechanisms by which the kidney acidifies the urine, research findings associated with the effects of corticosteroids and PTH on renal acidification will be discussed. A brief description of other hormonal effects related to calcitonin, adenosine, angiotensin-II, and α-adrenergic agonists will be provided. Tables summarizing the findings are provided after each section.

URINARY ACIDIFICATION MECHANISMS

Under most dietary conditions, a net accumulation of nonvolatile acid is generated at a rate of approximately 1 mEq/kg/day,[1] and the kidneys must excrete this net acid at the same rate as it is produced. In order for the kidneys to maintain normal plasma [HCO_3^-] levels, they must reabsorb all of the filtered HCO_3^- and generate new HCO_3^- to replace that which buffered nonvolatile acid. The kidney performs these functions via urinary acidification through H^+ secretion by the epithelial cells in different segments of the nephron. Alpern et al.[2] reviewed these mechanisms in detail. A brief overview will be provided here.

The nephron utilizes three primary cellular mechanisms to secrete H^+ ions into the urine: Na^+/H^+ exchange, K^+/H^+ exchange, and H^+-ATPase. The K^+/H^+ exchanger is not as well understood as the other two processes. Wingo[3] recently reviewed the significance of the K^+/H^+ exchange mechanism and other studies have documented its significance.[4-8]

The nephron exhibits considerable structural and functional heterogeneity.[9-12] For the purposes of this chapter, the key nephron segments that secrete H^+ will be considered. These include the proximal tubule (PT), the thick ascending limb (TAL), the distal convoluted tubule (DCT), and the collecting duct, which can be divided into the cortical collecting duct (CCD), outer medullary collecting duct (OMCD), and inner medullary collecting duct (IMCD) (see Figure 1). Although each H^+ secretory mechanism may be present in all nephron segments, evidence indicates that the early segments, i.e., the PT and TAL, secrete H^+ mostly via Na^+/H^+ exchange, and the collecting duct segments secrete H^+ via H^+-ATPase.

The PT reabsorbs 80–90% of the filtered HCO_3^- primarily by Na^+/H^+ exchange, although H^+-ATPase also participates[13-17] (see Figure 2). The H^+ ion moves from the cell into the lumen in exchange for Na^+ via the Na^+/H^+ antiporter in the apical membrane. The electrochemical gradient favoring Na^+ entry drives the antiporter. The secreted H^+ combines with a filtered HCO_3^- to form CO_2 and H_2O in the lumen. The CO_2 diffuses into the cell and the reaction is reversed to form a H^+ ion for secretion and a HCO_3^- ion, which leaves the cell via an electrogenic $3HCO_3^-/Na^+$ cotransporter or a Cl^-/HCO_3^- antiporter in the basolateral membrane.[13,18-20] Carbonic anhydrase, which exists in both the apical membrane and cell cytoplasm, is critical for maintaining a steady rate of acid secretion. The H^+ secretory mechanism in the TAL appears to be similar to that in the PT.[21,22]

From the late portion of the DCT to the late portion of the IMCD, most of the H^+ secretion occurs by H^+-ATPase, which is an electrogenic process.[7,23,24] The late portion of the DCT, the CCD, and the OMCD possess principal cells (PC) and intercalated cells (IC). The PC reabsorbs Na^+ and secretes K^+ via amiloride-sensitive and barium-sensitive ionic channels, respectively, in the apical membrane.[25,26] The IC can be subdivided into the α-IC and the β-IC. H^+ secretion in the α-IC occurs by H^+-ATPase in the apical membrane and HCO_3^-

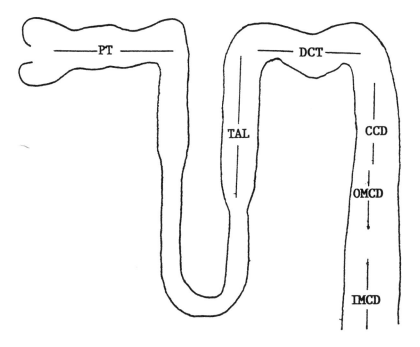

FIGURE 1. Basic structure of the nephron indicating the key nephron segments involved in H⁺ ion secretion. PT, proximal tubule; TAL, thick ascending limb; DCT, distal convoluted tubule; CCD, cortical collecting duct; OMCD, outer medullary collecting duct; IMCD, inner medullary collecting duct.

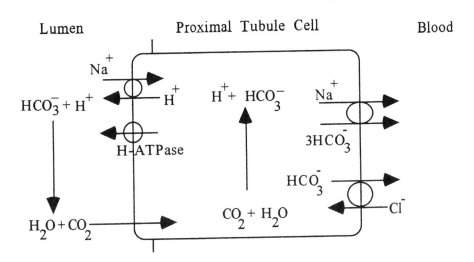

FIGURE 2. Basic mechanism of H⁺ secretion and HCO_3^- absorption in the proximal tubular cell. Not shown on this figure is the presence of carbonic anhydrase, which exists in both the apical membrane and cell cytoplasm. Also not shown is the Na⁺/K⁺-ATPase in the basolateral membrane which maintains a low [Na⁺] in the cell and supplies the energy for Na⁺/H⁺ antiporter in the apical membrane.

absorption occurs by Cl⁻/HCO_3^- exchange in the basolateral membrane (see Figure 3). The β-IC secretes HCO_3^- and absorbs H⁺ via opposite functional polarity of the α-IC.[27] Thus, the collecting duct has the capacity to acidify or alkalinize the luminal fluid, and this appears to depend on the acid-base status.[28,29] The IMCD contains a single cell type termed the IMCD cell that secretes H^+ primarily via electrogenic H^+-ATPase.[30,31]

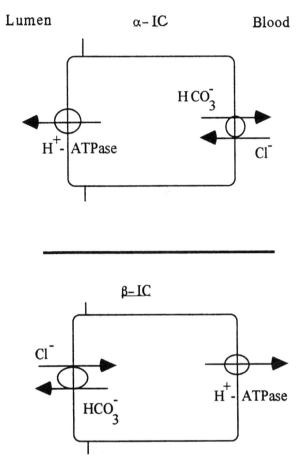

FIGURE 3. Basic mechanisms of H^+ and HCO_3^- transport in the α-IC and β-IC. IC, intercalated cell.

EFFECTS OF CORTICOSTEROIDS ON URINARY ACIDIFICATION

The effects of corticosteroids on urinary acidification and acid-base balance have been studied for many years. It is well recognized that patients with adrenal insufficiency or animals that have been adrenalectomized often exhibit metabolic acidosis and have an impaired ability to excrete the two major urinary buffers—phosphate and ammonia.[32-34] Thus, it certainly appears that the adrenal cortex is indeed essential for the kidneys to perform their role in acid-base homeostasis.

Aldosterone, the major mineralocorticoid, stimulates urinary acidification in the segments of the distal nephron including the DCT, CCD, OMCD, and IMCD.[35,36] The mechanism underlying this stimulation had long been questioned as to whether it was a direct or an indirect one. Aldosterone stimulates Na^+ absorption in principal cells and this results in a more lumen-negative transepithelial voltage, particularly in the CCD.[26,37,38] Consequently, the electrochemical gradient for H^+ secretion is elevated and urinary acidification is enhanced. This constitutes an indirect mechanism of aldosterone-stimulated H^+ secretion.

Numerous studies have also indicated that aldosterone directly stimulates the H^+-ATPase in the collecting duct as well as other H^+-secreting epithelia.[39-45] Stone et al.[45] reported that aldosterone increased HCO_3^- absorption (equivalent to H^+ secretion) in the inner stripe of the

OMCD and this process was independent of Na^+ absorption. (The OMCD can be divided into the outer stripe and inner stripe; the outer stripe follows the CCD and the inner stripe precedes the IMCD.[28,46]) Using the isolated perfused tubule technique, these investigators measured acidification in tubules from rabbits pretreated with the mineralocorticoid deoxycorticosterone acetate as well as in tubules from adrenalectomized rabbits where aldosterone was added directly to the isolated tubule segment. In both cases, mineralocorticoid treatment increased H^+ secretion. They also showed that acidification was unaffected by the replacement of Na^+ with tetramethylammonium in the lumen, indicating that H^+ secretion was independent of Na^+ transport. It should also be noted that the majority if not all of the cells in the inner stripe of the OMCD consists of the H^+-secreting α-IC; therefore, Na^+ transport does not occur to a major extent in this nephron segment.[47,48]

Interestingly, Garcia-Austt et al.[49] reported that pretreating rabbits with deoxycorticosterone elevated HCO_3^- secretion in the CCD. The CCD possesses both the α-IC and β-IC and can absorb or secrete HCO_3^-.[28,29] It was suggested that the HCO_3^- secretion resulted from the alkalosis produced by the deoxycorticosterone treatment rather than by a direct effect in the CCD, and that the HCO_3^- secretion in the CCD could represent a physiological defense mechanism against urinary acidification caused by elevated mineralocorticoids.

Garg and Narang[40] studied the effects of aldosterone in the late DCT, CCD, OMCD, and IMCD. They administered aldosterone to rabbits via a minipump implant device for 7 days, then harvested the renal tubules after sacrificing the animal. They reported that the aldosterone treatment increased NEM (*N*-ethylmaleimide)-sensitive ATPase activity in these segments. The NEM-sensitive ATPase is recognized as the H^+-ATPase.[15,50]

In addition to the indirect mechanism of H^+ secretion via Na^+ reabsorption and the direct mechanism via H^+-ATPase stimulation, another process by which aldosterone stimulates H^+ secretion involves the renal production of ammonia.[32,51] Along with stimulating Na^+ absorption, aldosterone stimulates K^+ secretion in the principal cells, and this can lead to K^+ deficiency which results in enhanced ammonia excretion.[51] Ammonia is the major urinary buffer and will yield a higher lumen pH which secondarily stimulates H^+ secretion in the collecting duct.

Along with these mineralocorticoid effects, considerable evidence demonstrates that glucocorticoids significantly influence urinary acidification mechanisms. Whereas in the study of mineralocorticoids investigators often used aldosterone or deoxycorticosterone, researchers have often used dexamethasone to study the effects of glucocorticoids.

Wilcox et al.[52] used both aldosterone and dexamethasone to study the effects of both corticosteroids on acid excretion in adrenalectomized rats. They found that aldosterone-treated rats consistently exhibited lower urinary pH than the dexamethasone-treated rats. Interestingly, they reported that the mineralocorticoids and glucocorticoids have dose-dependent and discrete actions on renal acid excretion in that aldosterone promoted urinary acidification whereas glucocorticoids promoted urinary buffer excretion in the form of phosphate and ammonia, and the glucocorticoids were more effective in augmenting net acid excretion.

Hulter et al.[53] reported that dexamethasone administered to adrenalectomized dogs elevated endogenous acid production, but this was fully compensated for by the elevation in renal net acid excretion so that metabolic acidosis was prevented. Glucocorticoids have been shown to regulate the production of ammonia in the kidney.[54] Thus, the evidence indicates that glucocorticoids enhance urinary acidification by elevating urinary buffer excretion.

Evidence also shows that glucocorticoids directly stimulate Na^+/H^+ exchange in the PT. Bidet et al.[55] reported that acute application of dexamethasone to isolated rabbit PT cells increased Na^+/H^+ exchange activity by increasing V_{max} of the carrier and this effect was consistent with an increase in the number of carriers in the membrane. Recently, Baum and Quigley[56] found that the addition of dexamethasone to the isolated, perfused rabbit PT stimulated acidification by approximately 30%, and the stimulation was blocked by actinomycin D and cycloheximide, indicating a dependence on protein synthesis. In another study,

Baum et al.[57] demonstrated that dexamethasone stimulated Na^+/H^+ antiporter activity in OKP cells (a clonal subline of the opossum kidney cell line often used to study PT function) in a dose- and time-dependent manner. This effect was also blocked by cycloheximide, again suggesting a regulatory role for glucocorticoids in the synthesis of the Na^+/H^+ exchanger.

Receptor identification studies have been conducted with variable results. Náray-Fejes-Toth et al.[58] demonstrated that the glucocorticoid agonist RU 28362 exerted mineralocorticoid-like effects in cultured rabbit CCD cells. Using specific glucocorticoid and mineralocorticoid antagonists, these authors showed that specific glucocorticoid receptors mediated the responses produced by RU 28362, and they speculated that the mineralocorticoids and glucocorticoids regulate the same gene.

Recently, Todd-Turla et al.,[59] using a competitive polymerase chain reaction technique, reported that corticosteroid mRNA was present in all nephron segments of the rat kidney but with a variable distribution. The mineralocorticoid receptor mRNA was 10-fold more abundant in the CCD, OMCD, and IMCD than in the PT and TAL. This evidence is certainly consistent with the known physiological effects of mineralocorticoids in the distal segments of the nephron. The glucocorticoid mRNA appeared to be higher in the PT than in the collecting duct segments, and this is consistent with glucocorticoid regulation on ammoniagenesis and H^+ secretion in the proximal tubule.[54,60,61] Therefore, the distribution pattern of glucocorticoid and mineralocorticoid receptor mRNA appeared consistent with reported corticosteroid function in the nephron.

Using immunostaining techniques with monoclonal, antiglucocorticoid receptor antibodies, Farman et al.[62] did not detect glucocorticoid receptors in the PT, although staining was positive in nephron segments beyond the PT. These authors suggested that the absence of staining in the PT could be related to an actual absence of glucocorticoid receptors, the presence of other glucocorticoid receptors that are insensitive to the immunostaining techniques, or non-receptor-mediated action of glucocorticoids in the PT.

Other investigations have focused on the natural corticosteroids, aldosterone, corticosterone, and 18-hydroxycorticosterone (18-OH-B), on urinary acidification in the rat. Ansaldo et al.[63] measured urine-to-blood (U-B) P_{CO_2} levels in adrenalectomized rats treated with the sodium channel blocker amiloride. Adrenalectomy reduced U-B P_{CO_2} levels, indicating a reduction in urinary acidification. Corticosterone or 18-OH-B treatment restored the U-B P_{CO_2} but aldosterone failed to do so. The authors reasoned that aldosterone acidified the urine primarily by a mechanism dependent upon the synthesis of Na^+ channels and consequently, enhanced Na^+ absorption, whereas corticosterone and 18-OH-B acted via other mechanisms such as those related to urinary buffers.

Damasco and Malnic[64] reported that each of these three natural hormones enhanced proximal and distal tubular acidification. This evidence is quite interesting particularly with respect to aldosterone—the major mineralocorticoid that acts primarily in distal nephron segments. The specific mechanism by which mineralocorticoids increase acidification in the PT is unclear, but two possibilities include a direct effect on Na^+/H^+ exchange or stimulation of Na^+/K^+-ATPase, which would increase the gradient favoring Na^+ entry and thus increase H^+ secretion.

In summary, the adrenal corticosteroids enhance urinary acidification by different mechanisms in different parts of the nephron, suggesting that they play a major role in acid-base homeostasis. The mineralocorticoids enhance acidification primarily in the collecting duct by three known mechanisms: (1) an indirect mechanism of stimulating Na^+ absorption which increases the electrochemical gradient for H^+ secretion by making the lumen more electrically negative; (2) directly stimulating H^+-ATPase in the apical membrane; and (3) stimulating K^+ secretion, which can lead to K^+ depletion and subsequent ammoniagenesis which increases buffer delivery to the distal tubule and secondarily stimulates H^+ secretion.

TABLE 1
Summary of the Effects of Corticosteroids on Urinary Acidification

Hormone	Effects	References
Aldosterone	↑ Acidification via an ↑ in electrochemical gradient for H^+ secretion via ↑ in Na^+ transport	26, 37, 38
Aldosterone	Direct stimulation of H^+-ATPase	39–45
Aldosterone	↑ Acidification via elevation in urinary buffer excretion	32, 51
Dexamethasone	↑ Acidification via elevation in urinary buffer excretion	53, 54
Dexamethasone	Stimulation of Na^+/H^+-ATPase	55–57
Aldosterone, corticosterone, and 18-hydroxycorticosterone	↑ Acidification PT and distal nephron shown by ↑ U-B P_{CO_2}	63, 64

The glucocorticoids also increase H^+ secretion. Evidence indicates that they directly enhance Na^+/H^+ exchange activity and increase urinary acidification by elevating the urinary buffers of phosphate and ammonia. The evidence of glucocorticoids producing mineralo-corticoid-like effects and the presence of glucocorticoid and mineralocorticoid receptors in the same nephron segments suggest interactive effects of corticosteroids on nephron function.

EFFECTS OF PARATHYROID HORMONE ON URINARY ACIDIFICATION

In addition to the corticosteroids, the effects of PTH on urinary acidification have been studied extensively. PTH is usually considered the calcium (Ca^{2+}) hormone. Whenever the body needs to increase plasma Ca^{2+} levels, PTH is released from parathyroid glands and stimulates the following: (1) Ca^{2+} resorption from the bone; (2) renal reabsorption of Ca^{2+} by acting on the DCT; and (3) production of vitamin D, which enhances Ca^{2+} absorption in the gastrointestinal tract.

It is well known now that PTH affects mechanisms of urinary acidification, and this subject was recently reviewed.[65] The accumulation of evidence suggests that PTH directly inhibits H^+ secretion in the PT, whereas it increases H^+ secretion in the distal nephron by enhancing urinary buffer excretion particularly in the form of phosphate. However, as with the evidence surrounding corticosteroid action, conflicting evidence exists and the physiological significance of PTH in urinary acidification is not completely understood.

In 1971, Muldowney et al.[66] suggested that metabolic acidosis caused by elevated PTH levels in hyperparathyroidism resulted from the inhibition of HCO_3^- reabsorption in the PT. Metabolic acidosis could be corrected by partial parathyroidectomy or vitamin D administration. Numerous studies with isolated perfused tubules, cultured cell lines, and brush border membrane vesicles have confirmed the inhibitory effect of PTH on HCO_3^- reabsorption in the PT.[67-70]

Evidence clearly indicates that the mechanism of action resulted from PTH stimulation of adenylate cyclase and the subsequent elevated cyclic-AMP (cAMP) levels that led to the inhibition of Na^+/H^+ antiporter by cAMP-dependent kinases.[68-71] Recent evidence now shows that the phosphatidylinositol cascade also plays a role in PTH action.[72,73] It is well established that phosphatidylinositol hydrolysis produces two products: inositol trisphosphate, which increases intracellular Ca^{2+}, and diacylglycerol, which stimulates protein kinase C (PKC).

Pastoriza-Munoz et al.[73] recently conducted a thorough investigation revealing that PTH alkalinized the cells of the rat PT via activation of the phosphatidylinositol cascade, which would suggest that PTH inhibits base exit across the basolateral membrane. They concluded that PTH alkalinized the cell via inhibition of HCO_3^- exit and that both arms of the phosphatidylinositol pathway played a role in the inhibitory mechanism. They also proposed an intriguing model of PTH-induced inhibition of urinary acidification in the PT cell, where a pool of PKC on the basolateral side regulated base exit and a pool of PKC on the apical side stimulated Na^+/H^+ exchange. This could reconcile the findings that indicate that PKC stimulates proximal tubular acidification by activating Na^+/H^+ exchange in the PT.[74,75] The model also includes the PTH-induced elevation of cAMP, which inhibits Na^+/H^+ exchange independently of phosphatidylinositol hydrolysis. Future studies will be required to confirm this model, but the cellular mechanism of PTH on proximal tubular acidification certainly involves second messengers other than cAMP.

Zaladek-Gil et al.[76] examined the effect of thyroparathyroidectomy (TPTX) on proximal tubular acidification, *in vivo,* in rats with and without Ca^{2+} supplementation. They suggested that PTH enhanced acidification in the PT and that Ca^{2+} played an important role in the process. They also found that TPTX significantly reduced the glomerular filtration rate, indicating that PTH acts as an important controller of glomerular hemodynamics, and that TPTX reduced titratable acid and ammonia excretion, indicating that PTH plays a role in the production of urinary buffers. This supports the findings of Bichara et al.,[77] who reported that in rats that received TPTX treatment PTH inhibited HCO_3^- reabsorption in the PT but stimulated H^+ secretion in the distal nephron via increased phosphate excretion. The net effect of PTH appeared to be to enhance net acid excretion.

Later, Zaladek-Gil et al.[78] again reported that the absence of PTH impaired acidification in the PT and found that the Ca^{2+} ionophore A23187 restored the acidification function. They concluded that proximal tubular acidification required both the normal concentration of PTH and adequate levels of Ca^{2+} and they noted that reduced and increased levels of PTH impaired H^+ secretion. The former effect was associated with Ca^{2+} and the latter with cAMP. It should be noted that these results contrast with those from studies of cultured renal cells, brush border membrane vesicles, and isolated perfused rabbit PT, where PTH inhibited Na^+/H^+ exchange.[67,69,70,79] Methodological differences between *in vivo* and *in vitro* studies could provide the explanation for this discrepancy.

Another possible explanation could be related to the findings from Cano et al.,[80] who demonstrated that cAMP had a dual effect on Na^+/H^+ exchange in OKP cells. They found that 8-bromoadenosine cAMP acutely inhibited Na^+/H^+ exchange, whereas the chronic application of cAMP increased antiporter activity. Thus, for hormones that have been shown to affect Na^+/H^+ exchange via cAMP metabolism in the PT such as PTH, acute effects may not predict chronic effects.

Good[81] reported that PTH inhibited HCO_3^- absorption in the isolated, perfused TAL. Inhibition was also caused by cAMP and forskolin, indicating that the PTH effect was a cAMP-dependent event. Recently, Borensztein et al.[82] supported these findings in tubule suspensions of the rat TAL. They reported that PTH elevated cAMP levels and lowered intracellular pH in the TAL cells. Arginine vasopressin (AVP), which is a well-known stimulator of adenylate cyclase produced the same effects as PTH. AVP at higher concentrations stimulated the phosphatidylinositol cascade mechanism but the physiological significance was questioned because of the required higher AVP levels.

Other evidence to indicate that PTH enhances acidification in the distal nephron segments comes from Mercier et al.,[83] who reported that PTH given to TPTX-treated rats increased urinary acidification by enhancing phosphate excretion, and from Bank and Aynedjian,[84] who showed that ammonia production contributes to the PTH-induced acidification in the distal nephron. One proposal is that the PTH-induced increase in acidification in the distal nephron could compensate for the PTH-induced inhibition of acidification in the PT. It has also been proposed that PTH contributes to the renal response made in metabolic acidosis by enhancing titratable acid excretion, and thus PTH could be a major player in acid-base disturbances.

TABLE 2
Summary of Effects of PTH on Urinary Acidification

Hormonal Effect	References
Inhibits Na^+/H^+ exchange in PT via cAMP metabolism	67–71
Inhibits Na^+/H^+ exchange in PT by phosphatidylinositol hydrolysis	72, 73
Stimulates acidification in distal nephron by elevating urinary buffer excretion	77, 83, 84
Stimulates Ca^{2+} acidification in PT	76, 78
Inhibits acidification and HCO_3^- absorption in TAL	81, 82

OTHER HORMONES AFFECTING URINARY ACIDIFICATION

There are some recent studies of other hormonal effects on renal acidification properties that deserve attention in this chapter. Bidet et al.[85] studied the effect of calcitonin in the DCT by measuring intracellular pH in primary cultures of rabbit DCT cells. They reported that calcitonin caused significant cellular acidification and they attributed this effect to a stimulation by the Cl^-/HCO_3^- exchanger in the apical membrane, which promotes HCO_3^- secretion in the DCT. The calcitonin-induced acidification was mimicked by dibutyryl cAMP and forskolin, indicating a cAMP-dependent mechanism. These findings suggest that calcitonin regulates intracellular pH and perhaps urinary acidification (or alkalinization) properties in the DCT by regulating Cl^-/HCO_3^- exchange.

Adenosine has received attention as a local hormone affecting numerous aspects of renal function such as glomerular filtration rate, renal blood flow, and renin release from the juxtaglomerular cell.[86,87] Takeda et al.[88] investigated the effect of adenosine on HCO_3^- transport in the isolated, perfused rabbit PT. They found that specific adenosine antagonists inhibited HCO_3^- exit across the basolateral membrane and that forskolin and cAMP derivatives had the same effect. They suggested that endogenous adenosine stimulates the basolateral $Na^+/3HCO_3^-$ cotransporter (see Figure 2) via an adenosine, receptor-mediated mechanism that inhibits cAMP production.

Angiotensin-II (AT-II) is another hormone known to affect renal acidification properties. Geibel et al.[89] found that AT-II increased both H^+ secretion and base exit in the rabbit PT by stimulating Na^+/H^+ exchange and $Na^+/3HCO_3^-$ cotransport, respectively. Liu and Cogan[90] reported that AT-II increased HCO_3^- absorption in the rat by inhibiting adenylate cyclase via a pertussis toxin-sensitive process, indicating the involvement of an inhibitory G protein. This is certainly consistent with other studies that indicated the significance of cAMP on H^+ secretion. Interestingly, Gomes and Mello Aires[91] reported that atrial natriuretic factor (ANF) inhibited the AT-II stimulation of HCO_3^- absorption, but ANF alone had no effect.

Finally, α agonists deserve some attention. It is not surprising that α_2-adrenergic agonists would stimulate H^+ secretion in the PT because of the known α_2-mediated inhibition of cAMP accumulation.[92,93] Indeed, Chan[94] and Nord et al.[95] have documented the stimulatory effect of α_2 agonists on PT acidification. It can be assumed that any hormone affecting cAMP metabolism will affect urinary acidification at least in the PT, and hormones affecting phosphatidylinositol metabolism will also affect acidification mechanisms.

TABLE 3
Other Hormones Affecting Urinary Acidification

Hormone	Effect	References
Calcitonin	Stimulates HCO_3^- secretion in DCT by stimulating Cl^-/HCO_3^- exchange	85
Adenosine	Stimulates $Na^+/3HCO_3^-$ cotransporter in PT	8
Angiotensin-II	Stimulates Na^+/H^+ exchange in PT	89, 90
α_2 Agonists	Stimulates Na^+/H^+ exchange in PT	94, 95

SUMMARY

The hormonal effects on urinary acidification mechanisms are numerous and complicated. Mineralocorticoids, glucocorticoids, and PTH affect these mechanisms in different ways, such as directly stimulating or inhibiting H^+ secretory processes in the nephron, indirectly affecting H^+ secretion by stimulating the renal transport of Na^+ and/or K^+, and influencing the production and excretion of ammonia and phosphate. Cellular mechanisms involved in these various hormonal effects involve cAMP metabolism, phosphatidylinositol hydrolysis, protein synthesis, and certainly other actions not yet known. Future goals should emphasize integrating *in vitro* studies with *in vivo* studies to distinguish better the simple hormonal effects from hormonal regulation of urinary acidification.

REFERENCES

1. **Laski, M. E. and Kurtzman, N. E.,** Characterization of acidification in the cortical and medullary collecting tubule of the rabbit, *J. Clin. Invest.*, 72, 2050, 1983.
2. **Alpern, R. J., Stone, D. K., and Rector, F. C. J.,** Renal acidification mechanisms, in *The Kidney*, 4th ed., Vol. 1, Brenner, B. M. and Rector, F. C., Eds., W. B. Saunders, Philadelphia, 1991, 318.
3. **Wingo, C. S.,** The renal H-K-ATPase: physiological significance and role in potassium homeostasis, *Annu. Rev. Physiol.*, 55, 323, 1993.
4. **Bello-Reuss, E.,** Characterization of acid-base transport mechanisms in the kidney cell line RCCT-28A, *Kidney Int.*, 43, 173, 1993.
5. **Fernandez, R., Lopes, M. J., De Lira, R. F., Dantas, W. F. G., Cragoe , E. J., Jr., and Malnic, G.,** Mechanism of acidification along cortical distal tubule of the rat, *Am. J. Physiol.*, 266 (Renal Fluid Electrolyte Physiol. 35), F218, 1994.
6. **Graber, M. and Pastoriza-Munoz, E.,** Regulation of cell pH by K^+/H^+ antiport in renal epithelial cells, *Am. J. Physiol.*, 265 (Renal Fluid Electrolyte Physiol. 34), F773, 1993.
7. **Wang, T., Malnic, G., Giebisch, G., and Chan, Y. L.,** Renal bicarbonate reabsorption in the rat: IV. Bicarbonate transport mechanisms in the early and late distal tubule, *J. Clin. Invest.*, 91, 2776, 1993.
8. **Wingo, C. S.,** Active proton secretion and potassium absorption in the rabbit outer medullary collecting duct, *J. Clin. Invest.*, 84, 361, 1989.
9. **Jacobson, H. R.,** Functional segmentation of the mammalian nephron, *Am. J. Physiol.*, 241 (Renal Fluid Electrolyte Physiol. 10), F203, 1981.
10. **Knepper, M. and Burg, M.,** Organization of nephron function, *Am. J. Physiol.*, 244 (Renal Fluid Electrolyte Physiol. 13), F579, 1983.
11. **Madsen, K. M. and Tisher, C. C.,** Structural-functional relationships along the distal nephron, *Am. J. Physiol.*, 250 (Renal Fluid Electrolyte Physiol. 19), F1, 1986.
12. **Ridderstrale, Y., Kashgarian, M., Koeppen, B., Giebisch, G., Stetson, D., Ardito, T., and Stanton, B.,** Morphological heterogeneity of the rabbit collecting duct, *Kidney Int.*, 34, 655, 1987.
13. **Alpern, R. J.,** Mechanism of basolateral membrane $H^+/OH^-/HCO_3$ transport in the rat proximal convolute tubule, *J. Gen. Physiol.*, 86, 613, 1985.
14. **Brown, D., Hirsch, S., and Gluck, S.,** Localization of proton-pumping ATPase in rat kidney, *J. Clin. Invest.*, 82, 2114, 1988.
15. **Kinne-Saffran, E., Beauwens, R., and Kinne, R.,** An ATP-driven proton pump in brush border membranes from rat renal cortex, *J. Membr. Biol.*, 64, 67, 1982.
16. **Sabolic, I., Haase, W., and Burckhardt, G.,** ATP-dependent H^+ pump in membrane vesicles from rat kidney cortex, *Am. J. Physiol.*, 248 (Renal Fluid Electrolyte Physiol. 17), F835, 1985.
17. **Ruiz, O. S. and Arruda, J. A. L.,** ATP-dependent renal H^+ translocation: regional localization, kinetic characteristics, and chloride dependence, *P.S.E.B.M.*, 200, 562, 1992.
18. **Alpern, R. J., Howlin, K. J., and Preisig, P. A.,** Active and passive components of chloride transport in the rat proximal convoluted tubule, *J. Clin. Invest.*, 85, 1360, 1985.
19. **Guggino, W. B., London, R., Boulpaep, E. L., and Giebisch, G.,** Chloride transport across the basolateral cell membrane of the Necturus proximal tubule: dependence on bicarbonate and sodium, *J. Membr. Biol.*, 71, 227, 1983.
20. **Yoshitomi, K., Burckhardt, B. C., and Frömter, E.,** Rheogenic sodium- bicarbonate cotransport in the peritubular cell membrane of rat renal proximal tubule, *Pflügers Arch.*, 405, 360, 1985.

21. **Good, D. W.,** Sodium dependent bicarbonate absorption by cortical thick ascending limb of rat kidney, *Am. J. Physiol.,* 250 (Renal Fluid Electrolyte Physiol. 17), F821, 1985.

22. **Krapf, R.,** Basolateral membrane H/OH/HCO$_3$ transport in the rat cortical thick ascending limb, *J. Clin. Invest.,* 82, 234, 1988.

23. **Capasso, G., Malnic, G., Wang, T., and Giebisch, G.,** Acidification in mammalian cortical distal tubule, *Kidney Int.,* 45, 1543, 1994.

24. **Schuster, V. L., Fejes-Toth, G., and Náray-Fejes-Toth, A.,** Colocalization of H$^+$-ATPase and band 3 anion exchanger in rabbit collecting duct intercalated cells, *Am. J. Physiol.,* 260 (Renal Fluid Electrolyte Physiol. 29), F506, 1991.

25. **Schlatter, E. and Schafer, J. A.,** Electrophysiological studies in principal cells of rat cortical collecting tubules. ADH increases the apical membrane Na$^+$-conductance, *Pflügers Arch.,* 409, 81, 1987.

26. **Tomita, K., Pisano, J. J., and Knepper, M. A.,** Control of sodium and potassium transport in the cortical collecting duct of the rat. Effects of bradykinin, vasopressin, and deoxycorticosterone, *J. Clin. Invest.,* 76, 132, 1985.

27. **Schuster, V. L.,** Organization of collecting duct intercalated cells, *Kidney Int.,* 38, 668, 1990.

28. **Lombard, W. E., Kokko, J. P., and Jacobson, H. R.,** Bicarbonate transport in cortical and outer medullary collecting tubules, *Am. J. Physiol.,* 244 (Renal Fluid Electrolyte Physiol. 13), F289, 1983.

29. **McKinney, T. D. and Burg, M. B.,** Bicarbonate transport by rabbit cortical collecting tubules, *J. Clin. Invest.,* 60, 766, 1977.

30. **Mankus, R., Schwartz, J. H., and Alexander, E. A.,** Acidification adaptation in cultured inner medullary collecting duct cells, *Am. J. Physiol.,* 264 (Renal Fluid Electrolyte Physiol. 33), F765, 1993.

31. **Schwartz, J. H., Masino, S. A., Nichols, R. D., and Alexander, E. A.,** Intracellular modulation of acid secretion in rat inner medullary collecting duct cells, *Am. J. Physiol.,* 266 (Renal Fluid Electrolyte Physiol. 35), F94, 1994.

32. **Hulter, H. N., Ilnicki, L. P., Harbottle, J. A., and Sebastian, A.,** Impaired H$^+$ secretion and NH$_3$ production in mineralocorticoid-deficient glucocorticoid-replete dogs, *Am. J. Physiol.,* 232 (Renal Fluid Electrolyte Physiol. 1), F136, 1977.

33. **Loeb, R. F.,** Chemical changes in the blood in Addison's disease, *Science,* 76, 421, 1932.

34. **Perez, G. O., Oster, J. R., and Vaamonde, C. A.,** Renal acidification in patients with mineralocorticoid deficiency, *Nephron,* 17, 461, 1976.

35. **Marver, D. and Kokko, J. P.,** Renal target sites and mechanism of action of aldosterone, *Miner. Electrolyte Metab.,* 9, 1, 1983.

36. **Sabatini, S., Hartsell, A., Meyer, M., Kurtzman, N. A., and Hierholzer, K.,** Corticosterone metabolism and membrane transport, *Miner. Electrolyte Metab.,* 19, 343, 1993.

37. **O'Neil, R. G. and Helman, S. I.,** Transport characteristics of renal collecting tubules: influences of DOCA and diet, *Am. J. Physiol.,* 233, F544, 1977.

38. **Reif, M. C., Troutman, S. L., and Schafer, J. A.,** Sodium transport by the rat cortical collecting tubule. Effects of vasopressin and deoxycorticosterone, *J. Clin. Invest.,* 77, 1291, 1986.

39. **Al-Awqati, Q., Norby, L. H., Mueller, A., and Steinmetz, P. R.,** Characteristics of stimulation of H transport by aldosterone in turtle urinary bladder, *J. Clin. Invest.,* 58, 351, 1976.

40. **Garg, L. C. and Narang, N.,** Effects of aldosterone on NEM-sensitive ATPase in rabbit nephron segments, *Kidney Int.,* 34, 13, 1988.

41. **Higasihara, E., Carter, N. W., Pucacco, L., and Kokko, J. P.,** Aldosterone effects on papillary collecting duct pH profile of the rat, *Am. J. Physiol.,* 246 (Renal Fluid Electrolyte Physiol. 15), F725, 1984.

42. **Khadouri, C., Marsy, S., Barlet-Bas, C., Cheval, L., and Doucet, A.,** Effect of metabolic acidosis and alkalosis on NEM-sensitive ATPase in rat nephron segments, *Am. J. Physiol.,* 262 (Renal Fluid Electrolyte Physiol. 31), F583, 1992.

43. **Mujais, S. K.,** Effects of aldosterone on rat collecting tubule N- ethylmaleimide-sensitive adenosine triphosphatase, *J. Lab. Clin. Med.,* 109, 34, 1987.

44. **Somchai, E. O., Kurtzman, N. A., and Sabatini, S.,** Regulation of collecting tubule adenosine triphosphatases by aldosterone and potassium, *J. Clin. Invest.,* 91, 2385, 1993.

45. **Stone, D. K., Seldin, D. W., Kokko, J. P., and Jacobson, H. R.,** Mineralocorticoid modulation of rabbit medullary collecting duct acidification, *J. Clin. Invest.,* 72, 77, 1983.

46. **Koeppen, B. M.,** Conductive properties of the rabbit outer medullary collecting duct: inner stripe, *Am. J. Physiol.,* 248 (Renal Fluid Electrolyte Physiol. 17), F500, 1985.

47. **Koeppen, B. and Giebisch, G.,** Cellular electrophysiology of potassium transport in the mammalian cortical collecting tubule, *Pflügers Arch.,* 405 (Suppl. 1), S143, 1985.

48. **Madsen, K. M. and Tisher, C. C.,** Structure-function relationships in H$^+$-secreting epithelia, *Fed. Proc.,* 44, 2704, 1985.

49. **Garcia-Austt, J., Good, D. W., Burg, M. B., and Knepper, M. A.,** Deoxycorticosterone-stimulated bicarbonate secretion in rabbit cortical collecting ducts: effects of luminal chloride removal and in vivo acid loading, *Am. J. Physiol.,* 249 (Renal Fluid Electrolyte Physiol. 18), F205, 1985.

50. **Gluck, S. and Al-Awquati, Q.,** An electrogenic proton-translocating ATPase from bovine kidney medulla, *J. Clin. Invest.,* 73, 1704, 1982.

51. **Tannen, R. L. and Kunin, A. S.,** Effect of potassium on ammoniagenesis by renal mitochondria, *Am. J. Physiol.,* 231, 44, 1976.

52. **Wilcox, C. S., Cemerikic, D. A., and Giebisch, G.,** Differential effects of acute mineralo- and glucocorticosteroid administration on renal acid elimination, *Kidney Int.,* 21, 546, 1982.

53. **Hulter, H. N., Sigala, J. F., and Sebastian, A.,** Effects of dexamethasone on renal and systemic acid-base metabolism, *Kidney Int.,* 20, 43, 1981.

54. **Welbourne, T. C.,** Glucocorticoid control of ammoniagenesis in the proximal tubules, *Semin. Nephrol.,* 10, 339, 1990.

55. **Bidet, M., Merot, J., Tauc, M., and Poujeol, P.,** Na^+-H^+ exchanger in proximal cells isolated from kidney. II. Short-term regulation by glucocorticoids, *Am. J. Physiol.,* 253 (Renal Fluid Electrolyte Physiol. 22), F945, 1987.

56. **Baum, M. and Quigley, R.,** Glucocorticoids stimulate rabbit proximal convoluted tubule acidification, *J. Clin. Invest.,* 91, 110, 1993.

57. **Baum, M., Cano, A., and Alpern, R. J.,** Glucocorticoids stimulate Na^+/H^+ antiporter in OKP cells, *Am. J. Physiol.,* 264 (Renal Fluid Electrolyte Physiol. 33), F1027, 1993.

58. **Náray-Fejes-Toth, A. and Fejes-Toth, G.,** Glucocorticoid receptors mediate mineralocorticoid-like effects in cultured collecting duct cells, *Am. J. Physiol.,* 259 (Renal Fluid Electrolyte Physiol. 28), F672, 1990.

59. **Todd-Turla, K. M., Schnermann, J., Fejes-Toth, A., Náray-Fejes-Toth, A., Smart, A., Killen, P. D., and Briggs, J. P.,** Distribution of mineralocorticoid and glucocorticoid receptor mRNA along the nephron, *Am. J. Physiol.,* 264 (Renal Fluid Electrolyte Physiol. 33), F781, 1993.

60. **Freiberg, J. M., Kinsella, J., and Sacktor, B.,** Glucocorticoids increase the Na^+-H^+ exchange and decrease the Na^+ gradient-dependent phosphate-uptake systems in the renal brush border membrane vesicles, *Proc. Natl. Acad. Sci. U.S.A.,* 79, 4932, 1982.

61. **Kinsella, J., Cujdik, T., and Sacktor, B.,** Na^+-H^+ exchange activity in renal brush border membrane vesicles in response to metabolic acidosis: the role of glucocorticoids, *Proc. Natl. Acad. Sci. U.S.A.,* 81, 630, 1984.

62. **Farman, N., Oblin, M. E., Lombes, M., Delahaye, F., Westphal, H. M., Bonvalet, J. P., and Gasc, J. M.,** Immunolocalization of gluco- and mineralocorticoid receptors in rabbit kidney, *Am. J. Physiol.,* 260 (Cell Physiol. 29), C226, 1991.

63. **Ansaldo, M., Damasco, M. C., de Lavallaz, M. S., Lantos, C. P., and Malnic, G.,** Role of corticosteroids in distal acidification of amiloride-treated rats, *Can. J. Physiol. Pharmacol.,* 70, 695, 1992.

64. **Damasco, M. C. and Malnic, G.,** Effect of corticosteroids on proximal tubular acidification in the rat, *Miner. Electrolyte Metab.,* 13, 26, 1987.

65. **Stim, J. A., Bernardo, A. A., and Arruda, J. A. L.,** The role of parathyroid hormone and vitamin D in acid excretion and extrarenal buffer mobilization, *Miner. Electrolyte Metab.,* 20, 60, 1994.

66. **Muldowney, F. P., Carroll, D. V., Donohoe, J. F., and Freaney, R. F.,** Correction of renal bicarbonate wastage by parathyroidectomy, *Q.J. Med.,* 40, 487, 1971.

67. **Iino, Y. and Burg, M. B.,** Effect of parathyroid hormone on bicarbonate absorption by proximal tubules in vitro, *Am. J. Physiol.,* 236 (Renal Fluid Electrolyte Physiol. 5), F387, 1979.

68. **Kahn, A. M., Dolson, G. M., Hise, M. K., Bennett, S. C., and Weinman, E. J.,** Parathyroid hormone and dibutyryl cAMP inhibit Na/H exchange in renal brush border vesicles, *Am. J. Physiol.,* 248 (Renal Fluid Electrolyte Physiol. 248), F212, 1985.

69. **McKinney, T. D. and Myers, P.,** Bicarbonate transport by proximal tubules: effect of parathyroid hormone and dibutyryl cyclic AMP, *Am. J. Physiol.,* 238 (Renal Fluid Electrolyte Physiol. 7), F166, 1980.

70. **Pollack, A. S., Warnock, D. G., and Strewler, G. J.,** Parathyroid hormone inhibition of Na^+-H^+ antiporter activity in a cultured renal cell line, *Am. J. Physiol.,* 250 (Renal Fluid Electrolyte Physiol. 19), F217, 1986.

71. **Weinman, E. J., Shenolikar, S., and Kahn, A. M.,** cAMP-associated inhibition of Na-H exchanger in rabbit kidney brush-border membranes, *Am. J. Physiol.,* 252 (Renal Fluid Electrolyte Physiol. 21), F19, 1987.

72. **Hruska, K. A., Moskowitz, D., Esbrit, P., Civitelli, R., Westbrook, S., and Huskey, M.,** Stimulation of inositol triphosphate and diacylglycerol production in renal tubular cells by parathyroid hormone, *J. Clin. Invest.,* 79, 230, 1987.

73. **Pastoriza-Munoz, E., Harrington, R. M., and Graber, M. L.,** Parathyroid hormone decreases HCO_3 reabsorption in the rat proximal tubule by stimulating phosphatidylinositol metabolism and inhibiting base exit, *J. Clin. Invest.,* 89, 1485, 1992.

74. **Mellas, J. and Hammerman, M. R.,** Phorbol ester-induced alkalinization of canine renal proximal tubular cells, *Am. J. Physiol.,* 250 (Renal Fluid Electrolyte Physiol. 27), F451, 1986.

75. **Weinman, E. J. and Shenolikar, S.,** Protein kinase C activates the renal apical membrane Na/H exchanger, *J. Membr. Biol.,* 93, 133, 1986.

76. **Zaladek-Gil, F., Costa-Silva, V. L., and Malnic, G.,** Effects of parathyroid hormone on urinary acidification in the rat, *Braz. J. Med. Biol. Res.,* 24, 1063, 1991.

77. **Bichara, M., Mercier, O., Paillard, M., and Leviel, F.,** Effects of parathyroid hormone on urinary acidification, *Am. J. Physiol.,* 251 (Renal Fluid Electrolyte Physiol. 20), F444, 1986.

78. **Zaladek-Gil, F., Silva, V. L. C., Cavanal, M. F., and Malnic, G.,** Effects of parathyroid hormone and calcium and their interrelationship on urinary acidification in the rat, *Clin. Sci.,* 83, 711, 1992.

79. **Sasaki, S. and Marumo, F.,** Mechanisms of inhibition of proximal acidification by PTH, *Am. J. Physiol.,* 260 (Renal Fluid Electrolyte Physiol. 29), F833, 1991.

80. **Cano, A., Preisig, P., and Alpern, R. J.,** Cyclic adenosine monophosphate acutely inhibits and chronically stimulates Na/H antiporter in OKP cells, *J. Clin. Invest.,* 92, 1632, 1993.

81. **Good, D. W.,** Inhibition of bicarbonate absorption by peptide hormones and cyclic adenosine monophosphate in rat medullary thick ascending limb, *J. Clin. Invest.,* 85, 1006, 1990.

82. **Borensztein, P., Juvin, P., Vernimmen, C., Poggioli, J., Paillard, M., and Bichara, M.,** cAMP-dependent control of Na^+/H^+ antiport by AVP, PTH, and PGE_2 in rat medullary thick ascending limb cells, *Am. J. Physiol.,* 264 (Renal Fluid Electrolyte Physiol. 33), F354, 1993.

83. **Mercier, O., Bichara, M., Paillard, M., and Prigent, A.,** Effects of parathyroid hormone and urinary phosphate on collecting duct hydrogen secretion, *Am. J. Physiol.,* 251 (Renal Fluid Electrolyte Physiol. 20), F802, 1986.

84. **Bank, N. and Aynedjian, H. S.,** A micropuncture study of the effect of parathyroid hormone on renal bicarbonate reabsorption, *J. Clin. Invest.,* 58, 336, 1976.

85. **Bidet, M., Tauc, M., Gastineau, M., and Poujeol, P.,** Effect of calcitonin on the regulation of intracellular pH in primary cultures of rabbit early distal tubule, *Pflügers Arch.,* 421, 523, 1992.

86. **Itoh, S., Carretero, O. A., and Murray, R. D.,** Possible role of adenosine in the macula densa mechanism of renin release in rabbits, *J. Clin. Invest.,* 76, 1412, 1985.

87. **Spielman, W. S. and Thompson, C. I.,** A proposed role for adenosine in the regulation of renal hemodynamics and renin release, *Am. J. Physiol.,* 242 (Renal Fluid Electrolyte Physiol. 11), F423, 1982.

88. **Takeda, M., Yoshitomi, K., and Imai, M.,** Regulation of Na^+-3HCO_3 cotransport in rabbit proximal convoluted tubule via adenosine A1 receptor, *Am. J. Physiol.,* 265 (Renal Fluid Electrolyte Physiol. 34), F511, 1993.

89. **Geible, J., Giebisch, G., and Boron, W. F.,** Angiotensin II stimulates both Na^+-H^+ exchange and Na^+/HCO_3 cotransport in the rabbit proximal tubule, *Proc. Natl. Acad. Sci. U.S.A.,* 87, 7917, 1990.

90. **Liu, F.-Y. and Cogan, M. G.,** Angiotensin II stimulates early proximal bicarbonate absorption in the rat by decreasing cyclic adenosine monophosphate, *J. Clin. Invest.,* 84, 83, 1989.

91. **Gomes, G. N. and Mello Aires, M.,** Interaction of atrial natriuretic factor and angiotensin II in proximal HCO_3 reabsorption, *Am. J. Physiol.,* 262 (Renal Fluid Electrolyte Physiol. 31), F303, 1992.

92. **Chabardés, D., Montegut, M., Imbert-Teboul, M., and Morel, F.,** Inhibition of α_2-adrenergic agonists on AVP-induced cAMP accumulation in isolated collecting tubule of the rat kidney, *Mol. Cell. Endocrinol.,* 37, 263, 1984.

93. **Garg, L. C.,** Actions of adrenergic and cholinergic drugs on renal tubular cells, *Pharm. Rev.,* 44, 81, 1992.

94. **Chan, Y. L.,** Adrenergic control of bicarbonate absorption in the proximal convoluted tubule of the rat kidney, *Pflügers Arch.,* 388, 159, 1980.

95. **Nord, E. P., Goldfarb, D., Michail, N., Moradeshagi, P., Hafezi, A., Vaystub, S., and Insel, P.,** $Alpha_2$-adrenergic agonists stimulate Na-H antiport activity in the rabbit proximal tubule, *J. Clin. Invest.,* 80, 1755, 1987.

Chapter 6

ENDOCRINOLOGY OF THE LUNG

Corinne G. Wong

CONTENTS

INTRODUCTION

Gas exchange in the lung and gas transport between the lung and other tissues are the major functions of the lung. In addition, pulmonary circulation results in profound effects on the functional capacities of other organ systems because only 2% of the systemic arterial blood bypasses the pulmonary capillaries. The epithelial layer of the extra- and intrapulmonary airways and the gas-exchange area of the lung possess a system of paracrine, neurocrine, or endocrine secretory cells that is known as the pulmonary neuroepithelial endocrine (PNEE) system. Moreover, the lung possesses a number of metabolic functions that include manufacturing of surfactant for local usage, filtration of small blood clots, removal of selected substances from the systemic venous blood that arrives via the pulmonary artery, and release of a variety of substances that enter the systemic arterial blood. Major pulmonary pathologies that arise include emphysema and lung cancer. In this chapter, two topics will be discussed: (1) hormonal regulation of surfactant protein gene expression in the fetal lung, and (2) molecular biology of the various peptides and neuropeptides that are located and synthesized in the PNEE system.

HORMONAL REGULATION OF SURFACTANT SYNTHESIS

Pulmonary surfactant is composed of a lipoprotein enriched in dipalmitoylphosphatidylcholine (DPPC), where the surfactant glycerophospholipids and proteins both function to reduce surface tension at the alveolar air-liquid interface[1] thereby stabilizing the terminal airway.[2-4] Pulmonary surfactant is synthesized by the type II cells of the lung alveolus, stored as lamellar bodies in the type II cells, and subsequently secreted into the alveolar space.[5-7]

Specifically, pulmonary surfactant is composed of approximately 90% lipids and 10% proteins. The major lipid components include DPPC, unsaturated phosphatidylcholines (PC), and phosphatidylglycerol (PG).[2,8-10] Four surfactant-associated proteins, each possessing a different structure and function, have been identified.[11,12] Surfactant-associated protein A (SP-A) is a highly glycosylated protein with molecular mass of 28 to 36 kDa and was the first of the surfactant proteins to be identified; SP-A is believed to play a role in the regulation of surfactant secretion and reuptake.[11] Numerous *in vitro* studies have shown that SP-A inhibits surfactant secretion, enhances reuptake perhaps by receptor-mediated endocytosis, and appears to be important for the formation of tubular myelin, which is a unique alveolar surfactant complex.[7,11] SP-B and SP-C are 4- to 8-kDa lipophilic proteins that appear to be important for the surface properties of surfactant; moreover, these two proteins seem to promote the adsorption of phospholipids to form a surface active monolayer and the squeeze-out of unsaturated components such as PG from the monolayer, thereby resulting in an enrichment of DPPC.[7,11] Finally, SP-D appears to be a lectin-like protein; both its structure and function have yet to be completely clarified.[12]

In the fetal lung, the capacity to synthesize surfactant occurs relatively late in gestation; surfactant synthesis and secretion are initiated after completion of 85 to 90% of gestation in all mammalian species studied thus far.[13] Secretion of surfactant into the amniotic fluid in the human fetus can be detected only after 30 to 32 weeks of gestation, although synthesis can be identified at 20 to 22 weeks of gestation.[14,15] SP-A expression occurs in fetal lung tissue after 75 to 85% of gestation is completed in all mammalian species studied thus far.[13] In the human fetal lung, expression of the SP-B and SP-C genes can be detected prior to midgestation. Moreover, the SP-A gene is expressed only in type II cells, whereas SP-B gene expression is detectable in the bronchioalveolar epithelial cells also.[13]

Multifactorial regulation of surfactant glycerophospholipid synthesis occurs as determined by studies utilizing fetal lung in organ culture as a model system because the preservation of tissue architecture and cellular interactions appears essential for the initiation and maintenance of type II cellular differentiation.[16,17] Surfactant-associated messenger RNAs for SP-A, SP-B, and SP-C have been examined by Northern blot analysis in the developing rabbit lung *in vivo*.[7] The genes for the surfactant-associated proteins are independently regulated and expressed in a lung-specific manner, although various factors affecting the mRNAs appear to result in a coordination of mRNA levels during normal perinatal development. Glucocorticoids in combination with other hormones and factors play a major role in the regulation of surfactant-associated protein expression.[13] Either additive or synergistic effects of glucocorticoids and triiodothyronine on PC synthesis have been shown in the rat, rabbit, and human fetal lung *in vitro*.[18-20] Overall, the synthesis of surfactant glycerophospholipids and proteins is under multifactorial control and is regulated by numerous hormones and factors such as glucocorticoids, prolactin, growth factors, thyroid hormones, estrogens, androgens, insulin, cAMP, and catecholamines acting through β-adrenergic receptors.[8,20,21]

PULMONARY ENDOCRINE CELL

The epithelial layer of both the extra- and intrapulmonary airways and the gas-exchange area of the human lung, mammals, and other animal groups harbor an apparently well-organized system of paracrine, neurocrine, or endocrine secretory cells known as the PNEE cells.[22,23] These cells are located around bifurcations of airways at or near the basement membranes of the bronchial epithelium.[24] Several studies have demonstrated that the PNEE cells share histochemical and ultrastructural features with cells of the APUD (amine-precursor uptake and decarboxylation) series,[25] which generally is comprised of the peptide hormone-producing cells in the epithelial lining of the gastrointestinal tract, the endocrine pancreas, the parafollicular cells of the thyroid, and the corticotropic and melanotropic cells of the anterior pituitary.

The human PNEE system appears to harbor the largest spectrum of bioactive mediators.[23] The distribution patterns of bioactive substances in the various human subpopulations of either solitary neuroepithelial endocrine cells or neuroepithelial bodies and in different cells of a single neuroepithelial body demonstrate great complexity, which currently is under intense study.[23] Serotonin immunoreactivity is demonstrated in almost all species studied thus far in the PNEE cells. Regulatory peptides have been found in a subpopulation of PNEE cells. In normal lung tissues, calcitonin gene-related peptide (CGRP), calcitonin, bombesin and gastrin-releasing peptide (GRP), enkephalin, somatostatin, substance P, cholecystokinin (CCK), and polypeptide YY have been found, whereas adrenocorticotropic hormone (ACTH) and a number of other bioactive substances should be regarded as ectopic.[23] The following section will describe in greater detail some of these pulmonary hormones, their origins, and their physiologic effects.

PULMONARY ENDOCRINE MOLECULES

ANGIOTENSIN-II

The conversion of angiotensin-I (AT-I) to angiotensin-II (AT-II) occurs in both the pulmonary circulation[26] and the luminal portion of the pulmonary endothelial cell,[27,28] by angiotensin converting enzyme (ACE), which is known also by a variety of other names that include kininase II, dipeptide hydrolase, and bradykininase.[29,30] ACE generally is released in response to lung injury.[29,31] The lung releases AT-II into the general circulation, although local production in other organs such as the brain, heart, lung, kidney, testis, and blood vessels appears possible.[30,32-36] Moreover, the colocalization of mRNA for the peptides renin and angiotensin confirms that local synthesis is possible.[37-39] In addition, both peripheral and central AT-II regulate the expression of genes of the renin-angiotensin system.[40,41]

AT-II is an octapeptide that exerts a variety of physiologic effects that include fluid homeostasis, aldosterone production, renal function, and contraction of vascular smooth muscle.[42] In the lung, AT-II contributes to regional vasomotor tone.[30] Binding of AT-II to specific receptors results in intracellular calcium mobilization through the stimulation of phospholipase C and subsequent production of inositol triphosphate, activation of calcium channels, inhibition of adenylate cyclase through pertussis toxin-sensitive G proteins,[43-45] and putative regulation of cellular growth.[46] Two pharmacologically distinct subtypes of AT-II receptors (type 1 [AT_1] and type 2 [AT_2]) have been characterized by the use of sensitivity to dithiothreitol,[47,48] by their ability to bind nonpeptide antagonists, and by cDNA cloning and expression of AT-II type 1 and type 2 receptors.[49-52] AT-II also has been shown to elevate cytosolic free calcium via activation of AT_1 receptors in human non–small cell lung cancer cells,[53] although the functional significance of this free calcium surge is not known presently.

Currently, the classical biochemical functions that are mediated by AT-II are assigned to the type 1 receptor, whereas the functions of the type 2 receptor remain to be clarified; however, evidence suggests that the type 2 receptor may be involved in cyclic guanosine monophosphate (cGMP) metabolism and prostaglandin synthesis.[52,54,55] One study has demonstrated that the AT_2 receptor is highly abundant and transiently expressed in the developing rat fetus, thereby suggesting a role of AT-II acting as a peptide hormone via the AT_2 receptor in fetal development.[52] Further studies have shown the existence of two subtypes (AT_{1A} and AT_{1B}) of the type 1 receptor. Isolation of DNA clones that encode the type 1 receptors has been performed from bovine adrenal, rat vascular, rat kidney, human liver, and human adrenal cDNA libraries, and a human genomic library.[51,56-59] These type 1 receptors are highly conserved at the amino acid level and display typical features of G-protein-coupled receptors such as the seven transmembrane-spanning segments.[57,60] In the rat, mouse, and human, at least two subtypes of the type 1 receptors have been identified that are expressed in a tissue-specific fashion and may play different functional roles in the cardiovascular system.[61-67] The AT_1 receptor appears to be the only subtype present in either vascular smooth muscle or rat lung tissue.[57,68,69] A recent report described the cloning and functional expression of an amphibian AT-II receptor that pharmacologically is unlike the mammalian AT_1 and AT_2 receptors.[70] These xAT receptors are present in *Xenopus* lung, liver, kidney, spleen, and heart, but not in adrenal, intestine, and smooth muscle.

BRADYKININ

Bradykinin is a peptide hormone (Arg-Pro-Pro-Gly-Phe-Ser-Pro-Phe-Arg) that is produced in response to tissue damage by the action of kallikrein proteases on the high-molecular-weight precursors known as kininogens.[71,72] Bradykinin is generated proteolytically from kininogen precursors in both the circulation and interstitial tissue fluids; local concentration is increased rapidly following tissue injury. The main degradation pathway of bradykinin in the lung is through the action of kininase II at the carboxy terminus and sequential cleavage by aminopeptidase P followed by dipeptidylaminopeptidase IV at the amino terminus.[73] Physiologic effects that are mediated by bradykinin include smooth muscle contraction, vasodilatation, increased vascular permeability, neurotransmitter release, neuronal transmission of pain or irritant messages, and altered vasomotor tone that are prominent features of the inflammatory process.[71] These bradykinin receptors also regulate mitogenesis and protein production in fibroblasts, thereby initiating repair steps that restore both normal tissue structure and function after injury.[74-76]

These physiologic effects are due to bradykinin binding to specific receptors that are found in a number of tissues.[74,77,78] Bradykinin receptors belong to the G-protein-coupled family, and pharmacologically different bradykinin receptor subtypes have been described recently. The B_1 receptor possesses a higher affinity for [des-Arg⁹]bradykinin than for bradykinin, has a limited tissue distribution in normal tissues and has been found primarily in vascular tissues.[71,79] Following either tissue trauma or insult, expression of the B_1 receptor has been reported.[80,81] In addition, the human lung fibroblast cell line WI38 mRNA encodes both B_1 and B_2 receptor subtypes, which were expressed in *Xenopus* oocytes.[82]

The B_2 receptor possesses a high affinity for bradykinin, but, in contrast to the B_1 receptor, has a low affinity for [des-Arg⁹]bradykinin; moreover, the B_2 receptor can be blocked by low concentrations of selective B_2 antagonists.[74] The B_2 receptor is found on a wide variety of tissue types including peripheral neuronal cells.[74] The B_3 receptor subtype has been proposed recently in trachea and lung due primarily to a lack of activity of B_2 antagonists.[83] Both the bradykinin receptor that has been cloned from rat uterus utilizing a *Xenopus* oocyte expression assay[84] and a human bradykinin receptor that has been cloned from the fibroblast cell line CCD-16L[85] and from the human gene[86] exhibit B_2 receptor characteristics. The deduced amino acid sequences of both the rat and human receptors show extensive similarity, which is consistent with their belonging to the superfamily of receptors containing seven membrane-spanning regions.[87] Recently, comparison on the pharmacology of the bradykinin B_2 receptors from the mouse, rat, and human was performed.[87] The human and rat receptors bound bradykinin and related ligands with pharmacology indicative of a B_2 subtype, whereas the expressed mouse receptor clone produced two populations where one possesses the pharmacology of B_2 receptors and the other has properties that are consistent with B_1-like properties. Finally, human bradykinin B_2 receptors that have been isolated by receptor-specific monoclonal antibodies are tyrosine phosphorylated, which may be involved in certain types of regulatory function; moreover, tyrosine kinase activity appears essential for bradykinin-mediated signal transduction leading to arachidonic acid release.[88]

NITRIC OXIDE (ENDOTHELIUM-DERIVED RELAXING FACTOR)

Nitric oxide (NO), which apparently is endothelium-derived relaxing factor, is a potent vascular smooth muscle dilator.[89-91] The mechanism for production of vasodilation occurs through the activation of guanylate cyclase and increased guanosine 3′,5′-cyclic monophosphate.[92] Inhalation of NO may be useful as a vasodilator with selectivity to the pulmonary circulation.[93-97] Specifically, inhalation of NO can reverse pulmonary vasoconstriction that was produced by either a thromboxane analogue or hypoxia in sheep.[93,94] The selectivity of inhaled NO in the pulmonary circulation may be due to its rapid combination with hemoglobin.[94,98-100] Such a reaction may limit availability of free NO within the pulmonary and systemic circulations. However, one study demonstrated that inhaled NO enters the circulation, but red blood cells prevented both systemic vasodilation and a significant amount of pulmonary vasodilation.[101] In addition, NO may contribute to the decrease of pulmonary vascular resistance that occurs at birth,[102] and evidence suggests that NO plays a regulatory role in pulmonary vascular resistance in the isolated neonatal guinea pig lung.[103] Finally, regulation of the NO-producing enzyme appears to be dependent on calcium and calmodulin.[104,105]

ENDOTHELIN

Endothelin-1 is a 21-residue peptide with vasoconstrictor properties, which was isolated and sequenced first from the culture medium of porcine endothelial cells.[106] Endothelin-like immunoreactivity has been localized in systemic tissue that include the brain, atrium, aorta, and uterus in addition to the pulmonary endocrine cells, airway epithelia, pulmonary tumors, and the developing and adult human lung.[107-109] Endothelin appears to be synthesized in the endocrine cells of the human lung,[109] and endothelin binding sites have been identified in the respiratory tracts of various mammals.[110-112]

Furthermore, three distinct genes encoding endothelins (ET-1, -2, -3) have been identified in various mammalian species including man.[106,107,113] These three isoforms may have different biological activities and different receptors.[113] Functional evidence exists for the existence of different endothelin receptors in the adult lung.[114] ET-1, -2, and -3 each consists of 21 amino acids, and their putative precursors are expressed as translational products from the human genome.[106,107,115,116] More comprehensive and detailed reviews have been provided elsewhere with regard to the biological actions of the naturally occurring endothelin isopeptides.[117,118] Evidence indicates that the ET-1 gene is induced by the vasoactive hormones angiotensin and vasopressin in cultured bovine carotid artery endothelial cells through receptor-mediated mobilization of intracellular calcium and activation of protein kinase C.[119,120]

In addition to its putative vasoactive role in the human lung, endothelin also induces bronchoconstriction and enhances cellular growth.[121-125] Its presence in the pulmonary endocrine cells and bronchial epithelium,[108,126] along with its suggested role in promoting cellular growth and/or differentiation, indicates that endothelin is a local hormone with diverse actions in the respiratory tract.

BIOACTIVE NEUROPEPTIDES

Subsets of both the nerves and endocrine cells that form the pulmonary neuroendocrine system in the airway epithelium are known to contain bioactive regulatory peptides that can act locally either as hormones or as possible neurotransmitters/modulators.[127] Such neuropeptides include substance P[128] and other tachykinins such as neurokinin A;[129] CGRP, which also is found in endocrine cells;[130] vasoactive intestinal polypeptide (VIP);[131] peptide histidine isoleucine or methionine (PHI/M);[132] galanin;[133] and neuropeptide Y (NPY).[134,135] All of these peptides possess strong actions on both vascular and airway smooth muscle and glandular secretion.[136,137] Of the neuropeptides that are found in the respiratory tract, both CGRP and substance P are found predominantly in the sensory nervous system.[138] The following sub-sections will describe in greater detail some of the functions assigned to the bioactive regulatory neuropeptides that have been found in the respiratory tract.

Tachykinins

Over the past decade, a class of neuropeptides known as tachykinins has been found to perform a vast array of biological functions in both the central and peripheral nervous systems as well as in the immune system.[139-142] The three mammalian tachykinins—substance P, neurokinin A (substance K), and neurokinin B (neuromedin K)—appear to be involved in numerous processes such as transmission of sensory information, smooth muscle contraction, nociception, inflammation, sexual behavior, and possibly wound healing and nerve regeneration.[143-146] The tachykinin receptors have been classified with respect to their preferred ligands in the following order: NK-1, substance P; NK-2, neurokinin A (substance K); NK-3, neurokinin B (neuromedin K). Because the tachykinins share a common C-terminal amino acid sequence that is essential for biological activity, cross-reactivity among the tachykinin receptors and their respective ligands does occur.[147,148]

Presently, only pharmacologic methods can distinguish between involvement of one or more of the tachykinins. However, current molecular characterization of the tachykinin receptors themselves will provide new approaches in the study on the various tachykinin functions. Substance P is a neuropeptide that is contained within the C fiber nerves that are localized primarily in the airways.[149] The human substance P receptor (NK-1) has been cloned[150] in addition to the bovine, rat, and human NK-2 receptors[151-153] and the rat NK-1 and NK-3 receptors.[154-156] Moreover, characterization of both the NK-1 and NK-2 tachykinin receptors in both the guinea pig and rat bronchopulmonary and vascular systems has been accomplished.[157] What role substance P and the other tachykinins play in airway responsiveness following ozone inhalation also is being investigated.[158,159]

Calcitonin and Calcitonin Gene-Related Peptide

Calcitonin (CT) and CGRP are derived from preprohormones that are encoded by three mRNAs (calcitonin, α-CGRP, and β-CGRP) derived from two genes (CALC1 and CALC2) that are located on chromosome 11.[160] The variety of expression of the three peptides in different cell lines derived from the same cell type is providing a useful system for studying the control of the expression of these peptides and their functional roles in various tissues.[160]

CT is a 32-amino acid peptide that is synthesized and secreted by the C cells of the mammalian thyroid gland, and also has been reported in the NEE cells of the human lung of all ages in both health and disease.[161-165] Moreover, CT immunoreactivity has been detected in the PNEE of various species, including monkeys,[166] hyperplastic and cultured hamster lungs,[167-169] rats,[170,171] and lizards.[172] The functional significance of CT in the lung currently is under study. One report indicates that serum CT may be an important marker for the presence of inhalation injury as well as a prognostic indicator,[173] whereas another study demonstrates that serum CT is not useful as a tumor marker in the diagnosis of lung cancer due to low sensitivity.[174]

CGRP is a 37-amino acid-residue peptide that was identfed from the analysis of the cDNA sequence of the CT gene from rat medullary thyroid carcinoma.[175] CGRP appears to function as a neurotransmitter in various populations of peripheral sensory nerves.[176] Distribution of CGRP immunoreactivity in the lung has been examined in a number of mammalian species[177-179] where CGRP immunoreactivity has been localized in both nerve fibers and endocrine cells. In general, much remains unknown about the arrangement of CGRP-immunoreactive nerves and cells within the respiratory epithelium, the frequency of their occurrence, and the morphologic relationship of these nerves to endocrine cells. One recent study indicates that pulmonary epithelial nerve fibers and endocrine-like cells exhibiting CGRP immunoreactivity form a morphological interrelationship, and most likely a possible functional complex, throughout the rat respiratory epithelium.[180] CGRP in the lung is a potent vasodilator and airway constrictor.[23,181]

Bombesin and Gastrin-Releasing Peptide

Bombesin is a tetradecapeptide that was first isolated from the skin of the frog *Bombina bombina*.[182] Similar peptides have been described since then in other species that include fish, avians, mammals, and invertebrates.[183] These bombesin-like peptides are defined by a region of homology at the carboxyl terminus, where their biologic activity is defined; this structural homology leads to the overlap in both physiologic and immunologic properties of the peptides. Bombesin binds to a cell surface receptor and initiates a number of early events, including inositol triphosphate and diacylglycerol accumulation, protein kinase C activation, Ca^{2+} mobilization, Na^+ influx and Na^+/H^+ antiport, arachidonic acid release, cAMP accumulation, elevation of both c-*myc* and c-*fos* mRNA levels, growth regulation, and modulation of neural activity.[184,185] Both bombesin and its mammalian homologue, GRP, have interesting actions that include mitogenesis for fibroblasts, epithelial cells, and small cell lung cancer (SCLC), bronchoconstriction, vasodilation, promotion of mucus secretion, regulation of gastrin release, monocyte chemotaxis, and appetite suppression.[186-188]

In humans, GRP and/or bombesin-like peptides are synthesized in isolated neuroendocrine cells as well as in the nervous system.[183] These bombesin-like peptides are a major product of pulmonary neuroendocrine cells.[189] To clarify the functional significance of GRP expression in the lung, GRP mRNA and immunoreactivity have been studied in human fetal lung development where GRP mRNA expression is detectable.[190-192] The pattern of GRP expression suggests a role in fetal lung development,[183] and GRP has been implicated as a growth factor toward human bronchial epithelial cells[193,194] with involvement in the stimulatory responses that lead to hyperplasia and development of premalignant cells in the lung.[188,195] Interestingly, pulmonary neuroendocrine cells, which produce and secrete GRP, are the first differentiated cell type to emerge in the fetal lung, and their appearance precedes the growth of the lung buds.[196]

In addition, the effects of bombesin administration on fetal lung demonstrated that this peptide accelerates fetal lung maturation (in terms of surfactant production) and also increases fetal lung growth both *in vivo* and *in vitro*.[192] Further studies indicate that hyperplasia of GRP-immunoreactive pulmonary neuroendocrine cells is found in certain pediatric lung diseases, most notably bronchopulmonary dysplasia,[197] and that bombesin-like peptides have been implicated as autocrine growth factors in the pathogenesis of some human SCLCs.[188] Also, tobacco smoke exposure appears to be involved in the increased GRP expression in adult human lung, and a strong association has been demonstrated experimentally in an animal model.[198]

Currently, human bronchial epithelial cells have been shown to express[199,200] the three known human receptors for GRP-like peptides: the GRP receptor,[201] the neuromedin B receptor,[201] and the bombesin receptor subtype 3.[202] The GRP receptor is a member of the guanine nucleotide (G)-binding protein-coupled receptor superfamily with the seven predicted hydrophobic transmembrane domains.[203] Additional studies utilizing newly developed GRP antagonists[204] and detailed molecular characterization of the known bombesin receptors[201-203] will clarify what significant functional roles GRP and other novel bombesin-like peptides from the normal lung[189] may play in lung development, pulmonary response to injury, and carcinogenesis.

Somatostatin

Somatostatin (somatotropin release-inhibiting factor) is a cyclic tetradecapeptide initially isolated from hypothalamic extracts.[205] Subsequent studies have demonstrated that somatostatin is distributed widely in diverse tissues such as the central nervous system and peripheral tissues including stomach, intestine, and pancreas. A wide array of biologic functions for somatostatin has been described that involve modulation on various endocrine and exocrine secretion processes which include inhibition of growth hormone, insulin, gastrin, glucagon, and secretion release.[206] In the central nervous system, somatostatin functions as a neurotransmitter and may be an important regulator of motor activity and cognitive processes.[207] In the human lung, somatostatin functions as an inhibitor of bronchoconstriction and, thus far, has been detected only in pathological tissues.[208] In monkeys, somatostatin-immunopositive pulmonary neuroepithelial bodies have been observed.[209]

As with the other biologic active peptides, somatostatin exerts its biological effects by binding to specific membrane receptors.[210-212] These membrane receptors are coupled to GTP-binding proteins or G proteins.[213,214] High-affinity somatostatin receptors have been demonstrated in various tissues such as different brain regions, pancreas, adrenal cortex, and brain, endocrine breast, and lung tumors.[215-218] Pharmacologic studies indicate the existence of at least two different human somatostatin receptor subtypes, and molecular cloning indicates the existence of four human somatostatin receptors[219] with confirmation that all four receptors are members of the G-binding protein-coupled seven-helix transmembrane-spanning receptor superfamily.[219] Finally, somatostatin analogs that are targeted to selective receptor subtypes appear to be promising for the diagnosis and treatment of different types of cancer.[220]

Cholecystokinin

The neuropeptide CCK, a member of the gastrin family, is a potent constrictor of tracheobronchial smooth muscle and has been reported to be present in diseased human lung,[208] in neuroepithelial bodies of the fetal monkey,[221] and in single NEE cells of the frog.[222] CCK is derived from a 115-amino acid precursor protein.[223] Posttranslational processing of the precursor protein results in four different amino acid forms[224] of which the 58, 39, and 33 amino acid forms contain CCK-8, which has a sulfated tyrosine amino acid residue.[225] CCK-8 possesses the full spectrum of biological activity that is seen with the longer forms.[225] Based on pharmacologic studies, there appear to be at least two CCK receptors.[226-229] Evidence exists for a third CCK receptor with a preference for gastrin.[225] Recent studies indicate that CCK binds to a single class of sites on SCLC cells[230] and that SCLC cells possess various types of CCK receptors as determined by their ability to interact with various CCK antagonists.[225] The significance of CCK receptors on SCLC cells remains to be clarified.

Opioid Peptides

Lung cancer cell lines of diverse histologies express multiple opioid receptors in addition to receptors for nicotine and α-bungarotoxin.[231] Different classes of opioid agonists have been shown to inhibit lung cancer growth *in vitro*.[231] Growth-inhibitory effects of opioids also have been shown from both *in vivo* and *in vitro* studies of other tumor types.[232-236] Further studies indicate that both the opioid and nicotine receptors affect growth regulation of human lung cancer cell lines, with the opioids possibly functioning as part of a tumor suppressor system and nicotine perhaps functioning in the circumvention of the tumor suppressor system as a pathway in the pathogenesis of lung cancer.[231] Additional reports suggest the existence of an antagonism between opioid- and nicotine-stimulated pathways on both behavioral and physiological processes in humans and whole animals.[237-239] Future studies may clarify the importance of opioids and nicotine in cellular growth along with the potential therapeutic value of opioids for the inhibition of cellular proliferation in bronchial epithelial cells that are destined to become lung cancer cells.

Vasoactive Intestinal Peptide

A number of neuropeptides located in both the central and peripheral nervous system have been found recently to stimulate the growth of normal cells in culture.[240] These peptides include bombesin, vasopressin, bradykinin, and VIP.[241,242] Studies indicate that VIP may function as a growth factor both in various tissues and in tumor cells that include several murine Lewis lung carcinoma cell lines and a human lung adenocarcinoma cell line.[241,243,244] Overall, however, results have been disparate on the studies of VIP effects on tumor cell growth.[245,246] Future studies will determine whether VIP may be a natural growth factor for tumor cells and whether a potential therapeutic utility exists for the use of VIP receptor antagonists in the treatment of selected lung tumors.

SEROTONIN

The biogenic monoamine serotonin (5-HT) is the most frequently reported bioactive substance in the PNEE cells and is known to be a potent broncho- and vasoconstrictor.[23] Serotonin is believed to be involved in the synthesis, storage, or release of co-stored regulatory bioactive peptides. Immunoreactivity for 5-HT can be found in the PNEE cells of the human lung of all ages, appearing initally in the eighth week of gestation, in both health and disease.[247-251] In addition, serotonin has been detected in other animal species that include the monkey,[252] pig, cat,[253] rabbit,[254] rat,[255] and *Protopterus* lung.[256] Finally, the human serotonin transporter that is expressed on human neuronal, platelet, placental, and pulmonary membranes has been cloned and expressed.[257] This transporter may mediate behavioral and/or toxic effects of both cocaine and amphetamines.

HISTAMINE

Histamine is present in large quantities in the lung where it is stored in the mast cells and has a number of pulmonary physiologic effects that include bronchoconstriction, increased pulmonary vascular permeability, and increased mucus secretion.[258] Histamine seems to represent a key factor in the functional link between mast cells and sensory nerves[259,260] based on pharmacologic studies utilizing receptor antagonists.[261] A functional relationship appears possible among mast cells, leukocytes, and sensory nerves.[261] Histamine release can be induced by tachykinins such as substance P in some mast cell populations such as those in the human skin.[261] Activation of H_1 receptors is associated strongly with pulmonary tachykinin release,[262] by direct action of histamine itself on the sensory nerves and/or indirectly by plasma protein leakage and formation of bradykinin.[263] Sensory nerve activation and neuropeptide release by bradykinin[262] may be through a direct effect by bradykinin receptors.

ECTOPIC BIOACTIVE PEPTIDES

Pathological human lung tissues that contain neoplastic counterparts of PNEE cells have been investigated for the presence of the various bioactive peptides. Apparently, the NEE cells in these neoplastic lung tissues express a larger spectrum of neuropeptides in comparison to healthy human lung.[23,264-266] Such neuropeptides include ACTH, neurotensin, motilin, glicentin, corticotropin-releasing factor, growth hormone-releasing factor, and VIP.[266] The significance of elevated neuropeptides in diseased lung tissues remains an important research topic.

CONCLUSIONS

The field of pulmonary endocrinology has exploded into a large and vast arena for research due to the introduction of both molecular biology and immunocytohistochemistry techniques. Many topics can now be addressed and studied in great detail that could only be speculative several decades ago. The data that have been published in recent years indicate the rapid accumulation of knowledge in which receptors for the neuropeptides that are located in the lung have been characterized; the pulmonary functions of these peptides have been described; and the development of pharmacological probes has occurred for dissecting out the various receptor functions in the lung. Overall, the significance of hormones that are present in both the healthy lung and pathologic pulmonary lesions can be defined more clearly now. The molecular relationships between hormonal malfunctions and pulmonary diseases can be determined more readily, which could lead to therapeutic treatment and amelioration of selected pulmonary disorders.

REFERENCES

1. **Clements, J.A. and King, R.J.,** Composition of surface-active material, in *The Biochemical Basis of Pulmonary Function,* Crystal R.G., Ed., Dekker, New York, 1976, 363.
2. **Van Golde, L.M.G., Batenburg, J.J., and Robertson, B.,** The pulmonary surfactant system: biochemical aspects and functional significance, *Physiol. Rev.,* 68, 374, 1988.
3. **Jobe, A. and Ilkegami, M.,** Surfactant for the treatment of respiratory distress syndrome, *Am. Rev. Respir. Dis.,* 136, 1256, 1987.
4. **Robertson, B. and Lachmann, B.,** Experimental evaluation of surfactant for replacement therapy, *Exp. Lung Res.,* 14, 279, 1988.
5. **Battenburg, J.J. and van Gold, L.B.G.,** Formation of pulmonary surfactant in whole lung and in isolated type II cells, *Rev. Perinat. Med.,* 3, 73, 1979.
6. **Auten, R.L., Watkins, R.H., Shapiro, D.L., and Horowitz, S.,** Surfactant apoprotein (A) is sythesized in airway cells, *Am. J. Respir. Cell. Mol. Biol.,* 3, 491, 1990.
7. **Connelly, I.H., Hammond, G.L., Harding, P.G.R., and Possmayer, F.,** Levels of surfactant-associated protein messenger ribonucleic acids in rabbit lung during perinatal development and after hormonal treatment, *Endocrinology,* 129, 2583, 1991.
8. **Rooney, S.A.,** The surfactant system and lung phospholipid biochemistry, *Am. Rev. Respir. Dis.,* 131, 439, 1985.
9. **Possmayer, F.,** Pulmonary perspective: a proposed nomenclature for pulmonary surfactant-associated proteins, *Am. Rev. Respir. Dis.,* 138, 990, 1988.
10. **Post, M. and Van Golde, L.M.G.,** Metabolic and developmental aspects of the pulmonary surfactant system, *Biochim. Biophys. Acta,* 947, 249, 1988.
11. **Possmayer, F.,** The role of surfactant-associated proteins, *Am. Rev. Respir. Dis.,* 142, 749, 1990.
12. **Nichols, K.V., Floros, J., Dynia, D.W., Veletza, S.V., Wilson, C.M., and Gross, I.,** Regulation of surfactant protein A mRNA by hormones and butyrate in cultured fetal rat lung, *Am. J. Physiol.,* 259 (Lung Cell. Mol. Physiol. 3), L488, 1990.
13. **Mendelson, C.R. and Boggaram, V.,** Hormonal control of the surfactant system in fetal lung, *Annu. Rev. Physiol.,* 53, 415, 1991.
14. **Hallman, M., Kulovich, M., Kirkpatrick, E., Sugarman, R.G., and Gluck, L.,** Phosphatidylinositol and phosphatidylglycerol in amniotic fluid: indices of lung maturity, *Am. J. Obstet. Gynecol.,* 125, 613, 1976.
15. **Quirk, J.G., Bleasdale, J.E., MacDonald, P.C., and Johnston, J.M.,** A role for cytidine monophosphate in the regulation of the glycerophospholipid composition of surfactant in developing lung, *Biochem. Biophys. Res. Commun.,* 95, 985, 1980.
16. **Masters, J.R.W.,** Epithelial-mesenchymal interaction during lung development: the effect of mesenchymal mass, *Dev. Biol.,* 51, 98, 1976.
17. **Sorokin, S.,** A study of development in organ cultues of mammalian lungs, *Dev. Biol.,* 3, 60, 1961.
18. **Gross, I. and Wilson, C.M.,** Fetal lung in organ culture, IV, Supra-additive hormone interactions, *J. Appl. Physiol.,* 52, 1420, 1982.
19. **Ballard, P.L., Hovey, M.L., and Gonzales, L.K.,** Thyroid hormone stimulation of phosphatidylcholine synthesis in cultured fetal rabbit lung, *J. Clin. Invest.,* 74, 898, 1984.
20. **Gonzales, L.W., Ballard, P.L., Ertsey, R., and Williams, M.C.,** Glucocorticoids and thyroid hormones stimulate biochemical and morphological differentiation of human fetal lung in organ culture, *J. Clin. Endocrinol. Metab.,* 62, 678, 1986.
21. **Ballard, P.L.,** Hormones and lung maturation, *Monogr. Endocrinol.,* 28, 1, 1986.
22. **Richardson, J.B.,** Nerve supply to the lungs, *Am. Rev. Respir. Dis.,* 119, 785, 1979.

23. **Scheuermann, D.W., Adriaensen, D., Timmermans, J.P., and De Groodt-Lasseel, M.H.A.,** Comparative histological overview of the chemical coding of the pulmonary neuroepithelial endocrine system in health and disease, *Eur. J. Morphol.*, 30, 101, 1992.

24. **Hage, E.,** Electron microscopic identifications of several types of endocrine cells in the bronchial epithelium of human features, *Z. Zellforsch. Mikrosk. Anat.*, 141, 401, 1972.

25. **Pearse, A.G.E.,** The cytochemistry and ultrastructure of polypeptide hormone-producing cells of the APUD series and the embryologic, physiologic and pathologic implications of the concept, *J. Histochem. Cytochem.*, 17, 303, 1969.

26. **Ng, K.K.F. and Vane, J.R.,** Conversion of angiotensin I to angiontensin II, *Nature*, 216, 762, 1967.

27. **Ryan, J.W., Ryan, U.S., Schultz, D.R., Whitaker, C., Chung, A., and Dorer, F.E.,** Subcellular localization of pulmonary angiotensin-converting enzyme (kininase II), *Biochem. J.*, 146, 497, 1975.

28. **Ryan, U.S., Ryan, J.W., Whitaker, C., and Ohio, A.,** Localization of angiotensin-converting enzyme (kinase II), II, Immunocytochemistry and immunofluorescence, *Tissue Cell*, 8, 125, 1976.

29. **Kelley, J.,** Lavage angiotensin converting enzyme as a marker of lung injury, *Am. Rev. Respir. Dis.*, 137, 531, 1988.

30. **Lees K.R., MacFadyen, R.J., and Reid, J.L.,** Tissue angiotensin converting enzyme inhibition: relevant to clinical practice? *Am. J. Hypertens.*, 3, 266S, 1990.

31. **Hollinger, M.A., Giri, S.N., Patwell, S., Zuckerman, J.E., Gorin, A., and Parsons, G.,** Effect of acute lung injury on angiotensin converting enzyme in serum, lung lavage, and effusate, *Am. Rev. Respir. Dis.*, 121, 373, 1980.

32. **Caldwell, P.R.B., Seegal, B.C., Hsu, K.C., Das, M., and Soffer, R.L.,** Angiotensin-converting enzymes: vascular endothelial localization, *Science*, 191, 1050, 1976.

33. **Campbell, D.J.,** Circulating and tissue angiotensin systems, *J. Clin. Invest..*, 79, 1, 1987.

34. **Cohen, S., Taylor, J.M., Murakami, K., Michelakis, A.M., and Inagami, T.,** Isolation and characterization of renin-like enzymes from mouse submaxillary glands, *Biochemistry*, 11, 4286, 1972.

35. **Ryan, J.W.,** Renin-like enzyme in the adrenal gland, *Science*, 158, 1589, 1976.

36. **Nakamaru, M., Jackson, E.K., and Inagami T.,** Beta-adrenoreceptor-mediated release of angiotensin II from mesenteric arteries, *Am. J. Physiol.*, 250, H144, 1986.

37. **Deschepper, C.F., Mellor, S.H., Cumin, F., Baxter, J.D., and Ganong, W.F.,** Analysis by immunocytochemistry and in situ hybridization of renin and its mRNA in kidney, testis, adrenal and pituitary of the rat, *Proc. Natl. Acad. Sci. U.S.A.*, 83, 7552, 1986.

38. **Dzau, V.J., Ellison, K.E., Brody, T., Ingelfinger, J., and Pratt, R.E.,** A comparative study of the distributions of renin and angiotensin messenger ribonucleic acids in rat and mouse tissues, *Endocrinology*, 120, 2334, 1987.

39. **Lynch, K.R., Simnad, V.I., Ben-Ari E.T., and Garrison, J.C.,** Localization of preangiotensinogen mRNA sequences in the rat brain, *Hypertension*, 8, 540, 1986.

40. **Kohara, K., Brosnihan, K.B., Ferrario, C.M., and Milsted, A.,** Peripheral and central angiotensin II regulates expression of genes of the renin-angiotensin system, *Am. J. Physiol.*, 262, E651, 1992.

41. **Ferrario, C.M.,** The renin-angiotensin system: importance in physiology and pathology, *J. Cardiovasc. Pharmacol.*, 15 (Suppl. 3), S1, 1990.

42. **Peach, M.J.,** Renin-angiotensin system: biochemistry and mechanisms of action, *Physiol. Rev.*, 57, 313, 1977.

43. **Griedling, K.K., Rittenhouse, S.E., Brock, T.A., Ekstein, L.S., Gimbrone, M.A., Jr., and Alexandre, R.W.,** Sustained diacylglycerol formation from inositol phospholipids in angiotensin II-stimulated vascular smooth muscle cells, *J. Biol. Chem.*, 261, 5901, 1986.

44. **Hescheler, J., Rosenthal, W., Hinsche, K.D., Wulfern, M., Trautwein, W., and Schultz, G.,** Angiotensin II-induced stimulation of voltage-dependent Ca^{+2} currents in an adrenal cortical cell line, *EMBO J.*, 7, 619, 1988.

45. **Crane, J.K., Campanile, C.P., and Garrison, J.C.,** The hepatic angiotensin II receptor, II, Effect of guanine nucleotides and interaction with cyclic AMP production, *J. Biol. Chem.*, 257, 4959, 1982.

46. **Schelling, P., Fischer, H., and Ganten, D.,** Angiotensin and cell growth: a link to cardiovascular hypertrophy? *J. Hypertens.*, 9, 3, 1991.

47. **Whitebread, S., Mele, M., Kamber, B., and De Gasparo, M.,** Preliminary biochemical characterization of two angiotensin II receptor subtypes, *Biochem. Biophys. Res. Commun.*, 163, 284, 1989.

48. **Chiu, A.T., McCall, D.E., Nguyen, T.T., Carini, D.J., Duncia, J.V., Herblin, W.F., Uyeda, R.T., Wong, P.C., Wexler, R.R., Johnson, A.L., and Timmermans, P.B.M.W.M.,** Discrimination of angiotensin II receptor subtypes by dithiothreitol, *Eur. J. Pharmacol.*, 170, 117, 1989.

49. **Chiu, A.T., Herblin, W.F., McCall, D.E., Ardecky, R.J., Carini, D.J., Duncia, J.V., Pease, L.J., Wong, P.C., Wexler, R.R., Johnson, A.L., and Timmermans, P.B.M.W.M.,** Identification of angiotensin II receptor subtypes, *Biochem. Biophys. Res. Commun.*, 165, 196, 1989.

50. **Timmermans, P.B.M.W.M., Wong, P.C., Chiu, A.T., and Herblin, W.F.,** Nonpeptide angiotensin II receptor antagonists, *Trends Pharmacol. Sci.*, 12, 55, 1991.

51. **Konishi, H., Kuroda, S., Inada Y., and Fujisawa, H.,** Novel subtype of human angiotensin II type 1 receptor: cDNA cloning and expression, *Biochem. Biophys. Res. Commun.*, 199, 467, 1994.
52. **Grady, E.F., Sechi, L.A., Griffin, C.A., Schambelan, M., and Kalinyak, J.E.,** Expression of AT_2 receptors in the developing rat fetus, *J. Clin. Invest.*, 88, 921, 1991.
53. **Batra, V.K., Gopalakrishnan, V., McNeill, J.R., and Hickie, R.A.,** Angiotensin II elevates cytosolic free calcium in human lung adenocarcinoma cells via activation of AT_1 receptors, *Cancer Lett.*, 76, 19, 1994.
54. **Bumpus, F.M., Catt, K.J., Chiu, A.T., De Gasparo, M., Goodfriend, T., Husain, A., Peach, M.J., Taylor, D.G., Jr., and Timmermans, P.B.M.W.M.,** Nomenclature for angiotensin receptors, A report of the Nomenclature Committee of the Council for High Blood Pressure Research, *Hypertension*, 17, 720, 1991.
55. **Timmermans, P.B., Chiu, A.T., Herblin, W.F., Wong, P.C., and Smith, R.D.,** Angiotensin II receptor subtypes, *Am. J. Hypertens.*, 5, 406, 1992.
56. **Sasaki, K., Yamano, Y., Bardhan, S., Iwai, N., Murray, J.J., Hasegawa, M., Matsuda, Y., and Inagami, T.,** Cloning and expression of a complementary DNA encoding a bovine adrenal angiotensin II type-1 receptor, *Nature*, 351, 230, 1991.
57. **Murphy, T.J., Alexdander, R.W., Griendling, K.K., Runge, M.S., and Bernstein, K.E.,** Isolation of a cDNA encoding the vascular type-1 angiotensin II receptor, *Nature*, 351, 233, 1991.
58. **Furuta, H., Guo, D.F., and Inagami, T.,** Molecular cloning and sequencing of the gene encoding human angiotensin II type 1 receptor, *Biochem. Biophys. Res. Commun.*, 183, 8, 1992.
59. **Curnow, K.M., Pascoe, L., and White, P.C.,** Genetic analysis of the human type-1 angiotensin II receptor, *Mol. Endocrinol.*, 6, 1113, 1992.
60. **Iwai, N., Yamano, Y., Chaki, S., Konishi, F., Bardhan, S., Tibbetts, C., Sasaki, K., Hasegawa, M., Matsuda, Y., and Inagami, T.,** Rat angiotensin II receptor: cDNA sequence and regulation of the gene expression, *Biochem. Biophys. Res. Commun.*, 177, 299, 1991.
61. **Iwai, N. and Inagami, T.,** Identification of two subtypes in the rat type I angiotensin II receptor, *FEBS Lett.*, 298, 257, 1992.
62. **Kakar, S.S., Sellers, J.C., Devor, D.C., Musgrove, L.C., and Neill, J.D.,** Angiotensin II type-1 receptor subtype cDNAs: differential tissue expression and hormonal regulation, *Biochem. Biophys. Res. Commun.*, 183, 1090, 1992.
63. **Sandberg, K., Ji, H., Clark, A.J.L., Shapira, H., and Catt, K.J.,** Cloning and expression of a novel angiotensin II receptor subtype, *Biol. Chem.*, 267, 9455, 1992.
64. **Sasamura, H., Hein, L., Krieger, J.E., Pratt, R.E., Kobilka, B.K., and Dzau, V.J.,** Cloning, characterization, and expression of two angiotensin receptor (AT-1) isoforms from the mouse genome, *Biochem. Biophys. Res. Commun.*, 185, 253, 1992.
65. **Takayanagi, R., Ohnaka, K., Sakai, Y., Nakao, R., Yanase, T., Haji, M., Inagami, T., Furuta, H., Gou D.F., Nakamuta, M., and Nawata, H.,** Molecular cloning, sequence analysis, and expression of a cDNA encoding human type-1 angiotensin II receptor, *Biochem. Biophys. Res. Commun.*, 183, 910, 1992.
66. **Mauzy, C.A., Hwang, O., Egloff, A.M., Wu, L.H., and Chung, F.Z.,** Cloning, expression, and characterization of a gene encoding the human angiotensin II type 1A receptor, *Biochem. Biophys. Res. Commun.*, 186, 277, 1992.
67. **Kitami, Y., Okura, T., Marumoto, K., Wakamiya, R., and Hiwada, K.,** Differential gene expression and regulation of type-1 angiotensin II receptor subtypes in the rat, *Biochem. Biophys. Res. Commun.*, 188, 446, 1992.
68. **Wienen, W., Mauz, A.B.M., Van Meel, J.C.A., and Entzeroth, M.,** Different types of receptor interaction of peptide and nonpeptide angiotensin II antagonists revealed by receptor binding and functional studies, *Mol. Pharmacol.*, 41, 1081, 1992.
69. **Entzeroth, M. and Hadamovsky, S.,** Angiotensin II receptors in the rat lung are of the AT-II-1 subtype, *Eur. J. Pharmacol.*, 206, 237, 1991.
70. **Ji, H., Sandberg, K., Zhang, Y., and Catt, K.J.,** Molecular cloning, sequencing, and functional expression of an amphibian angiotensin II receptor, *Biochem. Biophys. Res. Commun.*, 194, 756, 1993.
71. **Regoli, D. and Barabe, J.,** Pharmacology of bradykinin and related kinins, *Pharmacol. Rev.*, 32, 1, 1980.
72. **Baccaglini, P. and Hogan, P.,** Some rat sensory neurons in culture express characteristics of differentiated pain sensory neurons, *Proc. Natl. Acad. Sci. U.S.A.*, 80, 594, 1983.
73. **Pesquero J.B., Jubilut, G.N., Lindsey, C.J., and Paiva, A.C.M.,** Bradykinin metabolism pathway in the rat pulmonary circulation, *J. Hypertens.*, 10, 1471, 1992.
74. **Steranka, L.R., Manning, D.C., DeHaas, C.J., Ferkany, J.W., Borosky, S.A., Connor, J.R., Vavrek, R.J., Stewart, J.M., and Snyder, S.H.,** Bradykinin as a pain mediator: receptors are localized to sensory neurons, and antagonists have analgesic actions, *Proc. Natl. Acad. Sci. U.S.A.*, 85, 3245, 1988.
75. **Goldstein, R.H. and Wall, M.,** Activation of protein formation and cell division by bradykinin and des-Arg9-bradykinin, *J. Biol. Chem.*, 259, 9263, 1984.
76. **Becherer, P.R., Mertz, L.F., and Baenziger, N.L.,** Regulation of prostaglandin synthesis mediated by thrombin and B2 bradykinin receptors in a fibrosarcoma cell line, *Cell*, 30, 243, 1982.

77. **Odya, C., Goodfriend, T., and Pena, C.,** Bradykinin receptor-like binding studied with iodinated analogues, *Biochem. Pharmacol.*, 29, 175, 1980.

78. **Innis, R., Manning, D., Stewart, J., and Snyder, S.,** ^{3}H-bradykinin receptor binding in mammalian tissues, *Proc. Natl. Acad. Sci. U.S.A.*, 78, 2630, 1981.

79. **Regoli, D., Barabe, J., and Park, W.,** Receptors for bradykinin in rabbit aorta, *Can. J. Physiol. Pharmacol.*, 55, 855, 1977.

80. **Regoli, D., Marceau, F., and Lavigne, J.,** Induction of B1 receptors for kinins in the rabbit by a bacterial lipopolysaccharide, *Eur. J. Pharmacol.*, 71, 105, 1981.

81. **Bouthillier, J., deBlois, D., and Marceau, F.,** Studies on the induction of pharmacological responses to des-Arg[9]-bradykinin *in vitro* and *in vivo*, *Br. J. Pharmacol.*, 105, 257, 1987.

82. **Phillips, E., Conder, M., Bevan, S., McIntyre, P., and Webb, M.,** Expression of functional bradykinin receptors in *Xenopus* oocytes, *J. Neurochem.*, 58, 243, 1992.

83. **Farmer, S.G., Burch, R.M., Meeker, S.A., and Wilkins, D.E.,** Evidence for a pulmonary bradykinin B$_3$ receptor, *Mol. Pharmacol.*, 36, 1, 1989.

84. **McEachern, A., Shelton, E., Bhakta, S., Obernolte, R., Bach, C., Zuppan, P., Fujisaki, J., Aldrich, R., and Jarnagin, K.,** Expression cloning of a rat B$_2$ bradykinin receptor, *Proc. Natl. Acad. Sci. U.S.A.*, 88, 7724, 1991.

85. **Hess, J., Borkowski, J., Young, G., Strader, C., and Ransom, R.,** Cloning and pharmacological characterisation of a human bradykinin (bradykinin-2) receptor, *Biochem. Biophys. Res. Commun.*, 184, 260, 1992.

86. **Eggerickx, D., Raspe, E., Bertrand, D., Vassart, G., and Parmentier, M.,** Molecular cloning, functional expression, and pharmacological characterization of a human bradykinin B$_2$ receptor gene, *Biochem. Biophys. Res. Commun.*, 187, 1306, 1992.

87. **McIntyre, P., Phillips, E., Skidmore, E., Brown, M., and Webb, M.,** Cloned murine bradykinin receptor exhibits a mixed B$_1$ and B$_2$ pharmacological selectivity, *Mol. Pharmacol.*, 44, 346, 1993.

88. **Jong, Y.J.I., Dalemar, L.R., Wilhelm, B., and Baenziger, N.L.,** Human bradykinin B$_2$ receptors isolated by receptor-specific monoclonal antibodies are tyrosine phosphorylated, *Proc. Natl. Acad. Sci. U.S.A.*, 90, 10994, 1993.

89. **Furchgott, R.F.,** Studies on the relaxation of rabbit aorta by sodium nitrite: the basis for the proposal that the acid-activatable factor from bovine retractor penis is inorganic nitrite and the endothelium-derived relaxing factor is nitric oxide, in *Mechanisms of Vasodilation*, Vanhoutte, P.M., Ed., Raven Press, New York, 1988, 401.

90. **Ignarro, L.J.,** Endothelium-derived nitric oxide, Actions and properties, *FASEB J.*, 3, 31, 1989.

91. **Palmer, R.M.J., Ferrige, A.G., and Moncada, S.A.,** Nitric oxide release accounts for the biological activity of endothelium-derived relaxing factor, *Nature (London)*, 327, 524, 1987.

92. **Ignarro, L.J., Buga, G.M., Wood, K.S., Byrns, R.E., and Chaudhuri, G.,** Endothelium-derived relaxing factor produced and released from artery and vein is nitric oxide, *Proc. Natl. Acad. Sci. U.S.A.*, 84, 9265, 1987.

93. **Fratacci, M.D., Frostell, C.G., Chen, T.Y., Wain, J.C., Robinson, D.R., and Zapol, W.M.,** Inhaled nitric oxide: a selective pulmonary vasodilator of heparin-protamine vasoconstriction in sheep, *Anesthesiology*, 75, 990, 1991.

94. **Frostell, C., Fratacci, M.D., Wain, J.C., Jones, R., and Zapol, W.M.,** Inhaled nitric oxide: a selective pulmonary vasodilator reversing hypoxic pulmonary vasoconstriction, *Circulation*, 83, 2038, 1991.

95. **Girard, C., Lehot, J., Pannetier, J., Filley, S., French, P., and Estanove, S.,** Inhaled nitric oxide after mitral valve replacement in patients with chronic pulmonary hypertension, *Anesthesiology*, 77, 880, 1992.

96. **Pepke-Zaba, J., Higenbottam, T.W., Dinh-Xuan, A.T., Stone, D., and Wallwork, J.,** Inhaled nitric oxide as a cause of selective pulmonary vasodilation in pulmonary hypertension, *Lancet*, 338, 1173, 1991.

97. **Rich, G.F., Murphy, G.D., Roos, C.M., and Johns, R.A.,** Inhaled nitric oxide: selective pulmonary vasodilation in cardiac surgical patients, *Anesthesiology*, 78, 1028, 1993.

98. **Gruetter, C.A., Barry, B.K., McNamara, D.B., Gruetter, D.Y., Kadowitz, P.J., and Ignarro, L.J.,** Relaxation of bovine coronary artery, and activation of coronary arterial guanylate cyclase by nitric oxide, nitroprusside, and a carcinogenic nitrosoamine, *J. Cyclic Nucleotide Res.*, 5, 211, 1979.

99. **Gruetter, C.A., Gruetter, D.Y., Lyon, J.E., Kadowitz, P.J., and Ignarro, L.J.,** Relationship between cyclic guanosine 3'5'-monophosphate formation and relaxation of coronary arterial smooth muscle by glyceryl trinitrate, nitroprusside, nitrite and nitric oxide, *J. Pharmacol. Exp. Ther.*, 219, 181, 1981.

100. **Ignarro, L.J., Buga, G.M., Wood, K.S., Byrns, R.E., and Chaudhuri, G.,** Endothelium-derived relaxing factor produced and released from artery and vein is nitric oxide, *Proc. Natl. Acad. Sci. U.S.A.*, 84, 9265, 1987.

101. **Rich, G.F., Roos, C.M., Anderson, S.M., Urich, D.C., Daugherty, M.O., and Johns, R.A.,** Inhaled nitric oxide: dose response and the effects of blood in the isolated rat lung, *J. Appl. Physiol.*, 75, 1278, 1993.

102. **Abman, S.H., Chatfield, B.A., Hall, S.L., and McMurtry, I.F.,** Role of endothelium-derived relaxing factor during transition of pulmonary circulation at birth, *Am. J. Physiol.*, 259, H1921, 1990.

103. **Davidson, D. and Eldemerdash, A.,** Endothelium-derived relaxing factor: evidence that it regulates pulmonary vascular resistance in the isolated neonatal guinea pig lung, *Pediatr. Res.*, 29, 538, 1991.

104. **Mayer, B., Schmidt, K., Humbert, P., and Bohme, E.,** Biosynthesis of endothelium-derived relaxing factor: a cytosolic enzyme in porcine aortic endothelial cells calcium-dependently converts L-arginine into an activator of soluble guanylate cyclase, *Biochem. Biophys. Res. Commun.*, 164, 678, 1989.

105. **Forstermann, U., Gorsky, L.D., Pollock, J.S., Ishii, K., Schmidt, H.H.H.W., Heller, M., and Murad F.,** Hormone-induced biosynthesis of endothelium-derived relaxing factor/nitric oxide-like material in N1E-115 neuroblastoma cells requires calcium and calmodulin, *Mol. Pharmacol.*, 38, 7, 1990.

106. **Yanagisawa, M., Kurihara, H., Kimura, S., Tomobe, Y., Kobayashi, M., Mitsui, H., Yasaki, Y., Goto, K., and Masaki, T.,** A novel potent vasoconstrictor peptide produced by vascular endothelial cells, *Nature*, 332, 911, 1988.

107. **Inoue, A., Yanagisawa, M., Kimura, S., Kasuya, Y., Miyauchi, T., Goto, K., and Masaki, T.,** The human endothelin family: three structurally and pharmacologically distinct isopeptides predicted by three separate genes, *Proc. Natl. Acad. Sci. U.S.A.*, 86, 2863, 1989.

108. **Rozengurt, N., Springall, D.R., and Polak, J.M.,** Endothelin-like immunoreactivity is localized in airway epithelium of rat and mouse lung, *J. Pathol.*, 160, 5, 1990.

109. **Giaid, A., Polak, J.M., Gaitonde, V., Hamid, Q.A., Moscoso, G., Legon, S., Uwanogho D., Roncalli, M., Shinmi, O., Sawamura, T., Kimura, S., Yanagisawa, M., Masaki, T., and Springall, D.R.,** Distribution of endothelin-like immunoreactivity and mRNA in the developing and adult human lung, *Am. J. Respir. Cell. Mol. Biol.*, 4, 50, 1991.

110. **Kanse, S.M., Ghatei, M.A., and Bloom S.R.,** Endothelin binding sites in porcine aortic and rat lung membranes, *Eur. J. Biochem.*, 182, 175, 1989.

111. **Koseki, C., Imai, M., Hirata, Y., Yanagisawa, M., and Masaki, T.,** Autoradiographic distribution in rat tissues of binding sites for endothelin, a neuropeptide, *Am. Physiol. Soc.*, 256, 858, 1989.

112. **Power, R.F., Wharton, J., Zhao, Y., Bloom, S.R., and Polak, J.M.,** Autoradiographic localization of endothelin-1 binding sites in the cardiovascular and respiratory systems, *J. Cardiovasc. Pharmacol.*, 13, 550, 1989.

113. **Itoh, Y., Kimura, C., Onda, H., and Fujino, M.,** Canine endothelin-2: cDNA sequence for the mature peptide, *Nucleic Acids Res.*, 17, 5389, 1989.

114. **Lippton, H.L., Hauth, T.A., Cohen, G.A., and Hyman, A.L.,** Functional evidence for different endothelin receptors in the lung, *J. Appl. Physiol.*, 75, 38, 1993.

115. **Yamada, H., Yoneyama, F., Satoh, K., and Taira, H.,** Specific but differential antagonism by glybenclamide of the vasodepressor effects of cromakalim and nicorandil in spinal-anesthetized dogs, *Br. J. Pharmacol.*, 100, 413, 1990.

116. **Yanagisawa, M., Inoue, A., Ishikawa, T., Kasuya, Y., Kimura, S., Kumagaye, S., Nakajima, K., Watanabe, T., Sakakibara, S., Goto, K., and Masaki, T.,** Primary structure, synthesis, and biological activity of rat endothelin, an endothelium-derived vasoconstrictor peptide, *Proc. Natl. Acad. Sci. U.S.A.*, 85, 6963, 1988.

117. **Le Monnier De Gouville, A.C., Lippton, H.L., Cavero, I, Summer, W.R., and Hyman, A.L.,** Endothelin—a new family of endothelium-derived peptides with widespread biological properties, *Life Sci.*, 45, 1499, 1989.

118. **Sakurai, T., Yanagisawa, M., and Masaki, T.,** Molecular characterization of endothelin receptors, *Trends Pharmacol. Sci.*, 13, 103, 1992.

119. **Emori, T., Hirata, Y., Ohta, K., Kanno, K., Eguchi, S., Imai, T. Shichiri, M., and Marumo, F.,** Cellular mechanism of endothelin-1 release by angiotensin and vasopressin, *Hypertension*, 18, 165, 1991.

120. **Imai, T., Hirata, Y., Emori, T., Yanagisawa, M., Masaki, T., and Marumo, F.,** Induction of endothelin-1 gene by angiotensin and vasopressin in endothelial cells, *Hypertension*, 19, 753, 1992.

121. **Maggi, C.A., Patacchini, R., Giuliani, S., and Meli, A.,** Potent contractile effect of endothelin in isolated guinea-pig airways, *Eur. J. Pharmacol.*, 160, 179, 1989.

122. **Lagente, V., Chabrier, P.E., Mencia-Huerta, J.M., and Braquet, P.,** Pharmacological modulation of the bronchopulmonary action of the vasoactive peptide, endothelin, *Biochem. Biophys. Res. Commun.*, 158, 625, 1989.

123. **Komuro, I., Kurihara, H., Sugiyama, T., Takaku, F., and Yazaki, Y.,** Endothelin stimulates c-fos and c-myc expression and proliferation of vascular smooth muscle cells, *FEBS Lett.*, 238, 249, 1988.

124. **Takuwa, N., Takuwa, Y., Yanagisawa, M., Yamashita, K., and Masaki, T.,** A novel vasoactive peptide endothelin stimulates mitogenesis through inositol lipid turnover in Swiss 3T3 fibroblasts, *J. Biol. Chem.*, 264, 7856, 1989.

125. **Nakaki, T., Nakayama, M., Yamamoto, S., and Kato, R.,** Endothelin-mediated stimulation of DNA synthesis in vascular smooth muscle cells, *Biochem. Biophys. Res. Commun.*, 158, 880, 1989.

126. **MacCumber, M.W., Ross, C.A., and Synder, S.H.,** Endothelin-visualisation of messenger RNAs by *in situ* hybridisation provides evidence for local action, *Proc. Natl. Acad. Sci. U.S.A.*, 86, 2785, 1989.

127. **Springall, D.R., Bloom, S.R., and Polak, J.M.,** The distribution, nature and origin of peptide-containing nerves in mammalian airways, in *The Airways: Neural Control in Health and Disease*, Kaliner, M.A. and Barnes, P.J., Eds., Marcel Dekker, New York, 1988, 299.

128. **Wharton, J., Polak, J.M., Bloom S.R., Will, J.A., Brown, M.R., and Pearse, A.G.E.,** Substance P-like immunoreactive nerves in mammalian lung, *Invest. Cell Pathol.*, 2, 3, 1979.

129. **Hua, X.Y., Theodorsson-Norheim, E., Brodin, E., Lundberg, J.M., and Hokfelt, T.,** Multiple tachykinins (neurokinin A, neuropeptide K and substance P) in capsaicin-sensitive neurons in the guinea pig, *Regul. Peptides,* 13, 1, 1985.

130. **Cadieux, A., Springall, D.R., Mulderry, P.K., Rodrigo, J., Ghatei, M.A., Terenghi, G., Bloom, S.R., and Polak, J.M.,** Occurrence, distribution and ontogeny of CGRP immunoreactivity in the rat lower respiratory tract: effect of capsaicin treatment and surgical denervations, *Neuroscience*, 19, 605, 1986.

131. **Uddman, R., Alumets, J., Deusert, O., Hakanson, R., and Sundler, F.,** Occurrence and distribution of VIP nerves in the nasal mucosa and tracheobronchial wall, *Acta Otolaryngol.*, 86, 443, 1978.

132. **Christofides, N.D., Yiangou, Y., Piper, P.J., Ghatei, M.A., Sheppard, M.N., Tatemoto, K., Polak, J.M., and Bloom, S.R.,** Distribution of peptide histidine isoleucine (PHI) in the mammalian respiratory tract and some aspects of its pharmacology, *Endocrinology*, 115, 1958, 1984.

133. **Cheung, A., Polak, J.M., Bauer, F.E., Cadieux, A., Christofides, N.D., Springall, D.R., and Bloom, S.R.,** Distribution of galanin immunoreactivity in the respiratory tract of pig, guinea pig, rat and dog, *Thorax*, 40, 889, 1985.

134. **Lundberg, J.M., Terenius, T., Hokfelt, T., and Goldstein, M.,** High levels of neuropeptide Y in peripheral noradrenergic neurons in various mammals including man, *Neurosci. Lett.*, 42, 167, 1983.

135. **Sheppard, M.N., Polak, J.M., Allen, J.M., and Bloom, S.R.,** Neuropeptide tyrosine (NPY): a newly discovered peptide is present in the mammalian respiratory tract, *Thorax*, 39, 326, 1984.

136. **Said, S.I. and Dey, R.D.,** VIP in the airway, in *The Airways: Neural Control in Health and Disease*, Kaliner, M.A. and Barnes, P.J., Eds., Marcel Dekker, New York, 1988, 395.

137. **Lundberg, J.M., Saria, A., Lundblad, L., Anggard, A., Martling, C.R., Theodorsson-Norheim, E., Stjarne, P., and Hockfelt, T.G.,** Bioactive peptides in capsaicin-sensitive C-fiber afferents of the airways: functional and pathophysiological implications, in *The Airways: Neural Control in Health and Disease*, Kaliner, M.A. and Barnes, P.J., Eds., Marcel Dekker, New York, 1988, 417.

138. **Springall, D.R., Edginton, J.A.G., Price, P.N., Swanston, D.W., Noel, C., Bloom, S.R., and Polak, J.M.,** Acrolein depletes the neuropeptides CGRP and substance P in sensory nerves in rat respiratory tract, *Environ. Health Perspect.*, 85, 151, 1990.

139. **Lundberg, J.M., Brodin, E., and Saria, A.,** Effects and distribution of vagal capsaicin-sensitive substance P neurons with special reference to the trachea and lungs, *Acta Physiol. Scand.,* 119, 243, 1983.

140. **Coleridge, J.C.G. and Coleridge, H.M.,** Efferent vagal C fibre innervation of the lungs and airways and its functional significance, *Rev. Physiol. Biochem. Pharmacol.,* 99, 1, 1984.

141. **Lee, C.M., Campbell, N.J., Williams, B.J., and Iverson, L.L.,** Multiple tachykinin binding sites in peripheral tissues and in brain, *Eur. J. Pharmacol.*, 130, 209, 1986.

142. **Maggio, J.E.,** Tachykinins, *Annu. Rev. Neurosci.*, 11, 13, 1988.

143. **Pernow, B.,** Substance P, *Pharmacol. Rev.*, 35, 85, 1983.

144. **Mantyh, P.W., Mantyh, C.R., Gates, T., Vigna, S.R., and Maggio, J.E.,** Receptor binding sites for substance P and substance K in the canine gastrointestinal tract and their possible role in inflammatory bowel disease, *Neuroscience*, 25, 817, 1988.

145. **Karlsson, J.A. and Persson, C.G.A.,** Novel peripheral neurotransmitters and control of the airways, *Pharmacol. Ther.,* 43, 397, 1989.

146. **Skerrett, P.J.,** Substance P causes pain—but also heals, *Science*, 249, 625, 1990.

147. **Burcher, E., Buck, S.H., Lovenberg, W., and O'Donohue, T.L.,** Characterization and autoradiographic localization of multiple tachykinin binding sites in gastrointestinal tract and bladder, *J. Pharmacol. Exp. Ther.,* 236, 819, 1986.

148. **Martling, C.R., Theodorsson-Norheim, E., and Lovenberg, J.M.,** Occurrence and effects of multiple tachykinins; substance P, neurokinin A and neuropeptide K in human lower airways, *Life Sci.*, 40, 1633, 1987.

149. **Lundberg, J., Hokfelt, T., Martling, C., Saria, A., and Cuello, C.,** Substance P-immunoreactive sensory nerves in the lower respiratory tract of various mammals including man, *Cell Tissue Res.*, 235, 251, 1984.

150. **Gerard, N.P., Garraway, L.A., Eddy, R.L., Shows, T.B., Iijima, H., Paquet, J.L., and Gerard, C.,** Human substance P receptor (NK-1): organization of the gene, chromosome localization, and functional expression of cDNA clones, *Biochemistry*, 30, 10640, 1991.

151. **Masu, Y., Nakayama, K., Tamaki, H., Harada, Y., Kuno, M., and Nakanishi, S.,** cDNA cloning of bovine substance-K receptor through oocyte expression system, *Nature*, 329, 836, 1987.

152. **Sasai, Y. and Nakanishi, S.,** Molecular characterization of rat substance K receptor and its mRNAs, *Biochem. Biophys. Res. Commun.*, 165, 695, 1989.

153. **Gerard, N.P., Eddy, R.L., Shows, T.B., and Gerard, C.,** The human neurokinin A (substance K) receptor, Molecular cloning of the gene, chromosome localization, and isolation of cDNA from tracheal and gastric tissues, *J. Biol. Chem.*, 265, 20455, 1990.

154. **Yokota, Y., Sasai, Y., Tanaka, K., Fujiwara, T., Tsuchida, K., Shigemoto, R., Kakizuka, A., Ohkubo, H., and Nakanishi, S.,** Molecular characterization of a functional cDNA for rat substance P receptor, *J. Biol. Chem.,* 264, 17649, 1989.

155. **Hershey, A.D. and Krause, J.E.,** Molecular characterization of a functional cDNA encoding the rat substance P receptor, *Science,* 247, 958, 1990.

156. **Shigemoto, R., Yokota, Y., Tsuchida, K., and Nakanishi, S.,** Cloning and expression of a rat neuromedin K receptor cDNA, *J. Biol. Chem.,* 265, 623, 1990.

157. **Floch, A., Fardin, V., and Cavero, I.,** Characterization of NK-1 and NK-2 tachykinin receptors in guinea pig and rat bronchopulmonary and vascular systems, *Br. J. Pharmacol.,* 111, 759, 1994.

158. **Murlas, C., Murphy, T., and Chodimella, V.,** Ozone-induced mucosa-linked airway muscle hyperresponsiveness in the guinea pig, *J. Appl. Physiol.,* 69, 7, 1990.

159. **Hazbun, M.E., Hamilton, R., Holian, A., and Eschenbacher, W.L.,** Ozone-induced increases in substance P and 8-epi-prostaglandin $F_2\alpha$ in the airways of human subjects, *Am. J. Respir. Cell. Mol. Biol.,* 9, 568, 1993.

160. **Kelley, M.J., Snider, R.H., Becker, K.L., and Johnson, B.E.,** Small cell lung carcinoma cell lines express mRNA for calcitonin and alpha- and beta-calcitonin gene-related peptides, *Cancer Lett.,* 81, 19, 1994.

161. **Sheppard, M.N., Marangos, P.J., Bloom, S.R., and Polak, J.M.,** Neuron specific enolase: a marker for the early development of nerves and endocrine cells in the human lung, *Life Sci.,* 34, 265, 1984.

162. **Gosney, J.R., Sissons, M.C.J., and O'Malley, J.A.,** Quantitative study of endocrine cells immunoreactive for calcitonin in the normal adult human lung, *Thorax,* 40, 866, 1985.

163. **Gomez-Pascual, A., Martin-Lacave, I., Fernandez Rodriguez, A., Moreno, A., and Davidson, H.G.,** Histochemical and immunohistochemical study on the neuroendocrine cells in the human fetal lung, *Histol. Med.,* 2, 33, 1986.

164. **Ito, T., Nakatani, Y., Nagahara, N., Ogawa, T., Shibagaki, T., and Kanisawa, M.,** Quantitative study of pulmonary endocrine cells in anencephaly, *Lung,* 165, 297, 1987.

165. **Tsutsumi, Y.,** Immunohistochemical analysis of calcitonin and calcitonin gene-related peptide in human lung, *Hum. Pathol.,* 20, 896, 1989.

166. **Becker, K.L., Silva, O.L., Gazdar, A.F., Snider, R.H., and Moore, C.F.,** Calcitonin and small cell cancer of the lung, in *The Endocrine Lung in Health and Disease,* Becker, K.L. and Gazdar, A.F., Eds., W.B. Saunders, Philadelphia, 1984, 528.

167. **Gould, V.E., Linnoila, R.I., Memoli, V.A., and Warren, W.H.,** Neuroendocrine components of the bronchopulmonary tract: hyperplasias, dysplasias, and neoplasms, *Lab. Invest.,* 49, 519, 1983

168. **Linnoila, R.I., Becker, K.L., Silva, O.L., Snider, R.H., and Moore, C.F.,** Calcitonin as a marker for diethylnitrosamine-induced pulmonary endocrine cell hyperplasia in hamsters, *Lab. Invest.,* 51, 39, 1984.

169. **Nylen, E.S., Linnoila, R.I., Snider, R.H., Tabassian, A.R., and Becker, K.L.,** Comparative studies of hamster calcitonin from pulmonary endocrine cells in vitro, *Peptides,* 8, 977, 1987.

170. **Gosney, J.R. and Sissons, M.C.J.,** Widespread distribution of bronchopulmonary endocrine cells immunoreactive for calcitonin in the lung of the normal adult rat, *Thorax,* 40, 194, 1985.

171. **Gomez-Pascual, A., Martin-Lacave, I., Moreno, A.M., Fernandez, A., and Galera, H.,** Neuroendocrine (NE) cells in rat neonatal lungs, A histochemical and immunocytochemical study, *Anat. Histol. Embryol.,* 19, 158, 1990.

172. **Ravazzola, M., Orci, L., Girgis, S.I., Galan, F., and McIntyre, I.,** The lung is the major organ source of calcitonin in the lizard, *Cell. Biol. Int. Rep.,* 5, 937, 1981.

173. **O'Neill, W.J., Jordan, M.H., Lewis, M.S., Snider, R.H., Moore, C.F., and Becker, K.L.,** Serum calcitonin may be a marker for inhalation injury in burns, *J. Burn Care Rehabil.,* 13, 605, 1992.

174. **Nutini, S., Cappelli, G., Benucci, A., Catalani, C., and Nozzoli, F.,** Serum NSE, CEA, CT, CA 15-3 levels in human lung cancer, *Int. J. Biol. Markers,* 5, 198, 1990.

175. **Amara, S.G., Jonas, V., Rosenfeld, M.G., Ong, E.S., and Evans, R.M.,** Alternative RNA processing in calcitonin gene expression generates mRNAs encoding different polypeptide products, *Nature,* 298, 240, 1982.

176. **Holzer, P.,** Local effector functions of capsaicin-sensitive sensory nerve endings: involvement of tachykinins, calcitonin gene-related peptide and other neuropeptides, *Neuroscience,* 24, 739, 1988.

177. **Cadieux, A., Springall, D.R., Mulderry, P.K., Rodrigo, J., Ghat, Terenghi, G., Bloom, S.R., and Polak, J.M.,** Occurrence, distribution, and ontogeny of CGRP immunoreactivity in the rat lower respiratory tract: effect of capsaicin treatment and surgical denervations, *Neuroscience,* 19, 605, 1986.

178. **Martling, C.R., Saria, A., Fischer, J.A., Hokfelt, T., and Lundberg, J.M.,** Calcitonin gene-related peptide and the lung: neuronal coexistence with substance P, release by capsaicin and vasodilatory effect, *Regul. Peptides,* 20, 125, 1988.

179. **Uddman, R., Luts, A., and Sundler, F.,** Occurrence and distribution of calcitonin gene-related peptide in the mammalian respiratory tract and middle ear, *Cell Tissue Res.,* 241, 551, 1985.

180. **Shimosegawa, T. and Said, S.I.,** Pulmonary calcitonin gene-related peptide immunoreactivity: nerve-endocrine cell interrelationships, *Am. J. Respir. Cell. Mol. Biol.,* 4, 126, 1991.

181. **Adnot, S., Cigarini, I., Herigault, R., and Harf, A.,** Effects of substance P and calcitonin gene-related peptide on the pulmonary circulation, *J. Appl. Physiol.,* 70, 1707, 1991.

182. **Erspamer, V., Erspamer, G.F., and Inselvini, M.,** Some pharmacologic actions of alytensin and bombesin, *J. Pharm. Pharmacol.,* 22, 875, 1970.

183. **Miller, Y.E.,** Bombesin-like peptides: from frog skin to human lung, *Am. J. Respir. Cell. Mol. Biol.,* 3, 189, 1990.

184. **Rozengurt, E. and Sinnett-Smith, J.,** Bombesin stimulation of fibroblast mitogenesis: specific receptors, signal transduction and early events, *Philos. Trans. R. Soc. Lond. Ser. B,* 327, 209, 1990.

185. **Lebacq-Verheyden, A.M., Trepel, J., Sausville, E.A., and Battey, J.F.,** Bombesin receptors, in *Peptide Growth Factors and Their Receptors,* Vol. 2, Sporn, M.B. and Roberts, A.B., Eds., Springer, Berlin, 1990, 70.

186. **Sunday, M.E., Kaplan, L.M., Motoyama, E., Chin, W.W., and Spindel, E.R.,** Biology of disease: gastrin releasing peptide (mammalian bombesin) gene expression in health and disease, *Lab. Invest.,* 59, 5, 1988.

187. **Moody, T.W., Pert, C.B., Gazdar, A.F., Carney, D.N., and Minna, J.D.,** High levels of intracellular bombesin characterize human small-cell lung carcinoma, *Science,* 214, 1246, 1981.

188. **Cuttitta, F., Carney, D.N., Mulshine, J., Moody, T.W., Fedorko, J., Fischler, A., and Minna, J.D.,** Bombesin-like peptides can function as autocrine growth factors in human small cell lung cancer, *Nature,* 316, 823, 1985.

189. **Geraci, M.W., Miller, Y.E., Escobedo-Morse, A., and Kane, M.A.,** Novel bombesin-like peptide binding proteins from lung, *Am. J. Respir. Cell. Mol. Biol.,* 10, 331, 1994.

190. **Spindel, E.R., Sunday, M.E., Hofler, H., Wolfe, H.J., Habener, J.F., and Chin, W.W.,** Transient elevation of messenger RNA encoding gastrin-releasing peptide, a putative pulmonary growth factor in human fetal lung, *J. Clin. Invest.,* 80, 1172, 1987.

191. **Stahlman, M.T., Kasselberg, A.G., Orth, D.N., and Gray, M.E.,** Ontogeny of neuroendocrine cells in human fetal lung, II, An immunohistochemical study, *Lab. Invest.,* 52, 52, 1985.

192. **Sunday, M.E., Hua, J., Dai, H.B., Nusrat, A., and Torday, J.S.,** Bombesin increases fetal lung growth and maturation *in. utero* and in organ culture, *Am. J. Respir. Cell. Mol. Biol.,* 3, 199, 1990.

193. **Willey, J.C., Lechner, J.F., and Harris, C.C.,** Bombesin and the C-terminal tetradecapeptide of gastrin-releasing peptide are growth factors for normal human bronchial epithelial cells, *Exp. Cell Res.,* 153, 245, 1984.

194. **Siegfried, J.M., Guentert, P.J., and Gaither, A.L.,** Effects of bombesin and gastrin-releasing peptide in human bronchial epithelial cells from a series of donors: individual variation and modulation by bombesin analogues, *Anat. Rec.,* 236, 241, 1993.

195. **Weber, S., Zuckerman, J.E., Bostwick, D.G., Bensch, K.G., Sikic, B.I., and Raffin, T.A.,** Gastrin-releasing peptide is a selective mitogen for small cell lung carcinoma *in vitro, J. Clin. Invest.,* 75, 306, 1985.

196. **Hoyt, R.F., McNelly, N.A., and Sorokin, S.P.,** Dynamics of neuroepithelial body (NEB) formation in developing hamster lung: light microscopic autoradiography after ^{3}H-thymidine labeling *in vivo, Anat. Rec.,* 227, 340, 1990.

197. **Johnson, D.E., Loch, J.E., Elde, R.P., and Thompson, T.R.,** Pulmonary neuroendocrine cells in bronchopulmonary dysplasia and hyaline membrane disease, *Pediatr. Res.,* 16, 446, 1982.

198. **Tabassian, A.R., Nylen, E.S., Linnoila, R.I., Snider, R.H., Cassidy, M.M., and Becker, K.L.,** Stimulation of hamster pulmonary neuroendocrine cells and associated peptides by repeated exposure to cigarette smoke, *Am. Rev. Respir. Dis.,* 140, 436, 1989.

199. **DeMichele, M.A., Gaither Davis, A.L., Hunt, J.D., Landreneau, R.J., and Siegfried, J.M.,** Expression of mRNA for three bombesin receptor subtypes in human bronchial epithelial cells, *Am. J. Respir. Cell. Mol. Biol.,* 11, 66, 1994.

200. **Frankel, A., Tsao, M.S., and Viallet, J.,** Receptor subtype expression and responsiveness to bombesin in cultured human bronchial epithelial cells, *Cancer Res.,* 54, 1613, 1994.

201. **Corjay, M.H., Dobrzanski, D.J., Way, J.M., Viallet, J., Shapira, H., Worland, P., Sausville, E.A., and Battey, J.F.,** Two distinct bombesin receptor subtypes are expressed and functional in human lung carcinoma cells, *J. Biol. Chem.,* 266, 18771, 1991.

202. **Fathi, Z., Corjay, M.H., Shapira, H., Wada, E., Benya, R., Jensen, R., Viallet, J., Sausville, E.A., and Battey, J.F.,** A novel bombesin receptor subtype selectively expressed in testis and lung carcinoma cells, *J. Biol. Chem.,* 268, 5979, 1993.

203. **Battey, J.F., Way, J.M., Corjay, M.H., Shapira, H., Kusano, K., Harkins, R., Wu, J.M., Slattery, T., Mann, E., and Feldman, R.I.,** Molecular cloning of the bombesin/gastrin-releasing peptide receptor from Swiss 3T3 cells, *Proc. Natl. Acad. Sci. U.S.A.,* 88, 395, 1991.

204. **Leban, J.J., Kull, F.C., Landavazo, A., Stockstill, B., and McDermed, J.D.,** Development of potent gastrin-releasing peptide antagonists having a D-Pro-(CH_2NH)-Phe-NH_2 C terminus, *Proc. Natl. Acad. Sci. U.S.A.,* 90, 1922, 1993.

205. **Brazeau, P., Vale, W., Burgus, R., Ling, N., Butcher, M., Rivier, J., and Guillemin, R.,** Hypothalamic polypeptide that inhibits the secretion of immunoreactive pituitary growth hormone, *Science,* 179, 77, 1973.

206. **Reichlin S.,** Somatostatin, *N. Engl. J. Med.,* 309, 1495, 1983.

207. **Epelbaum, J.,** Somatostatin in the central nervous system: physiology and pathological modifications, *Prog. Neurobiol.*, 27, 63, 1986.

208. **Chejfec, G., Cosnow, I., Gould, N.S., Husain, A.N., and Gould, V.E.,** Pulmonary blastoma with neuroendocrine differentiation in cell morules resembling neuroepithelial bodies, *Histopathology*, 17, 353, 1990.

209. **Dayer, A.M., De Mey, J., and Will, J.A.,** Localization of somatostatin, bombesin, and serotonin-like immunoreactivity in the lung of the fetal Rhesus monkey, *Cell Tissue Res.*, 239, 621, 1985.

210. **Reubi, J.C., Perin, M.H., Rivier, J.E., and Vale, W.,** High affinity binding sites for a somatostatin-28 analog in rat brain, *Life Sci.*, 28, 2191, 1981.

211. **Zeggari, M., Viguerie, N., Susini, C., Esteve, J.P., Vaysse, N., Rivier, J., Wuensch, E., and Ribet, A.,** Characterization of pancreatic somatostatin binding sites with a 125I-somatostatin-28 analog, *Peptides*, 7, 953, 1986.

212. **Reubi, J.C., Perrin, M.H., Rivier, J.E., and Vale, W.,** High affinity binding sites for somatostatin to rat pituitary, *Biochem. Biophys. Res. Commun.*, 105, 1538, 1982.

213. **He, H.T., Rens-Domiano, S., Martin, J.M., Law, S.F., Borislow, S., Woolkalis, M., Manning D., and Reisine, T.,** Solubilization of active somatostatin receptors from rat brain, *Mol. Pharmacol.*, 37, 614, 1990.

214. **Law, S.F., Manning, D., and Reisine, T.,** Identification of the subunits of GTP-binding proteins coupled to somatostatin receptors, *J. Biol. Chem.*, 266, 17885, 1991.

215. **Srikant, C.B. and Patel, Y.C.,** Characterization of pituitary membrane receptors for somatostatin in the rat, *Endocrinology*, 110, 2138, 1982.

216. **Maurer, R. and Reubi, J.C.,** Somatostatin receptors in the adrenal, *Mol. Cell. Endocrinol.*, 45, 81, 1986.

217. **Srikant, C.B. and Patel, Y.C.,** Somatostatin receptors: identification and characterization in rat brain membranes, *Proc. Natl. Acad. Sci. U.S.A.*, 78, 3930, 1981.

218. **Sakamoto, C., Goldfine, I.D., and Williams, J.A.,** The somatostatin receptor on isolated pancreatic acinar cell plasma membranes. Identification of subunit structure and direct regulation by cholecystokinin, *J. Biol. Chem.*, 259, 9623, 1984.

219. **Rohrer, L., Raulf, F., Bruns, C., Buettner, R., Hofstaedter, F., and Schule, R.,** Cloning and characterization of a fourth human somatostatin receptor, *Proc. Natl. Acad. Sci. U.S.A.*, 90, 4196, 1993.

220. **Weckbecker, G., Raulf, F., Stolz, B., and Bruns, C.,** Somatostatin analogs for diagnosis and treatment of cancer, *Pharmacol. Ther.*, 60, 245, 1993.

221. **Will, J.A., Rademakers, A., and Dayer, A.M.,** Cholecystokinin-like immunoreactivity in neuroepithelial bodies (NEB) of the fetal Rhesus monkey lung, *Fed. Proc.*, 44, 917, 1985.

222. **Cutz, E., Goniakowska-Witalinska, L., and Chan, W.,** An immunohistochemical study of regulatory peptides in lungs of amphibians, *Cell Tissue Res.*, 244, 227, 1986.

223. **Takahashi, Y., Kato, K., Hayashizaki, Y., Wakabayashi, T., Ontsuka, E., Matsuki, S., Ikehara, M., and Matsubara, K.,** Molecular cloning of the human cholecystokinin gene by use of a synthetic probe containing deoxyinosine, *Proc. Natl. Acad. Sci. U.S.A.*, 82, 1931, 1985.

224. **Dockray, G.J.,** Immunoreactive component resembling cholecystokinin octapeptide in intestine, *Nature*, 270, 359, 1977.

225. **Staley, J., Jensen, R.T., and Moody, T.W.,** CCK antagonists interact with CCK-B receptors on human small cell lung cancer cells, *Peptides*, 11, 1033, 1990.

226. **Hays, S.M., Beinfeld, M.C., Jensen, R.T., Goodwin, F.K., and Paul, S.M.,** Demonstration of a putative receptor site for cholecystokinin in rat brain, *Neuropeptides*, 1, 53, 1980.

227. **Moran, T.H., Robinson, P.H., and McHugh, P.R.,** The pyloric cholecystokinin receptor: a site of mediation for satiety, *Ann. N.Y. Acad. Sci.*, 448, 621, 1985.

228. **Saito, A., Sankaran, H., Goldfine, E.C., and Williams, J.A.,** Cholecystokinin receptors in the brain: characterization and distribution, *Science*, 208, 1155, 1980.

229. **Steigerwalt, R.W., Goldfine, I.D., and Williams, J.A.,** Characterization of cholecystokinin receptors on bovine gallbladder membranes, *Am. J. Physiol.*, 247, 6709, 1984.

230. **Yoder, D. and Moody, T.W.,** High affinity binding of cholecystokinin to small cell lung cancer cells, *Peptides*, 8, 103, 1987.

231. **Maneckjee, R. and Minna, J.D.,** Opioid and nicotine receptors affect growth regulation of human lung cancer cell lines, *Proc. Natl. Acad. Sci. U.S.A.*, 87, 3294, 1990.

232. **Zagon, I. and McLaughlin, P.,** Naltrexone modulates tumor response in mice with neuroblastoma, *Science*, 221, 671, 1983.

233. **Murgo, A.,** Modulation of murine melanoma growth by naloxone, *Cancer Lett.*, 44, 137, 1989.

234. **Scholar, E., Violi, L., and Hexum, T.,** The antimetastic activity of enkephalin-like peptides, *Cancer Lett.*, 35, 133, 1987.

235. **Kumakura, K., Karoum, F., Guidotti, A., and Costa, E.,** Modulation of nicotinic receptors by opiate receptor agonists in cultured adrenal chromaffin cells, *Nature*, 283, 489, 1980.

236. **Eiden, L., Giraud, P., Dave, J., Hotchkiss, A., and Affolter, H.U.,** Nicotinic receptor stimulation activates enkephalin release and biosynthesis in adrenal chromaffin cells, *Nature*, 312, 661, 1984.

237. **Karras, A. and Kane, J.,** Naloxone reduces cigarette smoking, *Life Sci.*, 27, 1541, 1980.

238. **Beleslin, D., Krstic, S., Stefanovic-Denic, K., Strbac, M., and Micic, D.,** Inhibition by morphine and morphine-like drugs of nicotine-induced emesis in cats, *Brain Res. Bull.*, 6, 451, 1981.

239. **Kamerling, S., Wettstein, J., Sloan, J., Su, T.P., and Martin, W.R.,** Interaction between nicotine and endogenous opioid mechanisms in the unanesthetized dog, *Pharmacol. Biochem. Behav.*, 17, 733, 1982.

240. **Dalsgaard, C.J., Hutgardh-Nilsson, A., Haegerstrand, A., and Nilsson, J.,** Neuropeptides as growth factor: possible roles in human diseases, *Regul. Peptides*, 25, 1, 1989.

241. **Scholar, E.M. and Paul, S.,** Stimulation of tumor cell growth by vasoactive intestinal peptide, *Cancer*, 67, 1561, 1991.

242. **Bologna, M., Festuccia, C., Muzi, P., Biordi, I., and Ciomei, M.V.,** Bombesin stimulates growth of human prostatic cancer cells in vitro, *Cancer*, 63, 1714, 1989.

243. **Iishi, H., Tatsuta, M., Baba, M., Okuda, S., and Taniguchi, H.,** Enhancement by vasoactive intestinal peptide of experimental carcinogenesis induced by azoxymethane in rat colon, *Cancer Res.*, 47, 4890, 1987.

244. **Mitsuhashi, M. and Payan, D.G.,** The mitogenic effects of vasoactive neuropeptides on cultured smooth muscle cell lines, *Life Sci.*, 40, 853, 1987.

245. **Murakani, H. and Masui, H.,** Hormonal control of human colon carcinoma cell growth in serum-free medium, *Proc. Natl. Acad. Sci. U.S.A.*, 77, 3464, 1989.

246. **Kobori, O., Vuillot, M.T., and Martin, F.,** Growth responses of rat stomach cancer cells to gastro-entero pancreative hormones, *Int. J. Cancer*, 30, 65, 1982.

247. **Cutz, E., Gillan, J.E., and Track, N.S.,** Pulmonary endocrine cells in the developing human lung and during neonatal adaptation, in *The Endocrine Lung in Health and Disease*, Becker, K.L and Gazdar, A.F., Eds., W.B. Saunders, Philadelphia, 1984, 210.

248. **Takahashi, S. and Yui, R.,** Gastrin-releasing peptide (GRP) and serotonin in the human fetal lung: an immunohistochemical study, *Biomed. Res.*, 4, 315, 1983.

249. **Stahlman, M.T., Kasselberg, A.G., Orth, D.N., and Gray, M.E.,** Ontogeny of neuroendocrine cells in human fetal lung. II. An immunohistochemical study, *Lab. Invest.*, 52, 52, 1985.

250. **Gould, V.E., Linnoila, R.I., Memoli, V.A., and Warren, W.H.,** Neuroendocrine components of the bronchopulmonary tract: hyperplasias, dysplasias, and neoplasms, *Lab. Invest.*, 49, 519, 1983.

251. **Johnson, D.E., Kulik, T.J., Lock, J.E., Elde, R.P., and Thompson, T.R.,** Bombesin-, calcitonin-, and serotonin-immunoreactive pulmonary neuroendocrine cells in acute and chronic neonatal lung disease, *Pediatr. Pulmonol.*, 1 (Suppl.), S13, 1985.

252. **Will, J.A., Rademakers, A., and Dayer, A.M.,** Cholecystokinin-like immunoreactivity in neuroepithelial bodies (NEB) of the fetal Rhesus monkey lung, *Fed. Proc.*, 44, 917, 1985.

253. **Scheuermann, D.W., Timmermans, J.P., Adriaensen, D., and De Groodt-Lasseel, M.H.A.,** Immunoreactivity for calcitonin gene-related peptide in neuroepithelial bodies of the newborn cat, *Cell Tissue Res.*, 249, 337, 1987.

254. **Cho, T., Chan, W., and Cutz, E.,** Distribution and frequency of neuro-epithelial bodes in post-natal rabbit lung: quantitative study with monoclonal antibody against serotonin, *Cell Tissue Res.*, 255, 353, 1989.

255. **Adriaensen, D., Scheuermann, D.W., Timermans, J.P., and De Groodt-Lasseel, M.H.A.,** Calcitonin-gene-related peptide, enkephalin, and serotonin coexist in neuroepithelial bodies of the respiratory tract of the red-eared turtle, *Pseudemys scripta elegans*. An immunocytochemical study, *Histochemistry*, 95, 567, 1991.

256. **Zaccone, G., Goniakowska-Witalinska, L., Lauweryns, J.M., Fasulo, S., and Tagliafierro, G.,** Fine structure and serotonin immunohistochemistry of the neuroendocrine cells in the lungs of the bichirs *Polypterus delhezi* and *P. ornatipinnis*, *Basic Appl. Histochem.*, 33, 277, 1989.

257. **Ramamoorthy, S., Bauman, A.L., Moore, K.R., Han, H., Yang-Feng, T., Chang, A.S., Ganapathy, V., and Blakely, R.D.,** Antidepressent- and cocaine-sensitive human serotonin transporter: molecular cloning, expression, and chromosomal localization, *Proc. Natl. Acad. Sci. U.S.A.*, 90, 2542, 1993.

258. **Gass, G.H. and Kaplan, H.M., Eds.,** *CRC Handbook of Endocrinology*, CRC Press, Boca Raton, FL, 1982.

259. **Nilsson, G., Alving, K., Ahlstedt, S., Hokfelt, T., and Lundberg, J.M.,** Peptidergic innervation of rat lymphoid tissue and lung: relation to mast cells and sensitivity to capsaicin and immunization, *Cell Tissue Res.*, 262, 125, 1990.

260. **Alving, K., Matran, R., Lacroix, J.S., and Lundberg, J.M.,** Capsaicin and histamine antagonists-sensitive mechanism in the immediate allergic reaction of pig airways, *Acta Physiol. Scand.*, 138, 49, 1990.

261. **Lundberg, J.M., Alving, K., and Matran, R.,** Pulmonary physiology and pharmacology of neuropeptides, *Ann. N.Y. Acad. Sci.*, 550, 332, 1991.

262. **Saria, A., Martling, C.R., Yan, Z., Theodorsson-Norheim, E., Gamse, R., and Lundberg, J.M.,** Release of multiple tachykinins from capsaicin-sensitive sensory nerves in the lung by bradykinin, histamine, dimethylphenyl piperazinium and vagal nerve stimulation, *Am. Rev. Respir. Dis.*, 137, 1330, 1988.

263. **Svensson, C., Baumgarten, C.R., Pipkorn, U., Alkner, U., and Persson, C.G.A.,** Reversibility and reproducibility of histamine-induced plasma leakage in nasal airways, *Thorax*, 44, 13, 1989.

264. **Tsutsumi, Y., Osamura, R.Y., Watanabe, K., and Yanaihara, N.,** Immunohistochemical studies on gastrin-releasing peptide- and adrenocorticotropic hormone-containing cells in the human lung, *Lab. Invest.*, 48, 623, 1983.

265. **Polak, J.M. and Bloom, S.K.,** Regulatory peptides, Localization and measurement, in *The Endocrine Lung in Health and Disease*, Becker, K.L. and Gazdar, A.F., Eds., W.B. Saunders, Philadelphia, 1984, 300.

266. **Tsutsumi, Y.,** Immunohistochemical analysis of neuroendocrine substances in nonneoplastic lung and neuroendocrine lung tumors, in *Endocrine Pathology Update*, Vol. 1, Lechago, J. and Kameya, T., Eds., Field and Wood, Philadelphia, 1990, 189.

Chapter 7

STRUCTURE AND FUNCTION OF THE MAMMALIAN OVARY

John J. Peluso

CONTENTS

0-8493-9430-9/96/$0.00+$.50
© 1996 by CRC Press, Inc.

INTRODUCTION

The mammalian ovary is a very dynamic and complex organ. It is composed of three major structural elements: the stroma, the follicle, and the corpus luteum. In this chapter, the basic morphological and physiological aspects of each of these ovarian components will be reviewed. However, a complete discussion on each topic will not be presented. For topics where major reviews are available, individual research papers will generally not be cited but rather the review article.

The ovarian stroma is composed of two cell types. The first type of cells is connective tissue cells which provide a supportive function. The second cell type is interstitial cells. These interstitial cells possess steroidogenic enzymes and secrete progesterone and androgens. The interstitial cells also possess luteinizing hormone (LH) receptors and can respond to LH stimulation by increasing steroid output.[1] Although the amount of interstitium and steroid synthesis changes only slightly depending on the physiological state, such as pregnancy, the more dramatic changes in ovarian physiology are related to the development of follicular and luteal components.

FOLLICULAR FUNCTION

MORPHOLOGY AND PHYSIOLOGY OF OVARIAN FOLLICLES

The ovarian follicle is composed of thecal and granulosa cells separated by a basement membrane, and an oocyte surrounded by granulosa cells (Figure 1A). Ovarian follicles can be classified as either growing or degenerating. Each component of the follicle is altered during degeneration, which is referred to as atresia. The morphological and physiological changes associated with the atresia process will be discussed in detail later in the chapter.

Granulosa Cells
Structural and Functional Characteristics of Normal and Degenerating Granulosa Cells

A typical granulosa cell contains a large nucleus, oval mitochondria with lamellar cristae, Golgi apparati, multivesicular and lysosome-like bodies, rough endoplasmic reticulum, numerous ribosomes, and a scattering of lipid droplets in the basal granulosa[2] (Figure 1B). These ultrastructural features are characteristic of actively growing, protein-synthesizing cells,[3] but granulosa cells also are steroidogenic, producing estrogen, androgens, or progesterone depending on species and stage of follicular development.[4-6]

The granulosa cells are connected by various junctions, including "gap," "tight," or "nexus" junctions and "zona" occludens.[7,8] These intercellular connections function to (1) increase intercellular cohesion, (2) transport nutrients across the granulosa layer, (3) facilitate movement of follicular fluid to the antrum, and (4) permit the layers of granulosa cells to respond as a unit. These junctions may also allow a more uniform response to gonadotropin stimulation.[9]

The ultrastructure of the granulosa cell changes with the onset of atresia. These alterations occur in stages. Follicles in stage 1 of atresia exhibit pyknosis of the granulosa cells as the earliest morphological indication of atresia. Early atretic follicles also show a decrease in the number of granulosa cell contacts. As follicles undergo atresia, pyknotic nuclei are observed in the antrum and vacuoles (possibly dilated endoplasmic reticulum) become numerous in antral granulosa cells. Increased lipid within the granulosa cells, appearance of autophagic vacuoles, phagocyte-like cells invading the granulosa layer through a disrupted basement membrane, and disintegration of the granular cohesiveness are also characteristic of atretic follicles. These features are exaggerated as the atresia process continues[10] (Table 1).

Histochemical studies have further described alterations in follicular function as atresia progresses in large follicles. Granulosa cells of large preovulatory follicles normally contain small amounts of lipid. However, the lipid content in the granulosa cells increases as follicles

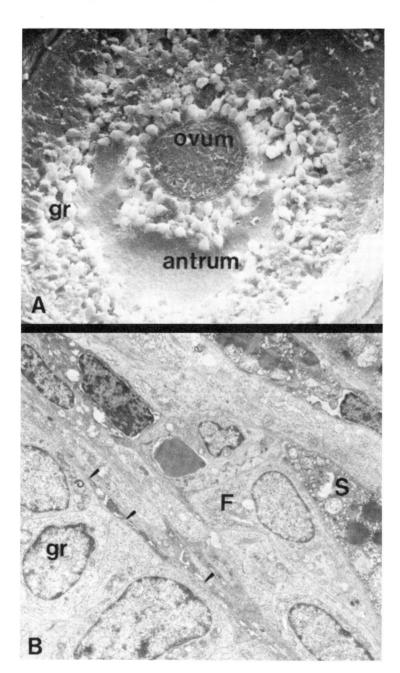

FIGURE 1. **(A)** A scanning electron micrograph of an antral follicle from an immature PMSG-primed rat. Note the presence of the granulosa cell layer (gr), ovum, and antrum ($\times$ 2500). **(B)** An electron micrograph showing the thecal and granulosa cells in a nonatretic follicle. Steroidogenic cells (S) of the theca interna contain lipid and vesicles of smooth endoplasmic reticulum. Fibroblastic-like cells (F) are found within the thecal cell layers. Granulosa cells (gr) are also identified. A basal lamina (arrows) separate the thecal and granulosa cell layers ($\times$ 42,500).

become atretic.[11,12] In addition, the content of lipid droplets in the granulosa changes from primarily phospholipid to triglycerides, cholesterol, and cholesterol esters. This conversion occurs before follicles possess the characteristics of atretic follicles[10] (Table 1). These changes appear to indicate an early alteration in steroid metabolism.[11] However, 3β-hydroxysteroid dehydrogenase (3β-HSD) activity, which is observed in mature follicles, remains even in late stages of atresia.[12,13] The presence of 3β-HSD, which converts pregnenolone to progesterone,

TABLE 1
Histological Changes Associated with Atretic Follicles

Follicular Component	Alteration	I	II	III	IV
Theca interna	Hypertrophy	–	–	+	+
	Radial arrangement of cells	–	+	++	++
Basement membrane	Hyalinization and thickening	–	+	++	+++
Granulosa	Pyknosis	+	++	absent	absent
	Decrease in cell divisions	+	++	absent	absent
Cumulus oophoros	Vascular ingrowth	+	++	absent	absent
	Pyknosis disintegration	+	++	absent	absent
Ova	Chromatolysis	+	++	++	–
	Shrinking	–	+	++	–
	Hyalinization of zona	+	++	+++	–

(Stage of Atresia: I, II, III, IV)

indicates that atretic follicles are still steroidogenically active. However, a recent report has demonstrated that 3β-HSD activity is reduced in atretic rat follicles.[14]

The activity of lactate dehydrogenase and glucose-6-phosphate dehydrogenase, important enzymes in carbohydrate metabolism, decreases in atretic follicles.[15] Concomitantly, the growth rate or mitotic index decreases[16,17] and acid phosphatase activity increases.[18] Using histochemical procedures, acid phosphatase, a hydrolytic enzyme of lysosome origin, is not demonstrable in healthy follicles. However, electron microscopic cytochemical studies of atretic preovulatory follicles demonstrate an increase in acid phosphatase activity in autophagic vacuoles. Also, in both healthy and atretic follicles, acid phosphatase activity is found in the Golgi complex and smooth endoplasmic reticulum of granulosa cells, indicating a possible role for acid phosphatase in steroidogenesis.[18,19] The presence of high acid phosphatase activity in degenerating follicles is predictable, but when it first appears and what triggers its activity in the atretic process is unknown.

Granulosa Cell Apoptosis

Although the mechanism responsible for follicular atresia has not been clearly defined, atresia seems to be initiated with the death of the granulosa cells.[20] Recent studies have shown that granulosa cell death is characterized by DNA fragmentation, suggesting that granulosa cells die through an active process referred to as programmed cell death or apoptosis.[21,22] In several nonovarian cell types, DNA fragmentation is triggered by an increase in $[Ca^{2+}]i$, which activates an endonuclease that eventually results in the cleavage of the DNA into multimers of about 180-bp nucleosomal units with 3'OH ends.[23,24] Because granulosa cells possess a calcium/magnesium-dependent endonuclease that is activated by the addition of calcium,[25] it has been proposed that an increase in $[Ca^{2+}]i$ initiates granulosa cell apoptosis.

Recent work has focused on the identification of hormonal factors that control granulosa cell DNA fragmentation. These studies have shown that hypophysectomy induces and estrogen prevents rat granulosa cell DNA fragmentation.[26] In addition, decreased levels of aromatase mRNA[27] and intrafollicular estrogen are associated with granulosa cell degeneration.[20] These studies support the concept that gonadotropins maintain estrogen biosynthesis within the follicle and that estrogen acts to prevent granulosa cell apoptosis.

Granulosa cells also undergo DNA fragmentation *in vitro* and this fragmentation is prevented by either epidermal growth factor (EGF) or basic fibroblast growth factor.[27] It is possible that estrogen, either acting directly on granulosa cells or indirectly by stimulating the production of intraovarian growth factors, controls $[Ca^{2+}]i$ levels and thus apoptotic DNA fragmentation. However, in rat granulosa cells, estrogen neither stimulates nor suppresses basal $[Ca^{2+}]i$ levels.[28] This observation supports the concept that estrogen prevents apoptosis indirectly by stimulating the synthesis of an intraovarian factor(s).

Thecal Cells

The thecal layer is divided into the theca externa, consisting of fibroblasts, connective tissue, and contractile elements, and the theca interna, which is composed of fibroblasts, transitional cells, thought to be undifferentiated gland cells,[29] and gland or steroidogenic-like cells, similar to steroid-secreting cells in other tissues.[29,30] Features of steroid-secreting cells include large quantities of lipid, abundant tubular smooth endoplasmic reticulum, dispersed Golgi elements, and vesicular mitochondria[30] (Figure 1B). Thecal cells are connected by gap junctions, although the junctions appear less frequently than in the granulosa cell layer.[31] During atresia, the thecal cells may show degenerative changes but only during later stages of atresia. These cells do not undergo apoptosis[22] but rather appear to evolve into interstitial tissue.[11]

The Oocyte

The two to four layers of granulosa cells that surround the oocyte are referred to as the cumulus oophorus and connect the oocyte to the membrana granulosa. The cumulus-oocyte integrity remains stable during atresia. The corona radiata, the layer of cells closest to the oocyte, send cytoplasmic projections through the zona pellucida, which contact microvilli on the oocyte (Figure 2). Gap junctions are often found at these points of contact.[30] This interaction between cumulus cells and the oocyte is thought necessary to provide nutrients and other materials to the oocyte.[2] It may also be of importance in maintaining the oocyte in meiotic arrest at the diplotene state.[32] During atresia, this close spatial relationship is lost when the coronal cell projections retract, the microvilli decrease in size and number, and the zona pellucida thickens. Concurrently, the germinal vesicle breaks down and an apparent resumption of meiosis occurs within the oocyte.[33] These degenerative changes are not seen, however, until late in atresia.

STEROIDOGENESIS IN HEALTHY AND ATRETIC FOLLICLE
Steroidogenic Pathways

Regardless of the physiological state, healthy and atretic ovarian follicles have the capacity to synthesize several steroid hormones. The main steriod synthesized is estradiol-17β (E_2). E_2 synthesis is a complex process; the primary substrate utilized for its synthesis is cholesterol. Cholesterol comes from three main sources: *de novo* synthesis from acetate; hydrolysis of sterol esters, which are stored within lipid droplets; and metabolism of free cholesterol from blood plasma. Esterfied cholesterol is the primary cholesterol used in ovarian steroid synthesis.[34]

The first step in steroid hormone synthesis is the side chain cleavage of cholesterol. This cleavage occurs within the mitochondria and is the rate-limiting step in steroid hormone biosynthesis. Side chain cleavage is an enzymatic reaction in which cholesterol is converted to pregnenolone, thus freeing a six-carbon fragment, isocaproate. This oxidative cleavage of cholesterol involves cytochrome P450, a flavoprotein, an iron sulfur protein, nicotinamide adenine dinucleotide phosphate (NADPH), and molecular oxygen. The actual enzymes involved in the conversion of cholesterol to pregnenolone are 20-hydroxylase, 20,22-desmolase, and 22-hydroxylase. The major regulator of this side chain cleavage reaction is the amount of available cholesterol. The availability is regulated by the nucleotide, cyclic AMP, and LH. These two substances enhance the availability of cholesterol, but do not influence cytochrome P450.

Once cholesterol has been converted to pregnenolone there are two main pathways that will lead to the production of E_2: a Δ^4 and a Δ^5 pathway. The Δ^4 pathway involves the conversion of pregnenolone to progesterone. This is controlled by the enzyme 3β-OH dehydrogenase and the Δ^5 isomerase. Progesterone is then hydroxylated at the C-17 position by NADPH and molecular oxygen yielding 17α-OH progesterone. The 17α-OH progesterone undergoes a side chain cleavage by the enzyme 17,20-desmolase, resulting in the formation of androstenedione.

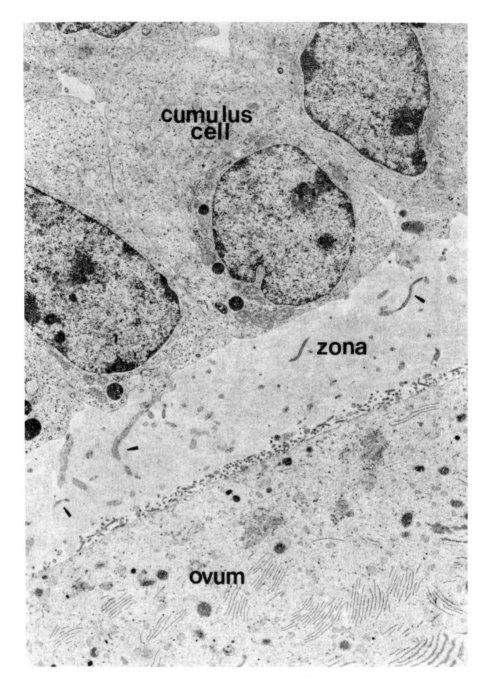

FIGURE 2. An electron micrograph illustrating the connection between the cumulus cells and ovum. Notice the cumulus cell projections (arrows) within the zona pellucida ($\times$ 6800).

The androgen is then aromatized by an aromatizing enzyme, aromatase, to estrone, which is then converted to estradiol-17β by 17β-hydroxysteroid dehydrogenase (Figure 3).

In the Δ^5 pathway, 17β-hydroxylase converts pregnenolone to 17α-pregnenolone by an enzymatic cleavage at the C-17 position. 17α-Pregnenolone then undergoes cleavage by the enzyme 17,20-desmolase, to yield the androgen, dihydroepiandrosterone. This androgen can be converted to androstenedione by 3β-OH dehydrogenase. Androstenedione may then undergo aromatization, yielding E_2 (Figure 3). For more details regarding these pathways as

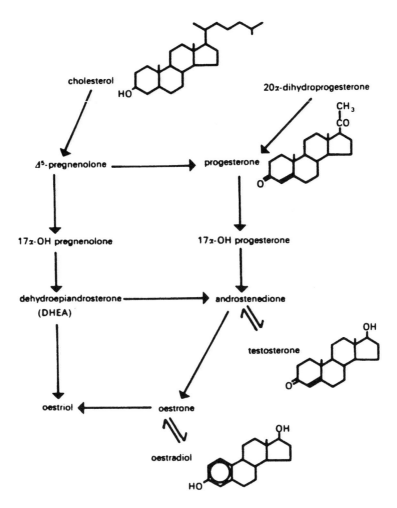

FIGURE 3. The major pathways of gonadal steroid synthesis. The route from pregnenolone to androstenedione via progesterone is known as the Δ^4 pathway, and that via dehydroepiandrosterone as the Δ^4 pathway.

well as the mechanism involved in controlling the expression of the steroidogenic enzymes refer to a recent review by Hum and Miller.[35]

Two Cell Theory

The process of cholesterol metabolism resulting in E_2 is influenced by the gonadotropins, follicle-stimulating hormone (FSH), and LH. FSH and LH are glycoprotein hormones secreted by the anterior pituitary. Steroidogenesis in the follicle is a complex process involving a synergism between these gonadotropins and the granulosa and theca cell layers of the follicle. These relationships are presented in greater detail in a review by Gore-Langton and Armstrong[34] and therefore only a brief review is presented below.

FSH and LH mediate their action through membrane receptors. The receptors for FSH are located exclusively on the granulosa cells and LH receptors are on theca cells. As the follicle develops, FSH induces LH receptor formation within the granulosa cells, thus granulosa cells in large preovulatory follicles contain both LH and FSH receptors.[36]

FSH affects steroidogenesis by enhancing the aromatization of androstenedione to E_2. LH affects several aspects of steriod biosynthesis by enhancing cholesterol side chain cleavage and stimulating extramitochondrial movement of cholesterol to a steroidogenic site, thereby increasing the quantity of cholesterol available for steroidogenesis. LH also elicits an increase in the aromatization of androstenedione to estrogen in the granulosa cell layer if FSH is present.[37]

Steroidogenesis and Atretic Follicles

Androgen, estrogen, and progesterone are also synthesized in atretic follicles. A comparison of follicular fluid steroid content in healthy and atretic follicles gives an indication of steroidogenic activity in the follicles of different stages (Table 2). In large atretic ovine follicles, total steroid secretion into follicular fluid is less than half the amount found in healthy follicles. Estrogen is the major steroid produced in normal follicles, whereas androgen is the prominent steroid found in fluid from atretic follicles. However, the total synthesis of androgen is decreased by 30–50% in atretic follicles.[5] Progesterone concentrations remain essentially the same.[5] Similar results were reported from studies on steroid production in granulosa cell cultures from healthy and atretic follicles.[6] It can be concluded from these data that one characteristic of atresia is a loss of aromatization ability in the granulosa cells. This loss is due to a decrease in the aromatase mRNA levels.[38]

TABLE 2
Steroid Hormone Concentrations (ng/ml) in the Fluid of Human Ovarian Follicles

Type of Tertiary Follicle	Testosterone	Estradiol	Progesterone
Nonovulatory	41	315	502
Preovulatory	22	1888	2013
Atretic	54	502	368

Receptors for FSH and LH are greatly decreased in the granulosa cells of atretic follicles[17,39] as a result of a decrease in mRNA levels.[38] This decline in gonadotropin receptors may explain the lack of estrogen and the build-up of testosterone in the follicular fluid. Whether the loss of FSH receptors occurs prior to a decline in estrogen levels has not been determined, but Moor and associates[5] suggest estrogen synthesis decreases very early in the atretic process.

GROWTH FACTOR SYNTHESIS WITHIN THE FOLLICLE

In addition to its well-characterized ability to synthesize steroids, the ovary produces numerous growth factors, which modulate and/or mediate the action of the gonadotropins. Over the last several years, numerous studies have been undertaken to elucidate the roles that these factors play. These individual studies are too numerous to be adequately reviewed and cited in this chapter. Therefore, only a brief summary will be presented and the reader referred to more detailed reviews.

There are many different growth factors produced within the ovary with new factors continually being identified. However, the more well-documented ovarian growth factors include epidermal growth factor (EGF) and its homolog, transforming growth factor-α (TGF-α), transforming growth factor-β (TGF-β), inhibin/activin, and insulin-like growth factor I (IGF-I).

Epidermal Growth Factor/Transforming Growth Factor-α

Although EGF and TGF-α are different compounds, they both bind and activate the EGF receptor. Thus, they have similar actions in terms of tyrosine kinase activity, EGF receptor autophosphorylation, and mitogenic activity. EGF/TGF-α have their major effects on the granulosa cells. These growth factors generally stimulate granulosa cell proliferation, but this effect has not been observed for rat granulosa cells. In addition, EGF has been shown to inhibit gonadotropin-induced granulosa cell differentiation.[40] Finally, recent studies have shown that EGF inhibits granulosa cells from undergoing apoptosis, thereby maintaining the follicle in a viable state.[27]

Transforming Growth Factor-β

TGF-β is a member of a large superfamily of growth factors that includes inhibin, activin, and mullerian inhibiting factor. In addition, there are multiple forms of TGF-β (i.e., β1, β2, and β3). Although only partial homology exists between the various TGF-βs, they frequently serve identical functions. TGF-β appears to be produced in both the granulosa and thecal cells, with its action being concentration, cell-type, and species dependent. In the granulosa cells, TGF-β modifies the action of FSH by increasing steroidogenesis and inducing LH, FSH, and EGF receptors. TGF-β1 has significant effects on thecal cells, inhibiting both steroidogenesis and proliferation. Consult the reviews by Knecht et al.[41] and Benahmed et al.[42]

Inhibin/Activin

Inhibin and activin were first isolated and purified from follicular fluid on the basis of their ability to inhibit (inhibin) or stimulate (activin) the release of FSH from pituitary cells *in vitro*. Inhibin is a 32-kDa heterodimeric glycoprotein composed of an α subunit and one of two β subunits, $β_A$ (inhibin-A) or $β_B$ (inhibin-B). Activins are homodimers of inhibin β subunits (i.e., activin-A or activin-B). In both primates and rodent ovaries, mRNA for inhibins/activins have been detected. Immature antral follicles express abundant amounts of inhibin/activin β subunits, while inhibin α subunits are expressed at higher levels in the larger more mature follicles. Thus, activin is present in immature follicles, with inhibin predominating in the preovulatory follicles.

Both inhibin and activin have direct effects on ovarian steroidogenesis. Activin inhibits LH-induced secretion of androgens from cultured thecal cells. Conversely, inhibin augments LH-stimuated androgen production. Activin also appears to act in an autocrine manner to regulate estradiol secretion from the granulosa cells. Specifically, activin enhances FSH-induced aromatase activity. Activin also promotes FSH-induced progesterone synthesis from immature, non-LH receptors containing granulosa cells. However, progesterone synthesis is inhibited by activin after the granulosa cells begin to express LH receptors. The role of inhibin in regulating granulosa cell steroidogenesis is not well defined and it is unlikely that it is a significant factor in regulating granulosa cell steroid synthesis.[43]

Insulin-Like Growth Factor I

IGF-I is expressed in relatively high levels within the ovary, with only the liver and uterus expressing more IGF-I. In the ovary, the granulosa cells are the source of IGF-I. Further, FSH has been shown to induce the expression of IGF-I. Both porcine and murine granulosa cells possess high-affinity, low-capacity binding sites for IGF-I. In addition, both FSH and LH are capable of up-regulating granulosa cell IGF-I binding. These studies suggest an autocrine/paracrine role for IGF-I in regulating granulosa cell function.

In vitro culture studies support this hypothesis by demonstrating that IGF-I enhances FSH-induced progesterone and estrogen synthesis, LH receptor expression, and inhibin biosynthesis. IGF-I action may be due to its ability to increase adenylate cyclase activity and thereby increase cAMP levels. Thecal cells may also be responsive to IGF-I, because these cells have IGF-I binding sites and IGF-I stimulates thecal androgen biosynthesis.[44]

OVULATION

Most ovarian follicles ultimately undergo atresia. In women, one follicle per cycle is "rescued" from the atresia process and develops into an ovulatory-sized follicle. This one follicle is destined to respond to the LH surge by ovulating. The ovulatory process is a complex phenomenon composed of three separate physiological events: oocyte (egg) maturation, preovulatory luteinization (steroidgenesis), and follicular rupture. The following comments will focus on these key events.

Oocyte Maturation

Once the primordial germ cells enter the fetal ovary, meiosis begins and progresses from leptotene to diplotene of the first meiotic division. Shortly thereafter, meiosis becomes arrested in the prophase or dictyate stage (first meiotic arrest). A few hours prior to follicular rupture, the oocyte within an ovulatory follicle resumes meiosis. This is accompanied morphologically by the breakdown of the oocyte nucleus, the germinal vesicle. Preovulatory oocyte maturation begins with the oocyte in the dictyate stage of the first meiotic division and ends at metaphase of the second meiotic division. At this stage the oocyte is ready to be fertilized.[45]

The surge of gonadotropic hormones which occurs prior to ovulation is necessary for the resumption of meiosis within the oocyte. During the preovulatory gonadotropin surge, both FSH and LH levels increase. However, there is much debate about which hormone is responsible for the resumption of meiosis within the oocyte. The possibility exists that both gonadotropins act synergistically to initiate ova maturation.[46]

Oocytes, released from follicles and placed in culture are capable of resuming meiosis spontaneously, in the absence of gonadotropic stimulation. Studies indicate that the ability of the oocyte to mature upon release from the follicle is acquired only at late stages of follicular maturation. In adult and immature mice, pigs, and hamsters, the ability of the oocyte to resume meiosis *in vitro* and to reach metaphase II is possible only if the oocyte is fully grown and contained in medium or large antral follicles.[45]

When oocytes are cultured within preovulatory follicles, oocyte maturation is dependent on stimulation by gonadotropic hormones. The gonadotropic hormone that is responsible for the resumption of meiosis within follicle-enclosed oocytes is not known and may be species specific, but in all mammals both FSH and LH play a key regulatory role. LH has previously been shown to be capable of inducing germinal vesicle breakdown (GVB) and completion of at least the first meiotic division in rat oocytes. Other investigations, however, clearly indicate that FSH is more effective in inducing preovulatory oocyte maturation in follicle-enclosed oocytes *in vitro*. Thus, the control of the induction of ova maturation is a complex event and cannot be interpreted as being the sole responsibility of FSH at this time.[45]

The role of surrounding cumulus cells in the preovulatory maturation of oocytes is also controversial. Initially, it was believed that the cumulus cells provided a beneficial effect for the maturing oocyte. This effect has been shown to be related to the specific energy requirements of the denuded oocyte maturing *in vitro*. When pyruvate is added to the culture medium containing denuded oocytes, maturation progresses readily and is indistinguishable from maturation of oocytes enclosed in the cumulus mass. The cumulus oophorus may actually have an inhibitory effect on the resumption of oocyte meiosis.[47]

Chang,[48] in 1955, first demonstrated that rabbit follicular fluid (FF) had an inhibitory effect on ova maturation. These observations were later confirmed and expanded largely through the efforts of Tsafriri.[45] These investigations initially involved the co-culture of liberated oocytes along with follicular constituents and demonstrated that an inhibitory substance (oocyte maturation inhibitor, OMI) is secreted from granulosa cells. This factor presumably is secreted into FF and arrests oocytes in the dictyate stage of meiosis. It was further suggested that gonadotropins were capable of overriding this inhibitory influence. The mode of action of this inhibitor could be mediated by cAMP. This inhibitor of oocyte maturation isolated from porcine FF has been partially characterized. Its inhibitory action could not be destroyed by heating to 60°C or repeated freezing and thawing and could not be extracted with charcoal. OMI has a molecular weight of about 2000 Da.

This inhibitor of ova maturation, partially purified and characterized in the pig and in the cow, does not appear to be species specific because FF from the pig interfered with ova maturation in the mouse. The addition of ovine LH to culture medium partially reversed the effect of this inhibitor, supporting the hypothesis that FF inhibitor and LH are both involved in the control of preovulatory oocyte maturation.[45]

It appears, therefore, that ova maturation is under the influence of several stimulatory and inhibitory factors and that some of their actions are mediated through secondary messengers such as cAMP. In the presence of gonadotropins, just prior to follicular rupture, the oocyte is capable of resuming meiosis, possibly as a result of previous exposure to steroid hormones. The gonadotropin surge, therefore, appears to be responsible for overcoming all inhibitory influence(s) on ova maturation, allowing the events necessary for ovulation to proceed normally, and to prepare the ovum for eventual fertilization.[46]

Preovulatory Steroid Synthesis

In addition to stimulating preovulatory oocyte maturation, the gonadotropin surge stimulates the synthesis and secretion of steroid hormones within the preovulatory follicle as well as the morphological alterations that eventually lead to the rupture of the follicle. Evidence suggests that the rate of progesterone, E_2, and testosterone synthesis changes during the preovulatory period. Steroid synthesis is a dynamic event that occurs only within follicles that have developed appropriate receptor populations.[46]

Throughout the reproduction cycle, there is a characteristic pattern of gonadotropin secretion and a corresponding pattern of ovarian steroid hormone production and secretion. In all species, prior to follicular rupture, there is a significant increase in serum LH concentration. LH binds to receptors on the granulosa cells of large preovulatory follicles and stimulates prostaglandin E_2 (PGE_2). PGE_2 stimulates progesterone production by human granulosa cells *in vitro*. It has been suggested that PGE_2-stimulated progesterone synthesis is essential for follicular rupture, because cyanoketone interferes with progesterone synthesis and inhibits ovulation. In addition, intrafollicular injection of progesterone antiserum blocks ovulation. A definite conclusion concerning the role of steroids and the disruption of the follicle wall has not been reached, but it has been demonstrated that progesterone can increase the distensibility of large follicular strips, supporting a putative role of progesterone in the process of ovulation.[49]

Follicular Rupture

The extrusion of the ovum is the culminating event in the process of ovulation and is dependent on sequential biochemical and morphological events that occur only within ovulatory follicles. Because an increase in intrafollicular pressure does not occur, the oocyte are not forcibly extruded from the follicle.[49] Rather the follicular wall thins and becomes distensible. These changes are responsible for follicle rupture and thinning.[49]

Preovulatory follicles require gonadotropic hormones (LH and FSH) in order to rupture.[46] In response to the preovulatory surge of LH and FSH the follicle undergoes a sequence of changes that culminate in rupture. Morphological changes that occur within the large preovulatory follicles of the rabbit, just prior to follicular rupture, have been extensively studied.[50-55] The following is a brief summary of these studies.

Surface cells within the germinal epithelium increase in size and many show large, round, dense cytoplasmic bodies, located predominantly in the apical region of the follicular wall. It has been suggested that these bodies secrete lytic substances which ensure with the degeneration of the collagen matrix of the surface covering. Then the number of gap junctions in the thecal layer decreases, and a small increase in vascularization and edema occurs within the thecal layer. This edema accounts for the preovulatory swelling within the follicle that occurs as a result of an increase in capillary circulation within the thecal layer.

Granulosa cells also begin to dissociate and thin out in the apical region. There is an increase in the number of granulosa cell projections that penetrate and fragment the basement membrane. The number of gap junctions present between the granulosa cells progressively decreases as rupture approaches. Just prior to follicular rupture, a stigma forms at the apex of the follicle and is the place from which the ovum will eventually extrude.

Collagen has been identified in many mammalian species and collagenolytic activity has been identified in follicles of the rat. Collagenase-like enzymes injected into the antra of mature follicles of the rabbit stimulate swelling, stigma formation, and ovulation. Thus, many of the changes that occur within the preovulatory follicle prior to rupture appear to be events that promote the secretion of an ovulatory enzyme, which may be a collagenase.

In summary, follicular rupture is a dynamic event that requires major morphological changes throughout the follicle wall. The integrity of the wall is upset as rupture nears, vascularization increases, and the follicle swells above the surface of the ovary. Just moments prior to rupture, as a result of structural changes within the follicular wall, the most apical portion of the follicle distends, the tissue loses its integrity, and the ovum, surrounding cumulus cells, and antral fluid are slowly expelled from the follicle.

FUNCTION OF THE CORPUS LUTEUM

STEROIDOGENIC CAPACITY OF THE CORPUS LUTEUM

After the follicle ruptures and releases its ovum, it differentiates into a corpus luteum. This transformation, called luteinization, is characterized by morphological differentiation of the granulosa cells and to some extent thecal cells into luteal cells. Luteinization is initiated by the preovulatory LH surge. The surge levels of LH stimulate cAMP and progesterone production as well as *de novo* RNA and protein synthesis.[56] For two to three days after the preovulatory LH surge, there is a decrease in progesterone secretion and a corresponding decrease in the number of LH receptors within the differentiating granulosa cells.[57] Thus, the luteinizing follicle becomes less responsive to LH accounting for the decrease in progesterone levels.

As the granulosa cells luteinize, the amount of cytoplasm increases, the mitochondria develop tubular cristae, the cytoplasm fills with smooth endoplasmic reticulum, the Golgi complexes enlarge, and numerous lipid droplets appear. As a result, granulosa cells differentiate into large luteal cells. The mature corpus luteum also contains small luteal cells. Two possibilities exist to explain the existence of two sizes of luteal cells. First, the thecal cells could undergo a similar morphological luteinization but do not become as large. Evidence supporting this concept has been developed for the bovine corpus luteum.[58] The second possibility is granulosa cells first differentiate into small and then large luteal cells, with the transition between each of these stages being regulated by LH.[59]

Regardless of the source or mechanism responsible for the existence of small and large luteal cells, there appear to be functional differences between the two types of luteal cells. These differences have been characterized to the greatest extent in the ovine corpus luteum by Niswender's laboratory.[60] Niswender's studies have shown that small luteal cells differ from large luteal cells in that the small luteal cells (1) have a lower basal rate of progesterone secretion, (2) possess LH receptors, and (3) secrete progesterone in response to either LH or cAMP stimulation. In contrast, large luteal cells have at least a twofold higher basal progesterone secretion rate but do not show enhanced progesterone secretion in response to either LH or cAMP. Due in part to this enhanced secretory rate, large luteal cells account for up to 80% of the progesterone secreted by the mature corpus luteum.

The progesterone secreted from both the small and large luteal cells accounts for the elevated progesterone levels throughout the luteal phase of the cycle. However, there is considerable species variation in the length of the luteal phase (Table 3). In women, the secretion of progesterone is maximum for 8 to 10 days then declines, reaching its nadir 14 days after ovulation.

TABLE 3
Characteristics of the Luteal Period of Various Mammalian Species

Species	Length of Cycle or Pregnancy (days)		Luteotropic Hormone[a]	Uterine Luteolysin	No. of Days that Pregnancy Is Dependent On	
	Cycle	Pregnant			CL	Pituitary
Cat	14–21	58–65		No	50	1st half
Cow	21–22	278–293	LH, PRL, E?	Yes—local	200	
Dog (beagle)	203–224	59–68		No	All	All
Ferret	None	42	PRL	No	All	All
Fox	None	51–54		No	All	All
Gerbil	4–6	24–26				
Goat	20–21	146–151			All	All
Guinea pig	16–17	67–68	LH, FSH, PRL	Yes—local	21–25	40
Hamster (golden)	4	16	FSH, PRL, LH, E	Yes—local	All	All
Horse	19–25	330–345	E	Yes—local	115–200	
Human	28	280	LH	No	40	40
Mink	8–9	40–75				All
Monkey (rhesus)	28–29	163	LH	No	27–28	32–40
Mouse	4–6	19–20	LH, PRL, E	Yes	All	11–12
Opossum	0.29	12–13		No	All	
Pig	20–21	112–115	LH, PRL	Yes—local	All	All
Rabbit	None	30–32	E	Yes	All	All
Rat	4–5	20–22	LH, PRL, E	Yes	All	12
Sheep	16–17	147–155	LH, PRL	Yes—local	55	50
Squirrel	16			No	All	

LH, luteinizing hormone; FSH, follicle-stimulating hormone; PRL, prolactin; E, estradiol; CL, corpus luteum.

The Corpus Luteum of the Menstrual Cycle and Pregnancy

The corpus luteum of both the menstrual cycle and pregnancy can synthesize seven different steroids. Progesterone is the major secretory product, but other secreted steroids include 17-hydroxyprogesterone, 20α-hydroxy-Δ4-pregnen-3-one, pregnenolone, andro-stenedione, estradiol, and estrone. LH uniformly increases the synthesis of all these steroids, suggesting that the rate-limiting step, which is influenced by LH, is the conversion of cholesterol into pregnenolone.

Although the same steroids are produced, the corpus luteum of the menstrual cycle synthesizes much more progesterone than the corpus luteum of pregnancy. Further, the luteal phase corpus luteum is very responsive to LH whereas luteal responsiveness to LH decreases as pregnancy continues. As pregnancy continues, the number of LH receptors on luteal cells decreases, thereby decreasing the ability to synthesis cAMP and progesterone.[61]

If conception occurs during the menstrual cycle, then the corpus luteum is maintained until the embryo has implanted. In order to prevent luteolysis, the trophoblastic cells of the human embryo secrete a glycoprotein hormone, human chorionic gonadotropin (hCG). hCG has LH-like properties and can maintain luteal progesterone secretion. Through this mechanism, luteal regression is postponed until the fetal-placental unit has developed the capacity to produce sufficient quantities of progesterone to allow pregnancy to continue.[62]

LUTEAL REGRESSION

The corpus luteum of the menstrual cycle has a finite life span but the mechanism responsible for luteal regression (luteolysis) is not well defined. It is known that the decrease in LH levels and luteal LH receptors, which occurs during the late luteal phase of the cycle, is not adequate to cause luteal regression. In many species other than primates, the uterus secretes a luteolytic factor, presumably prostaglandin $F_{2\alpha}$ ($PGF_{2\alpha}$). Receptors for $PGF_{2\alpha}$ have been identified in the corpus luteum of cows, hamsters, rats, sheep, and women, and administration of pharmacological doses of $PGF_{2\alpha}$ results in luteal regression.[63] It appears that $PGF_{2\alpha}$ activates phospholipase C, which causes hydrolysis of membrane phosphatidylinositol-4,5-biphosphate to inositol-1,4,5-triphosphate (IP_3), and 1,2-diacylglycerol. Diacylglycerol increases the affinity of protein kinase C for calcium and IP_3 releases calcium from the intracellular stores, resulting in an increase in free intracellular calcium.[60] This increase in intracellular calcium appears to activate an endonuclease, which in turn promotes the cleavage of the DNA into characteristic oligonucleosome-size fragments with the luteal cells dying via apoptosis.[60]

OVARIAN FUNCTION DURING VARIOUS PHYSIOLOGICAL STATES

THE IMMATURE OVARY
Fetal Life

The mammalian ovary differentiates throughout the first and second trimester of pregnancy. The germ cells migrate from the yolk sac and enter the gonadal ridge, while somatic cells arise from mesenchyme, the coelomic epithelium, and mesonephric tissue. The first small follicles appear during the fourth month of gestation. Around the sixth month, many preantral follicles develop, and antral follicles are often observed by the last two months of fetal life.[64] Although many follicles are found within the fetal ovary, most are atretic and are often morphologically different from the atretic follicles of adult ovaries. These differences include alterations within the basal lamina and hypertrophied or undifferentiated thecal cells.[64]

These alterations in follicular structure may be related to LH and FSH levels. The role of gonadotropins in controlling follicle development has been investigated in the fetal rhesus monkey. Fetuses were hypophysectomized when follicular growth was occurring and follicular development assessed at term. After fetal hypophysectomy, the ovaries contained one third the normal number of oocytes. Also the number of small follicles was reduced, indicating that gonadotropins stimulate follicular growth during fetal life.[65]

Follicular Development and Childhood

During childhood, the ovary is very active with follicles developing to antral size. However, these follicles become atretic and do not reach preovulatory size. Both serum gonadotropins and estrogen levels increase by 6 or 8 years of age. Because this increase in hormone levels corresponds to an increase in the number of antral follicles, it is postulated that the increase in serum gonadotropins is responsible for both the increase in estrogen levels and follicular development in the prepubertal ovary.[64]

THE MENSTRUAL CYCLE AND OVARIAN FUNCTION

Although follicles develop during fetal and pubertal stages of life, cyclic patterns of follicle growth and ovulation occur only after puberty. The pattern of follicular growth and atresia is regulated by a series of hormonal interactions. Follicular growth is a continuous process that occurs throughout the menstrual or estrous cycle. However, the pattern of follicular development differs in the follicular and luteal phases of the cycle.

Follicle Development During the Follicular Phase

Thecal cells differentiate and become associated with small preantral follicles, forming a follicle of approximately 150 μ in diameter. Once the thecal cells differentiate, the granulosa cells undergo a series of mitoses, resulting in the formation of large preantral follicles.

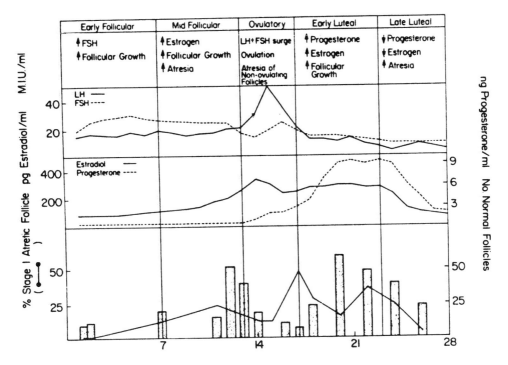

FIGURE 4. Changes in hormone levels and follicular growth (shaded bars) and atresia (-----) during the human menstrual cycle.

Follicular growth through the preantral stage appears to be gonadotropin independent and occurs throughout the menstrual cycle. However, when the follicle is about 250 μ in diameter, an antral cavity forms.[66] These follicles continue to grow by repeated granulosa cell mitoses, such that at the start of each menstrual cycle there are several small antral follicles (2 to 5 mm in diameter) present within the ovary.[67] During the first few days of the menstrual cycle, some of the granulosa cells within a "select" follicle express aromatase.[68] This increase in aromatase accounts for a slight increase in E_2 synthesis.[20] It is this increase in E_2 synthesis, however, that identifies this follicle as the one destined to ovulate.[69] In this "selected" follicle, granulosa cells continue to undergo mitoses and more granulosa cells express the aromatase. In women, the "selected" follicle can be identified by day 6–10 and will ovulate around day 14 of the cycle.[13] Conversely, granulosa cell mitoses in those follicles not destined to ovulate gradually decrease, with these follicles ultimately undergoing atresia (degeneration).[67] This generalized relationship between E_2 and follicle growth not only characterizes the events of the primate menstrual cycle, but also the estrous cycle of most other species (Figure 4).

Estradiol-17β Secretion and Granulosa Cell Mitoses

It is not known how the granulosa cells within the developing preovulatory follicle perform the diverse functions of mitosis and E_2 secretion. At least two mechanisms could explain this phenomenon. First, there could exist two "types" of granulosa cells. One type is undifferentiated and only undergoes mitosis, and a second type is partially differentiated (i.e., expresses aromatase and secretes E_2) but can still proliferate. It can be further theorized that when these aromatase-containing cells undergo mitosis their ability to secrete E_2 is temporarily inhibited. This hypothesis correlates well with the observation that there is an inverse relationship between E_2 secretion and granulosa cell DNA synthesis within follicles.[70,71] A careful analysis of the events during the menstrual or estrous cycles of several species reveals that there is temporal separation between the time of rapid follicular growth and maximum E_2 secretion.[66]

This relationship has not been completely described for the primate menstrual cycle, most likely due to the fact that a limited number of observations can be made during the preovulatory period. It must be pointed out that neither of these hypotheses can be directly tested *in vivo* due to various technical limitations.

Although there is a positive relationship between increasing E_2 and the development of the preovulatory follicle, there is also a negative relationship between E_2 and the rate of mitosis within follicles destined to become atretic. This temporal relationship suggest that the E_2 secreted from the developing preovulatory follicle influences mitosis within follicles destined to become atretic. Several investigators have attempted to address the role of E_2 in follicular growth and atresia using various *in vivo* models.[72] However, these *in vivo* studies have shown that E_2 can have both stimulatory and inhibitory actions.

Follicular Development During the Luteal Phase

Although the formation of the corpus luteum is the dominant event, there are two waves of follicular growth that occur during the luteal phase of the cycle.[67] The first wave occurs shortly after ovulation when both E_2 and progesterone (P_4) are secreted at low rates. This wave of follicular development is truncated by day 22, which corresponds to the time when both serum P_4 and E_2 levels are at their maximum. Similarly, follicular growth resumes as the corpus luteum begins to regress, as judged by a rapid decline in serum E_2 and P_4 level. One of the follicles that starts growing at this time eventually is selected to become the ovulatory follicle of the subsequent cycle.[67] The temporal relationship between elevated steroid levels and suppressed follicular growth, again, raises the possibility that steroids, most likely progesterone, have a negative effect on follicular growth. Progesterone has been shown to suppress cell proliferation in a number of cell types,[73,74] and, indeed, *in vivo* studies have shown that progesterone can suppress follicular development.[20]

AGING AND OVARIAN FUNCTION

Age dramatically affects ovarian function. In most species, the frequency of regular reproductive cycles decreases with age.[75] The number of oocytes and follicles also decreases with age, although the number of large preovulatory-sized follicles, ovulations, and corpus lutea remain normal until the end of fertile life. After ovulation ceases, follicular development continues until the oocytes are depleted from the ovary, but these follicles ultimately undergo atresia.[75]

In the human ovary, the number of follicles smaller that 100 μ and greater than 1 mm in diameter decreases with advancing age.[76] Similar trends are observed in all species. Some data indicates that the decreased number of follicles accounts for the suppressed function of the aged ovary. When most of the follicles are depleted, the human ovary becomes small and fibrous. The amount of interstitial tissue also becomes reduced because it is derived from atretic follicles. The remaining interstitial cells possess LH and FSH receptors and steroidogenic enzymes.[77] However, the functional capacity of the interstitial tissue of the aged ovary remains to be determined.

REFERENCES

1. **Ross, G., Vande Wiele, R., and Frantz, A.,** *The Ovary and Breast,* W. B. Saunders, Philadelphia, 1981.
2. **Zamboni, L.,** Fine morphology of the follicle wall and follicle cell-oocyte association, *Biol. Reprod.,* 10, 125, 1974.
3. **Guraya, S.,** Morhpology, histochemistry and biochemistry of follicular growth and atresia, *Ann. Biol. Anim. Biochem. Biophys.,* 13, 230, 1973.
4. **Makris, A. and Ryan, K.,** Progesterone, androstenedione, testosterone, esterone and estradiol synthesis in hamster ovarian follicle cells, *Endocrinology,* 96, 694, 1975.
5. **Moor, R., Hay, M., Dott, H., and Cran, D.,** Macroscopic identification and steroidogenic function of atretic follicles in sheep, *J. Endocrinol.,* 77, 309, 1978.
6. **McNatty, K., Makris, A., DeGrazia, C., Osathanondh, R., and Ryan, K.,** The production of progesterone, androgens and oestrogens by human granulosa cells *in vitro* and *in vivo, J. Steroid Biochem.,* 11, 775, 1979.
7. **Amsterdam, A., Josephs, R., Lieberman, E., and Lindner, H.,** Organization of intramembrane particles of granulosa cell gap junctions in rat ovarian follicles, *J. Cell. Biol.,* 63, 2, 1974.
8. **Merk, F., Albright, J.T., and Botticelli, C.R.,** The fine structure of granulosa cell nexuses in rat ovarian follicles, *Anat. Rec.,* 175, 107, 1973.
9. **Albertini, D. and Anderson, E.,** The appearance and structure of intercellular connections during the ontogeny of the rabbit ovarian follicle with particular reference to gap junctions, *J. Cell. Biol.,* 63, 234, 1974.
10. **Peluso, J., England-Charlesworth, C., Bolender, D., and Steger, R.,** Ultrastructural alterations associated with the initiation of follicular atresia, *Cell Tissue Res.,* 211, 105, 1980.
11. **Guraya, S. and Greenwald, G.,** A comparative histochemical study of interstitial tissue and follicular atresia in the mammalian ovary, *Anat. Rec.,* 149, 411, 1964.
12. **Motta, P. and Bourneva, V.,** A comparative histochemical study of -3B-hydroxysteroid dehydrogenase and lipid content in the rat ovary with special reference to the interstitial cells, *Acta Histochem.,* 38, 340, 1970.
13. **Bomsel-Helmrecih, O., Marik, J., Hulka, J., and Papiernik, E.,** Preovulatory morphology and steroid content of follicles, in *Human Ovulation,* Hafez, E.S.E., Ed., North-Holland, New York, 1979, 121.
14. **Teerds, K.J. and Dorrington, J.H.,** Immunohistochemical localization of 3 beta-hydroxysteroid dehydrogenase in the rat ovary during follicular development and atresia, *Biol. Reprod.,* 49, 989, 1993.
15. **Peluso, J., Breitenecker, G., and Hafez, E.,** Atresia of ovarian follicles and ova, in *Human Ovulation,* Hafez, E., Ed., North-Holland, New York, 1979, 177.
16. **Byskov, A.,** *Atresia,* Raven Press, New York, 1977.
17. **Peluso, J. and Steger, R.,** Role of FSH in regulating granulosa cell division and follicular atresia in rats, *J. Reprod. Fertil.,* 54, 275, 1978.
18. **Dimino, M., Malcom, S., and Elfont, E.,** Changes in acid hydrolase activities of ovarian subcellular fractions of immature rats after gonadotropic treatment, *Biol. Reprod.,* 17, 780, 1977.
19. **Elfont, E., Roska, J., and Dimino, M.,** Cytochemical studies of acid phosphatase in ovarian follicles: a suggested role for lysosomes in steroidogenesis, *Biol. Reprod.,* 17, 787, 1977.
20. **Greenwald, G. and Terranova, P.,** Follicular selection and its control, in *The Physiology of Reproduction,* Knobil, E. and Neill, J.D., Eds., Raven Press, New York, 1988, 387.
21. **Hughes, F.J. and Gorospe, W.C.,** Biochemical identification of apoptosis (programmed cell death) in granulosa cells: evidence for a potential mechanism underlying follicular atresia, *Endocrinology,* 129, 2415, 1991.
22. **Tilly, J.L., Kowalski, K.I., Johnson, A.L., and Hsueh, A.,** Involvement of apoptosis in ovarian follicular atresia and postovulatory regression, *Endocrinology,* 129, 2799, 1991.
23. **Schwartzman, R.A. and Cidlowski, J.A.,** Apoptosis: the biochemistry and molecular biology of programmed cell death, *Endocr. Rev.,* 14, 133, 1993.
24. **Hurwitz, A. and Adashi, E.Y.,** Ovarian follicular atresia as an apoptotic process: a paradigm for programmed cell death in endocrine tissues, *Mol. Cell. Endocrinol.,* 84, C19, 1992.
25. **Zeleznik, A., Ihrig, L., and Bassett, S.,** Developmental expression of Ca++/Mg++-dependent endonuclease activity in rat granulosa and luteal cells, *Endocrinology,* 125, 2218, 1989.
26. **Billig, H., Furuta, I., and Hsueh, A.,** Estrogens inhibit and androgens enhance ovarian granulosa cell apoptosis, *Endocrinology,* 133, 2204, 1993.
27. **Tilly, J.L., Billig, H., Kowalski, K.I., and Hsueh, A.,** Epidermal growth factor and basic fibroblast growth factor suppress the spontaneous onset of apoptosis in cultured rat ovarian granulosa cells and follicles by a tyrosine kinase-dependent mechanism, *Mol. Endocrinol.,* 6, 1942, 1992.
28. **Morley, P., Whitfield, J., Vanderhyden, B., Tsang, B., and Schwartz, J.,** A new, nongenomic estrogen action: the rapid release of intracellular calcium, *Endocrinology,* 131, 1305, 1992.
29. **Hiura, M. and Fujita, H.,** Electron microscopy of the cytodifferentiation of the theca cell in the mouse ovary, *Arch. Histol. Jpn.,* 40, 95, 1977.
30. **Christensen, A. and Gillim, S.,** *The Correlation of Fine Structure and Function in Steroid-Secreting Cells with Emphasis on Those of the Gonads,* Appleton-Century-Crofts, New York, 1969.

31. **Amsterdam, A. and Linder, H.,** *Incidence and Characterization of Gap Junctions in the Graafian Follicle,* Raven Press, New York, 1977.

32. **Tsafriri, A. and Channing, C.,** An inibitory influence of granulosa cells and follicular fluid upon porcine oocyte meiosis *in vitro, Endocrinology,* 96, 922, 1975.

33. **Vasquez-Nin, G. and Sotelo, J.,** Electron microscope study of the atretic oocytes of the rat, *Zellforsch. Z.,* 80, 518, 1967.

34. **Gore-Langton, R. and Armstrong, D.,** Follicular steroidogenesis and its control, in *The Physiology of Reproduction,* Knobil, E. and Neill, J.D., Eds., Raven Press, New York, 1988, 331.

35. **Hum, D.W. and Miller, W.L.,** Transcriptional regulation of human genes for steroidogenic enzymes, *Clin. Chem.,* 39, 333, 1993.

36. **Richards, J. and Hedin, L.,** Molecular aspects of hormone action in ovarian follicular development, ovulation and luteinization, *Annu. Rev. Physiol.,* 50, 441, 1988.

37. **Wang, C., Hsuesh, A., and Erickson, G.,** LH stimulation of estrogen secretion by cultured rat granulosa cells, *Mol. Cell. Endocrinol.,* 24, 17, 1981.

38. **Tilly, J.L., Kowalski, K.I., Schomberg, D.W., and Hsueh, A.,** Apoptosis in atretic ovarian follicles is associated with selective decreases in messenger ribonucleic acid transcripts for gonadotropin receptors and cytochrome P450 aromatase, *Endocrinology,* 131, 1670, 1992.

39. **Peluso, J., Steger, R., and Hafez, E.,** Sequential changes associated with the degeneration of preovulatory rat follicles, *J. Reprod. Fertil.,* 49, 215, 1977.

40. **May, J.V. and Schomberg, D.W.,** The potential relevance of epidermal growth factor and transforming growth factor-alpha to ovarian physiology, *Semin. Reprod. Endocrinol.,* 7, 1, 1989.

41. **Knecht, M., Feng, P., and Catt, K.J.,** Transforming growth factor-beta: autocrine, paracrine and endocrine effects in ovarian cells, *Semin. Reprod. Endocrinol.,* 7, 12, 1989.

42. **Benahmed, M., et al.,** Transforming growth factor-βs in the ovary, *Ann. N.Y. Acad. Sci.,* 687, 13, 1993.

43. **Hillier, S.G. and Miro, F.,** Inhibin, activin and follistatin, *Ann. N.Y. Acad. Sci.,* 687, 29, 1993.

44. **Adashi, E.Y.,** Intraovarian regulation: the proposed role of insulin-like growth factors, *Ann. N.Y. Acad. Sci.,* 687, 10, 1993.

45. **Tsafriri, A.,** Local nonsteroidal regulators of ovarian function, in *The Physiology of Reproduction,* Knobil, E.N. and Neill, J.D., Eds., Raven Press, New York, 1988, 567.

46. **Lipner, H.,** Mechanisms of mammalian ovulation, in *The Physiology of Reproduction,* Knobil, E.N. and Neill, J.D., Eds., Raven Press, New York, 1988, 447.

47. **Buccione, R., Schroeder, A.C., and Eppig, J.J.,** Interactions between somatic cells and germ cells throughout mammalian oogenesis, *Biol. Reprod.,* 43, 543, 1990.

48. **Chang, M.,** The maturation of rabbit oocyte in culture and their maturation, activation, fertilization, and subsequent development in fallopian tube, *J. Exp. Zool.,* 128, 378, 1955.

49. **Rondell, P.,** Role of steroid synthesis in the process of ovulation, *Biol. Reprod.,* 10, 199, 1974.

50. **Bjersing, L. and Cajander, S.,** Ovulation and the mechanism of follicle rupture. I. Light microscopic changes in rabbit ovarian follicles prior to induced ovulation, *Cell Tissue Res.,* 149, 287, 1974.

51. **Bjersing, L. and Cajander, S.,** Ovulation and the mechanism of follicle rupture. II. Scanning electron microscopy of rabbit germinal epithelium prior to induced ovulation, *Cell Tissue Res.,* 149, 301, 1974.

52. **Bjersing, L. and Cajander, S.,** Ovulation and the mechanism of follicle rupture. III. Transmission electron microscopy of rabbit germinal epithelium prior to induced ovulation, *Cell Tissue Res.,* 149, 313, 1974.

53. **Bjersing, L. and Cajander, S.,** Ovulation and mechanism of follicle rupture. IV. Ultrastructure of the membrana granulosa of rabbit Graafian follicles prior to induced ovulation, *Cell Tissue Res.,* 153, 1, 1974.

54. **Bjersing, L. and Cajander, S.,** Ovulation and the mechanism of follicular rupture. V. Ultrastructure of the tunica albuginea and theca externa of rabbit Graafian follicles prior to induced ovulation, *Cell Tissue Res.,* 153, 15, 1974.

55. **Bjersing, L. and Cajander, S.,** Ovulation and the mechanism of follicular rupture. VI. Ultrastructure of the theca interna and the inner vascular network surrounding rabbit Graafian follicles prior to induced ovulation, *Cell Tissue Res.,* 153, 31, 1974.

56. **Birnbaumer, L., Day, S., Hunzicker-Dunn, M., and Abramowitz, J.,** *Ontogeny of the Corpus Luteum: Regulatory Aspects in Rats and Rabbits,* Raven Press, New York, 1979.

57. **Hill, G.A., et. al.,** Use of individual human follicles to compare oocyte *in vitro* fertilization to granulosa cell *in vitro* luteinization, *Fertil. Steril.,* 48, 258, 1987.

58. **Filicori, M.,** Maintenance of the corpus luteum of the menstrual cycle: hypothalamo-pituitary-ovarian axis, *Semin. Reprod. Endocrinol.,* 8, 115, 1990.

59. **Chaffkin, L.M., Luciano, A.A., and Peluso, J.J.,** The role of progesterone in regulating human granulosa cell proliferation and differentiation *in vitro, J. Clin. Endocrinol. Metab.,* 76, 696, 1993.

60. **Niswender, G.D., Juengel, J.L., McGuire, W.J., Belfiore, C.J., and Wiltbank, M.C.,** Luteal function: the estrous cycle and early pregnancy, *Biol. Reprod.,* 50, 239, 1994.

61. **Marsh, J., Savard, K., and Lemaire, W.,** Steroidogenic capacities of the different compartments of the human ovary, in *The Endocrine Function of the Human Ovary,* James, V., Serio, M., Giusti, G., James, V., Serio, M., and Giusti, G., Eds., Academic Press, New York, 1976, 37.

62. **Gibori, G. and Miller, J.,** The ovary: follicle development, ovulation and luteal function, in *Biochemistry of Mammalian Reproduction,* Zaneveld, L. and Chatterton, R., Eds., John Wiley & Sons, New York, 1982.

63. **Auletta, F., Schofield, M., and Abae, M.,** The mechanisms controlling luteolysis in non-human primates and women, *Semin. Reprod. Endocrinol.,* 8, 122, 1990.

64. **Peters, H., Byskov, A., and Grinsted, J.,** Follicular growth in fetal and prepubertal ovaries of humans and other primates, *Clin. Endocrinol. Metab.,* 7, 469, 1978.

65. **Gulyas, B., Hodgen, G., Tullmer, W., and Ross, G.,** Effects of fetal or maternal hypophysectomy on endocrine organs and body weight in infant Rhesus monkeys (Macaca mulatta): with particular emphasis on oogenesis, *Biol. Reprod.,* 16, 216, 1977.

66. **Hirshfield, A.,** Development of follicles in the mammalian ovary, *Int. Rev. Cytol.,* 124, 43, 1991.

67. **Gougeon, A.,** Dynamics of follicular growth in the human: a model from preliminary results, *Hum. Reprod.,* 1, 155, 1986.

68. **Tamura, T., et al.,** Immunohistochemical localization of 17 alpha-hydroxylase/C17-20 lyase and aromatase cytochrome P-450 in the human ovary during the menstrual cycle, *J. Endocrinol.,* 135, 589, 1992.

69. **Bomsel-Helmreich, O., et al.,** Health and atretic human follicles in the preovulatory phase: differences in evolution of follicular morphology and steroid content of follicular fluid, *J. Clin. Endocrinol. Metab.,* 48, 686, 1979.

70. **Frishman, G., Luciano, A., and Peluso, J.,** Effect of the ratio of follicle-stimulating hormone to luteinizing hormone on rat granulosa cell proliferation and oestradiol-17β secretion, *Hum. Reprod.,* 7, 1073, 1992.

71. **Monniaux, D.,** Short-term effects of FSH *in vitro* on granulosa cells of individual sheep follicles, *J. Reprod. Fertil.,* 79, 505, 1987.

72. **Hutz, R.J.,** Disparate effects of estrogen on *in vitro* steroidogenesis by mammalian and avin granulosa cells, *Biol. Reprod.,* 40, 709, 1989.

73. **Clarke, C.L.,** Progestin regulation of cellular proliferation, *Endocr. Rev.,* 11, 266, 1990.

74. **Chaffkin, L.M., Luciano, A.A., and Peluso, J.J.,** Progesterone as an autocrine/paracrine regulator of human granulosa cell proliferation, *J. Clin. Endocrinol. Metab.,* 75, 1404, 1992.

75. **Butcher, R. and Page, R.,** *Role of the Aging Ovary in Cessation of Reproduction,* Raven Press, New York, 1981.

76. **Talbert, G.,** Effect of maternal age on reproductive capacity, *Am. J. Obstet. Gynecol.,* 102, 451, 1968.

77. **Peluso, J., Steger, R., Jaszozak, S., and Hafez, E.,** Gonadotropin binding sites in human postmenopausal ovaries, *Fertil. Steril.,* 27, 789, 1976.

Chapter 8

THE ESTROGEN RECEPTOR

Scott Lundeen, Iain Anderson, Wesley Gray, and Jack Gorski

CONTENTS

INTRODUCTION

The estrogen receptor (ER) is a nuclear protein that specifically binds to its ligand, estrogen, modulates the transcription of specific target genes, and ultimately leads to physiological and morphological changes in the target tissue. The mechanism by which estrogens exert their control on gene expression, however, is still poorly defined at the molecular level. The basic concept of the two-step model of estrogen action, initially proposed in the 1960s, has changed little since its inception. However, we now know that a specific receptor protein is located in the nucleus, that specific, known nucleotide sequences bind the receptor, and certain proteins that associate with the ER have been identified. Although these advances have added to and slightly modified the model of estrogen action, there is still much more that we do not understand. Moreover, there are still many areas of controversy, such as the multimeric state of ER binding to DNA, the dependence of ligand for DNA binding, and, even more recently, the dependence of the ligand for transcriptional activation. We wish to provide a basic review of the ER, highlight some of the more recent advances in the field that have changed our models of estrogen action, and point out areas of controversy that will require additional research to resolve.

HISTORICAL PERSPECTIVE

It has been known since the 1800s that substances produced by the gonads, now known as steroid hormones, influence the physiology of specific tissues. Estrogen, one such steroid hormone, is known to be involved in the development of secondary sex characteristics, female reproductive function, and fetal development. Although progress was made in identifying and purifying these substances, little was known about how they brought about the morphological changes in target tissues. Work by Mueller and co-workers in the 1950s[1] demonstrated that estrogen mediates its effects on the uterus by increasing total RNA and protein levels in the cells. That steroid hormones effect the transcription of specific target genes was first demonstrated in flies. It had been shown that "puffing" of the polytene chromosomes in insect salivary glands was due to transcriptional activity.[2] Analysis of the polytene chromosomes following treatment with the insect steroid hormone ecdysone showed that puffing occurred at specific locations in the chromosomes.[3] Moreover, there was a specific pattern of puffing; early puffs appeared within 5 min and were followed by late puffs several hours later.[4] These early studies demonstrated that cells treated with steroid hormones lead to the transcription of specific genes and that a cascade of transcription occurs in these cells. It is clear that in the target tissues for estrogen, such as the uterus, a similar cascade takes place. This cascade model of gene activation by steroid hormones was recently reviewed by Landers and Spelsberg.[5]

The synthesis of tritiated estrogens, labeled to high specific activity, led to some of the most significant advances in field ER research. Jensen and Jacobson[6] demonstrated that such estrogens accumulate in specific target tissues such as the uterus and vagina. Toft and Gorski[7,8] identified a protein in the rat uterus that specifically binds to ^{3}H-17β-estradiol (E$_2$). This was the first demonstration of a protein that could bind estrogen with high affinity, the first demonstration of the ER. Shortly thereafter the basic model of estrogen action was proposed.[9,10] In this two-step model, estrogen diffuses into the cell where it binds to a cytosolic ER. Upon binding the ligand, the receptor undergoes some undefined transformation and is translocated into the nucleus where it interacts with the DNA to alter transcription of specific genes. This is the basic model of ER action from which all current models have evolved as new data have become available. The most significant divergence of the current models from the two-step model is that it is now clear that the ER is a nuclear protein that interacts with nuclear components, such as chromatin, prior to binding the ligand; thus, there is no translocation step. In the current model (Figure 1), the estrogen diffuses into the cell and moves into the nucleus where it binds to the ER.[11] After binding the ligand, the ER undergoes a poorly defined conformational change, allowing it to interact with the other transcription factors and the basic transcription machinery, thereby altering the transcription of specific target genes. In the following sections we will detail the specific properties of the ER and highlight some of the experimental bases for this model.

STEROID/THYROID HORMONE RECEPTOR SUPERFAMILY

The ER is a member of a large family of nuclear receptor proteins called the steroid/thyroid hormone receptor superfamily, which has been the subject of many recent reviews.[12-16] These receptors are grouped into this family based on overall structural and specific sequence

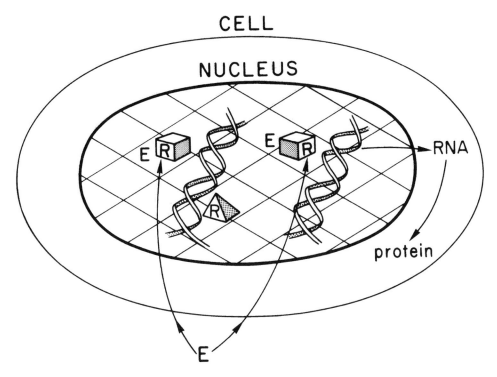

FIGURE 1. The basic model of estrogen action. R, receptor; E, estrogen; pyramid, unoccupied receptor; box, occupied receptor. (From Gorski, J. and Hansen, J.C., *Steroids*, 49, 461, 1987. With permission.)

similarity. The structure of the ER is shown in Figure 2. The overall structure for all members of the steroid/thyroid hormone receptor superfamily is very similar. They have a modular structure[16] containing an N-terminal transactivation domain (A/B domain), the length of which varies significantly between members of the superfamily; a DNA binding domain (C domain); a hinge region (D domain); a ligand binding domain (E domain); and a region at the C terminus of unknown function (F domain). Other members of this steroid receptor family include the progesterone (PR), androgen (AR), glucocorticoid (GR), mineralocorticoid (MR), and vitamin D (VDR) receptors. Cloning of the complementary DNAs (cDNA) encoding these receptors caused rapid advancement in our understanding of their structure and function, but also allowed for the isolation and identification of other genes encoding proteins that have structural and sequence similarity.[13,16] The thyroid hormone (TR) and retinoic acid receptors (RAR and RXR) were found to be related, showing striking sequence similarity.[17,18] Other so-called "orphan receptors" have also been identified that share homology with this family of receptors. They are referred to as orphan receptors because their ligands have not yet been identified. Members of this class of nuclear receptors include COUP, c-erb A, and many others (see review in Ref. 19). In fact, it has been estimated that about 50 such receptors exist.[19] It is possible that some of the orphan receptors may not actually be true receptors and therefore do not have specific ligands. However, because many receptors share high sequence similarity in the ligand binding domains with the other members of the superfamily, it seems likely that in most cases a ligand is required for function.

The entire gene encoding the ER receptor and most of the other steroid/thyroid hormone receptors have also been cloned.[20-23] A comparison of the genes for these receptors reveals a similar intron-exon structure, suggesting that they may have evolved from a common ancestor. The gene for the ER is greater than 140 kb and is encoded by 8 exons.[24] It is interesting that several of the specific functions of the steroid receptors are encoded by individual exons, which will be discussed in the coming sections.

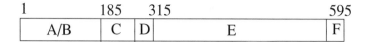

Domain	Associated Function
A/B	Transcriptional Activation (TAF 1) Protein-Protein Interactions
C	DNA Sequence Recognition DNA Binding Dimerization
D	Dimerization Nuclear Location
E	Ligand Binding Transcriptional Activation (TAF 2) Bind Sites for HSP 90 Nuclear Location Dimerization
F	Transcriptional Activation?

FIGURE 2. The modular structure of the ER and functions that have been associated with the regions.

The N-terminal A/B domain varies the most among superfamily members. It ranges in size from 25 amino acids (VDR) to 603 amino acids (MR).[16] The A/B domain in the ER is 185 amino acids and is encoded almost entirely by exon 1. This region is the least well-characterized region of the steroid receptors. One associated function is a transcripton activation factor (TAF).[25-28] In the ER this TAF, called TAF 1, is a constitutive transcriptional activator, which is tissue specific, functioning only in certain cell lines. Related to the transactivating activity, the N-terminal A/B domain is also involved in protein-protein interactions with specific transcription factors (see Ref. 29), thereby facilitating the transactivation activity of the receptor. This will be discussed further in a later section.

The other domains of these receptors are much more highly conserved and better characterized. The DNA binding domain (DBD) of the steroid receptors is the most highly conserved region among superfamily members and is absolutely required for transcriptional activation.[25] It is 66 to 68 amino acids long; in the ER it has 66 amino acids. This region of the ER binds to a specific 15-bp palindromic sequence termed the estrogen response element (ERE), AGGTCANNNTGACCT.[30] Crystal structure and footprint analysis suggest that the ER binds to the ERE as a homodimer.[30,31] However, unlike the vitellogenin ERE, almost all other identified EREs are not perfect palindromes, but rather contain one intact half site of AGGTCA with the other half site having one or more differences from the consensus. The ER can still bind these sequences, in some cases with properties similar to a homodimer and in other cases with different properties.[32-34] This suggests that the ER may not always bind to the DNA as a homodimer. This also will be discussed in detail later in the chapter.

The DBD in the ER contains nine invariant cysteine residues that are involved in the formation of two zinc finger-like structures. Interestingly, these are encoded by separate exons, exons 2 and 3. The two zinc fingers can also be separated into two functional subregions termed CI and CII. CI contains the first zinc finger, directly interacts with specific DNA sequences termed the hormone response element (HRE), and is involved in recognition of these sequences. Both the solution and crystal structure of the DBD of the ER have confirmed that the CI region contacts the DNA in the major groove.[31,35] The C terminus of the first zinc finger and the linker region between the two zinc coordination sites forms an α helix. Four amino acids in this helix (glu-203, lys-206, lys-210, and arg-211) directly hydrogen bond with the middle 4 bp of an ERE half site. Site-directed mutagenesis studies demonstrated that changing three amino acids on the C-terminal side of this first zinc finger in the ER to the corresponding three amino acids of the GR was sufficient to make the ER recognize the glucocorticoid response element (GRE) sequence instead of the ERE.[36] The second zinc finger, which is in the CII subregion, is involved in homodimer and probably heterodimer formation. Crystal structural analysis of the DBD revealed that three amino acids in the second zinc finger interact directly with a second DBD in homodimer formation. These data correspond well with the solution and crystal structure analysis of the GR DBD.[37,38]

The D or hinge region is also highly conserved among the nuclear receptors. This is part of the functional CII region that contains the second zinc finger, mentioned earlier. Therefore, one function of the hinge region is protein-protein interactions in homodimer and also probably heterodimer formation as well. The hinge region also contains the nuclear location signal (NLS) for many of the superfamily members, including the ER.[39-41] A more detailed analysis of the NLS is given in a later section.

The C-terminal ligand binding domain is also highly conserved among members of the receptor superfamily. As its name implies, one of the functions of this domain is ligand binding. The ligand binding domain is required for ligand-dependent transcription and this activity can be communicated by an amphipathic helix present in the protein. When the ligand binding domain of the GR is moved from the C terminus of the protein to the N terminus, ligand-dependent transcription is still achieved. Although it is clear that this domain of the protein is involved in ligand binding, the specific amino acids involved are not well defined. The affinity labeling compounds, E_2 aziridine and tamoxifen aziridine, both label the ER at cys-530, suggesting that this residue resides in the ligand binding pocket.[42] The neighboring amino acids of cys-530 may also be involved in ligand binding. Mutations of both lys-529 and -531 to glutamines reduce the affinity of the receptor for E_2.[43] Other amino acids in this region have also been associated with ligand binding, namely gly-525, met-521, and ser-522.[44] However, mutations in many parts of the ligand binding domain alter ligand interactions.[45] This suggests that the overall conformation of the ligand binding domain is critical for ligand interaction. Further research is needed to identify the amino acids in the ligand binding pocket of the ER and those that specifically interact with the ligand.

The ligand binding domain has several other specific functions. One of these is a second transcription activation function (TAF 2). TAF 2 requires amino acids 538–552 in the ER for function and differs from TAF 1 in that it is ligand dependent and functions in all cell types that have been examined, including yeast.[25,27,46,47] Moreover, TAF 1 and TAF 2 can act independently or synergistically to activate transcription.[28,48] In addition to TAF 2 in the ligand binding domain of the ER, another region has been identified that demonstrates constitutive transactivation activity in yeast.[49] This region, located between amino acids 302 and 339, is highly conserved among steroid receptors. Moreover, the corresponding region of the GR has been shown to have transactivating activity.[50] Another function of this region is protein-protein interactions of the receptor in dimerization[51] and in interactions with transcription factors, heat shock proteins (hsp90 and hsp70), and other unidentified proteins. Further analysis of these interactions is detailed in a later section.

ESTROGEN RECEPTOR IS A NUCLEAR PROTEIN
IN THE ABSENCE OF STEROID

Where the steroid/thyroid receptors reside in the cell when the ligand is not present is an area of contention among many researchers. There are some receptors in this family that have very high affinity for the nucleus in the absence of their ligand and for which there is little doubt regarding their subcellular location. These represent one extreme in this family and include the TR and retinoic acid receptor. At the other end of the spectrum and perhaps the most controversial regarding its location when unoccupied is the GR. Many groups have reported finding the GR in the cytoplasm when unliganded and is only found in the nucleus after it binds its ligand.[52,53] However, there are also many other studies that indicate the GR is localized in the nucleus even when unliganded.[54-56] A review of the current literature related to steroid receptor location was published recently and readers should consult this reference for further information on this topic.[57] The affinity of the ER for the nucleus when unliganded lies between these two extremes. Early experiments showed that extracts made with hypotonic solution from tissues not exposed to estrogen had ER in the cytosolic fraction. However, when estrogen was added to the cells prior to preparation of the cytosol, ER could not be extracted with low ionic strength buffer. Rather, high ionic strength buffer (0.6 M NaCl) was required to extract the receptor from the nucleus.[58] This is true for most, if not all, the steroid receptors. This was initially interpreted to indicate that the receptor is a cytosolic protein when unoccupied and is translocated to the nucleus upon addition of estrogen (or other ligand for the other receptors), where it then exerts its control on gene transcription. These experiments provided the basis for the translocation step in the two-step model of estrogen action. However, in 1984 this view of the ER changed, and for most other steroid receptors shortly thereafter as well. With two different techniques, it was clearly demonstrated that the receptor was a nuclear protein even in the absence of the steroid ligand. Welshons et al.[59] used enucleation with cytoclasin D to show that most of the receptor was located in the nucleoplast, whereas the cytoplast contained very low levels of ER. The same conclusion was reached using immunocytochemical staining with antibodies specific for the ER.[60,61] There is now evidence indicating that all the members of this family of receptors are nuclear proteins even when the ligand is absent.[55,56] This concept is fairly well accepted for most of the nuclear receptors, with the principal exception of the GR.

NUCLEAR LOCATION SIGNALS

The steroid receptors have specific amino acid sequences that direct them into the nucleus and keep them there. These sequences consist primarily of basic amino acids located in the receptors' hinge region. This region has a similar sequence to the NLS for the SV40 large T antigen[62] and is present in all nuclear receptors including the ER. That this sequence functions as an NLS was first demonstrated with the GR and was extended to demonstrate the presence of the sequence in ER and PR.[39-41] When amino acids 256–303 were fused with β-galactosidase (a nonnuclear protein), the chimeric protein localized to the nucleus.[40] More recent studies have identified three protonuclear location signals between amino acids 256 and 303.[41] These three protonuclear location signals cooperate to localize the ER to the nucleus; they are not sufficient individually. In addition, an estrogen-inducible NLS has also been identified. This sequence was detected when the three constitutive NLS sequences were deleted. It should be noted that DNA binding is not required to localize the ER in the nucleus. ER mutants created by deleting the DBD were still located in the nucleus.[41]

CONFORMATIONAL EFFECTS OF LIGANDS

ESTROGENS AND ANTIESTROGENS

Although the ER requires estrogen to regulate transcription, the functional effect of estrogen binding to its receptor is a matter of debate.[63] The ER, when extracted from tissues into a low ionic strength cytosol, is found in a complex with hsp90 and other heat shock proteins and/or chaperonins. It is unlikely that this complex exists within the cell because ERs are found in the nucleus (see previous sections), whereas hsp90 is exclusively cytoplasmic.[64,65] The ER cannot bind to DNA *in vitro* until it is released from this complex. The binding of estrogen to its receptor has been thought to cause release from heat shock proteins and induction of dimerization *in vivo*, leading to DNA binding of the receptor. A further conformational difference must exist between estrogen-ER and antiestrogen-ER complexes, because some antiestrogens still allow the receptor to bind to DNA *in vivo*[66] while blocking transcriptional activation. Several studies show that unoccupied ERs can also bind to DNA *in vivo*,[66-68] thereby requiring a model in which the receptor is bound to DNA in the absence of ligand, and estrogens simply cause a conformational change that allows the receptor to activate transcription.

A common element between these models is that transcription activation by the ER requires a conformational change brought about by estrogen binding. Fortunately, there is ample evidence to show that estrogen or antiestrogen binding changes the conformation of the receptor from the unbound state. It has also been shown that the various conformations of the receptor bound to estrogens and antiestrogens are different. A review by Nelson et al.[69] is a good source for older references on this subject.

Aqueous two-phase partitioning is a sensitive method for detecting conformational changes in proteins. The distribution of a protein between two aqueous polymer solutions is measured under varying conditions, and a change in distribution indicates a change in conformation. The application of this technique to steroid receptors was recently reviewed.[70] Hansen and Gorski[71] used an aqueous two-phase partitioning system containing polyethylene glycol (PEG) and dextran to show that the conformation of the ER from rat uterine cytosol was considerably altered after binding to the estrogen 17β-E_2 or the antiestrogen 4-hydroxy-tamoxifen (4-OHT) (Table 1). For further characterization of this conformational change, PEG-palmitate was substituted for PEG to make one phase more hydrophobic than the other. The unbound ER preferred the hydrophobic PEG-palmitate phase, whereas receptors bound to estrogen or antiestrogen were primarily found in the dextran phase, indicating that ligand binding reduces the hydrophobicity of the ER protein surface. If the cytosol is incubated with ligand at $4°C$, there is a large difference between the partitioning of the E_2-ER complex and the 4-OHT-ER complex. This difference is not due simply to the nonsteroidal nature of 4-OHT, however, because receptor bound to diethylstilbestrol (DES), a nonsteroidal estrogen, partitions similarly to receptor bound to E_2. Heating the ligand-ER complex to $30°C$ is believed to cause dissociation of the associated heat shock proteins. This treatment caused further changes in the partitioning behavior of the ligand-receptor complexes. However, after heating there was little difference between the partition coefficients of receptors bound to E_2 or 4-OHT.

Fritsch et al.[72] used two methods to show that the decrease in hydrophobicity is a property of the ligand binding domain of the ER. The ligand binding domain alone was produced in *Escherichia coli* or released from the N-terminal half of the rat uterine receptor by proteolysis. In both cases, PEG-palmitate/dextran partitioning showed that the hydrophobic surface of the ligand binding domain is dramatically reduced upon binding either E_2 or 4-OHT, whereas differences between both ligand-occupied forms are small. Heated ERs also showed a decrease in hydrophobicity upon binding ligands, thus proving that the change in hydrophobicity is a property of the ER ligand binding domain and is not caused by dissociation of associated proteins in response to ligand binding.

Recent proteolysis studies by Beekman et al.[73] provide further evidence of a conformational change between unbound and ligand-occupied ERs. *In vitro* translated ER was radioactively labeled and subjected to proteolysis. In the presence of estrogens or antiestrogens, a large piece of the ER was somewhat protected from proteolysis whereas the unoccupied ER was quickly digested. There was also a difference in fragment sizes protected by estrogens

TABLE 1
Partition Coefficients of Estrogen Receptor and
Antiestrogen Receptor Complexes

ER Form	PEG 1[a]		PEG 2[b]	
	17β-E_2	4-OHT	17β-E_2	DES
		K_{obs}[c]		
Unoccupied	1.09 ± 0.03	1.14 ± 0.20	0.94 ± 0.09	0.93 ± 0.09
	(10)	(10)	(8)	(12)
Nontransformed	0.54 ± 0.02	0.91 ± 0.06	0.48 ± 0.05	0.39 ± 0.02
	(16)	(12)	(8)	(12)
Transformed	0.09 ± 0.01	0.05 ± 0.02	0.05 ± 0.01	0.05 ± 0.01
	(13)	(13)	(8)	(12)

[a] PEG 8000 was obtained from Sigma.
[b] PEG 8000 was obtained from Koch-Light.
[c] Values represent the mean ± SE of partitionings performed in 5.4% dextran, 5.4% PEG, 0.1 M Li_2SO_4 phase systems buffered with TED, pH 8.0.

From Hansen, J.C., and Gorski, J., *J. Biol. Chem.*, 261, 13990, 1986. With permission.

and antiestrogens, with estrogens protecting a larger fragment. Deletion of the extreme C terminus of the ligand binding domain caused the peptides protected by both ligands to be equal in size. Therefore, the authors hypothesized that the conformation of the C terminus of the receptor is important for activation of transcription upon estrogen binding, whereas antiestrogens do not bring about the proper conformation in this region.

Another finding that suggests a modest conformational difference between ERs bound to different ligands is their migration pattern during a gel mobility shift assay. Numerous investigators have observed that when bound to estrogen, the receptor runs slightly faster than when bound to an antiestrogen, probably reflecting a difference in the shapes of the ER-ligand-ERE complexes.[43,44,74-76] The unoccupied receptor consistently has been observed to run intermediate between the other species. Sabbah et al.[76] provided convincing evidence that this change in mobility is due only to noncovalent binding of ligands: heating of E_2 occupied receptor in the presence of a large excess of ICI164,384 (ICI) or vice versa allowed ligand exchange to occur, and a corresponding change in mobility was observed. Interestingly, various mutations in the C-terminal part of the ligand binding domain can eradicate this phenomenon, providing further evidence that this region may be a site of important conformational differences between estrogen- and antiestrogen-occupied receptors.[43,44]

The studies discussed above have analyzed the overall physical properties of the receptor. Additional evidence for the existence of important differences between estrogen-occupied and antiestrogen-occupied receptors comes from site-directed mutagenesis and protein modification experiments. These show that although estrogens and antiestrogens presumably occupy the same hydrophobic pocket, they also interact differentially with some regions of the ligand binding domain.

Borgna and Scali[77] modified ER in lamb uterine cytosols with diethylpyrocarbonate (DEPC) before incubation using different ligands. DEPC-modified receptors showed a slightly reduced affinity for 4-OHT, but they had a much reduced affinity for E_2 and DES. Removal of the 17β hydroxyl group from E_2 produced a ligand that had similar affinity for wild type and DEPC-modified ER. DES contains a hydroxyl group that corresponds to the 17β hydroxyl of E_2, whereas 4-OHT has no corresponding hydroxyl. Thus, the residue modified by DEPC may play a role in the discrimination between estrogens and antiestrogens.

Site-directed mutagenic analysis has identified amino acids that are important for binding to estrogens but not to antiestrogens. Alteration of lysines 529 and 531 in the C terminus of the human ER ligand binding domain to glutamine produces a double mutant with reduced affinity for E_2, but affinity for 4-OHT is not affected.[43] When this receptor was tested for transcription activation in cells, much lower concentrations of antiestrogens were able to block estrogen-activated transcription as compared with the wild-type receptor. Mutation of an adjacent asparagine residue enhanced this effect. Danielian et al.[44] found several mutations in the same region of the mouse ER that severely reduced estrogen binding but did not reduce the partial agonist activity of 4-OHT.

The studies noted above demonstrated differences in the overall properties of the steroid binding domain upon binding to estrogens or antiestrogens. The C-terminal end of the ligand binding domain has been implicated in the discrimination between these two classes of ligands, although other regions of this domain may also be involved.

SPECIFIC DNA SEQUENCES

Estrogens and antiestrogens are not the only ligands that can alter the conformation of the ER. Binding of the receptor to its response element causes changes in both the DNA and the protein. An ER DBD peptide bends the DNA containing the ERE to an angle of 34°,[78] whereas the full-length ER produces a 56° bend.[79] The structure of the DBD of the ER has been described for the monomer peptide by nuclear magnetic resonance spectroscopy[35] and for the dimer bound to a consensus response element by X-ray crystallography.[31] Similar structural studies on the GR DBD preceded those for the ER DBD.[37,38] A comparison of the structures of the DBD free and bound to a response element shows that DNA binding changes the conformation of a region in the second zinc-binding motif. This region forms a dimerization interface between the two DBD peptides when they are bound to the response element. Thus, DNA binding and dimerization of the DBD peptide are coupled through a change in peptide conformation.

The domains of steroid receptors were shown to be functionally independent, although removal of the steroid binding domain reduces the affinity of the ER for a consensus ERE.[51] In addition, binding of the ER to a response element may produce a change in the ligand binding domain in addition to its previously mentioned effect on the DBD. Fritsch et al.[80] detected an increase in the dissociation rate of E_2 from rat uterine ER in response to specific DNA binding (Figure 3). Rat uterine cytosol was incubated with either an oligonucleotide containing the consensus ERE from the *Xenopus* vitellogenin A2 gene or a mutant of this sequence, which has about 1000-fold lower affinity for the ER.[63] The amount of oligonucleotide added was enough to saturate the receptor with the consensus ERE, but almost no receptor was bound to the mutant sequence under these conditions. The rate of E_2 dissociation from the receptor was faster in the presence of the consensus ERE than in the presence of the mutated ERE or no ERE, showing that this difference in estrogen binding was not merely due to the presence of DNA.

SUBUNIT COMPOSITION

Some of the most controversial aspects of ER action are the multimeric states of the receptor found in solution and bound to DNA, and the effect of ligands on these states. While the receptor has been shown to bind as a homodimer to a sequence for which it has high affinity, most EREs exhibit some modification to this sequence; therefore, we must consider the possibility that the ER may have more than one mode of DNA binding.

The sequence to which the ER binds with highest affinity contains two AGGTCA sites as an inverted repeat with a 3-bp spacer. The ER has been shown to bind to this sequence as a homodimer by gel shift assays,[75] and a symmetrical DNA footprint was found when the ER was bound to this sequence.[81] Dominant negative mutants of the ER have been identified that may act by forming dimers with wild-type receptors.[82] The crystal structure of the DBD

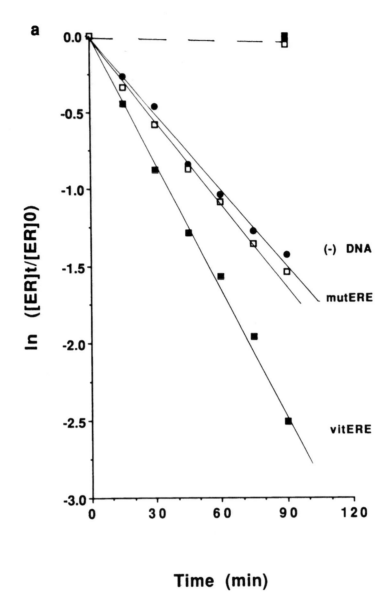

FIGURE 3. Dissociation kinetics of estrogen from the ER in the absence and presence of DNA. (**a**) Rat uterine cytosolic ER occupied with [³H]estradiol in TKM buffer was placed at 28°C for varying amounts of time either in the presence of 3 μM DES (solid lines) or in the absence of DES (dashed lines) with no DNA (closed circles), 20 nM mutERE (open squares) or 20 nM vitERE (closed squares). (**b**) The experiment was performed as in (**a**), except ER was occupied with [³H]E₃ and dissociation performed at 4°C for the indicated times. (From Fritsch et al., *J. Biol. Chem.*, 267, 1823, 1992. With permission.)

of the ER bound to the consensus ERE showed that two ER DBD peptides could bind and interact with each other on the consensus ERE.[31] The structural data on DNA binding are incomplete at present. The peptide used for the crystal structure has a much lower affinity for the ERE than it does for the full-length receptor. The addition of part of the ER's hinge region to this peptide reduces the dissociation rate of the receptor from the ERE considerably, indicating that important protein-protein or protein-DNA interactions have not yet been identified.[83] Also, the difference in the DNA bending angles induced by the ER DBD alone and the full-length ER[79] suggests that other domains of the ER contribute to DNA bending

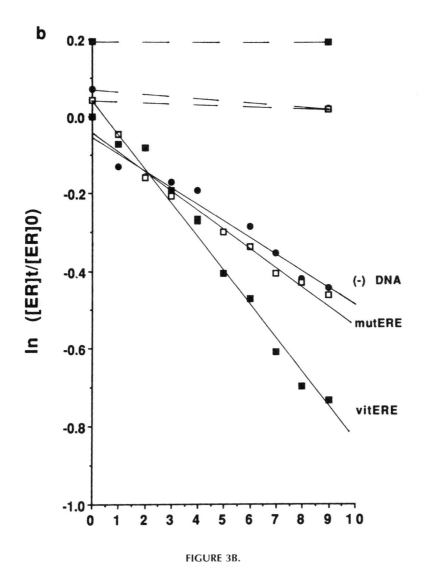

FIGURE 3B.

by influencing the interaction of the DBD with DNA or by contacting the DNA themselves. A full understanding requires the structure of the entire ER bound to an ERE.

Furlow et al.[84] sought to measure the amount of estrogen and consensus ERE bound by rat uterine ER saturated with both ligands. For this purpose, a DNA-receptor immunoprecipitation (DRIP) assay was developed in which ER was incubated with estrogen and an oligonucleotide containing the consensus ERE before precipitation with an anti-ER antibody and protein A-agarose beads. In multiple experiments, the ratio of estrogen to ERE was found to be about 1:1, suggesting that ER monomers or heterodimers represented the DNA-binding species in the experimental conditions used. Thus, dimerization may not be required for ER binding, even to the consensus ERE.

Most EREs contain at least one mutation from the consensus sequence, reducing the binding affinity for the receptor severalfold. Homodimers of ER have been shown to bind to the two nonconsensus EREs from the *Xenopus* vitellogenin B1 gene.[34] Gel shift assays have shown that other nonconsensus EREs form complexes with the ER identical in mobility to that of the consensus ERE.[32,85] In some cases, EREs having multiple mutations in one of the half sites appear to bind two species of ER, which could represent monomers and dimers (ERE Mut in Ref. 33, E2m1 and E2m4 in Ref. 86).

Some EREs have been identified that consist merely of half sites. Kato et al.[33] found that an upstream region of the chicken ovalbumin gene contained several AGGTCA sequences separated by at least 100 bp from each other. Estrogen was able to regulate gene expression from this region in HeLa cells when human ER was cotransfected, and mutation of any one of these half sites reduced gene expression. When gel shift assays were performed with these nonconsensus ERE sites, no band was seen that corresponded to an ER dimer unless an antibody was added, but a band corresponding to a lower molecular weight species was seen consistently. This band was eliminated when an antibody against the ER was present, suggesting that it represents a monomer or heterodimer of the receptor.

Dimerization of the ER on an ERE could proceed by two different pathways: either the receptor dimerizes before binding to the ERE or one monomer binds to DNA and is then stabilized by the binding of another monomer. The latter case has been observed for truncated PRs[87] and the DBDs of the GR[38,88] and ER,[31] indicating that dimerization is not a prerequisite for DNA binding. The gel shift results discussed above suggest this may also be the case for the full-length ER.

In solution, ERs have been reported to undergo dimerization upon binding estrogens as measured by cooperativity of estrogen binding.[89] Cooperativity was not observed immediately upon binding of estrogen, suggesting that the receptor was monomeric before it bound E_2. ER dimerization in the absence of an ERE was found to occur within the hormone binding domain,[51,75,90] which has very different properties in the unoccupied and ligand-occupied states (discussed in another section). Dimerization within this domain would therefore likely be influenced by the presence or absence of a ligand as well as the type of ligand. Concentration requirements for ER dimerization under these various conditions have not been determined. Hopefully, experiments using overexpressed and purified receptors will answer this important question.

The effect of estrogen and antiestrogen binding on the ability of the receptor to bind to DNA has been quite a controversial subject. Initially, Kumar and Chambon[75] reported that the ER requires estrogen for DNA binding, which was attributed to the induction of ER dimerization by estrogen. The receptor used in this study was subsequently found to have a point mutation that renders its estrogen-binding activity unstable in the absence of a ligand.[91] Since then many groups have shown that unoccupied ERs can bind to EREs *in vitro* with identical affinity to estrogen- or antiestrogen-occupied ERs (see Ref. 84, or review in Ref. 92). This occurs even at the low concentrations found in rat uterine cytosols. Unoccupied receptors have also been shown to bind to EREs *in vivo* by cross-linking and transcription interference studies.[66-68] Therefore, both *in vitro* and *in vivo*, the unoccupied ER is able to bind to an ERE, implying that either dimerization is occurring on the DNA, as shown for the DBD alone, or the unoccupied ER is able to dimerize under the conditions of these experiments. Currently, this issue is not settled.

ESTROGEN RECEPTOR INTERACTIONS

ESTROGEN RECEPTOR-CHROMATIN INTERACTION

The ER is a ligand-dependent transcriptional factor. As such, its ultimate action results in modulating transcription of specific genes. During transcription there is an ordered assembling of basic transcriptional factors (TF) on the promoter, resulting in the formation of an initiation component complex. This process begins with TF IID (a TATA-binding protein) binding to the TATA element in the promoter. Once TF IID binds to the DNA, TF IIB can then interact with this complex. This then interacts with RNA polymerase II and TF IIF. The final initiation complex is formed when TF IIE and TF IIH bind.[93,94] This assembly constitutes a complete transcriptional complex that is sufficient for basal level transcription.

As mentioned earlier, the ER modulates transcription by binding to its ERE, which is present in certain genes. These response elements are typically located at varying distances from the promoter. The degree to which ER modulates transcription depends on the gene, the promoter content, and cellular factors. The ability of the ER to regulate transcription from EREs located either 5′ or 3′ to the promoter and at distances 200 to 2000 bp away from the promoter (typical of enhancer sequences) suggests that the ER may be capable of regulating transcription via several mechanisms.

Figure 4 depicts our current view of how the ER regulates transcription. This model suggests that the ER's ability to regulate transcription may involve two mutually inclusive mechanisms.[11] In the first mechanism, the receptor interacts with chromatin, which alters the chromatin structure around specific genes. This results in a change in the transcription rate of these genes. The second mechanism would require an interaction between the ER and the basal transcription factor and/or accessory proteins.

The effect of chromatin structure on estrogen-dependent transcription remains controversial. Several investigators have reported that the chromatin around the ER-responsive gene is disrupted in an E_2-dependent manner, whereas others report that the mere binding of ER produces this effect.[95-97] Seyfred and Gorski[168] cloned the 5′ regulatory region of the prolactin (PRL) gene into the bovine papilloma virus (BPV) and stably transfected this chimera into GH_3 cells. This system was used as a model to study the effect of chromatin structure on estrogen-dependent transcription. Seyfred et al.[97] showed that the chromatin around the regions containing the EREs are altered following estrogen treatment, as revealed by increased DNase I sensitivity. Both E_2 and 4-OHT induced this alteration in the chromatin around the distal region of the PRL promoter. However, only E_2 was able to render the PRL promoter region hypersensitive to DNase I. The distal enhancer of the PRL gene contains two EREs at −1721 and −1581 bp relative to the promoter. This region is separated from the promoter by seven nucleosomes. Because the promoter of the PRL gene does not contain an ERE, the alteration in the chromatin at the promoter following estrogen administration may be facilitated by the interaction of the ER with the general transcriptional complex. This will be discussed further in another section.

Additional evidence that estrogens alter chromatin structure was provided by studies of Gilbert and colleagues.[95] Using a yeast cell containing an estrogen-responsive reporter gene, they were able to demonstrate an E_2-dependent alteration in the chromatin surrounding the reporter gene. Addition of E_2 to the system resulted in an increase in both ER-dependent transcription and DNase I hypersensitivity of the gene, demonstrating that the change in chromatin resulted from estrogen action. Although they were able to demonstrate the effect of E_2 on chromatin, when a mutant ER that does not bind E_2 was used in the assay, there was a low level of DNase hypersensitivity in the promoter. These data suggest that the binding of ER alone is sufficient to alter chromatin structure.

The regulation of the PRL gene illustrates the ER's ability to modulate transcription via chromatin alteration when the ERE is more than 1.5 kb from the promoter. However, ER can alter the chromatin when it is a few hundred base pairs away from the promoter, which was demonstrated by the *Xenopus* vitellogen B1 gene. This gene contains an ERE in a nucleosome-free region at −300 bp relative to the promoter. Schild et al.,[98] using reconstituted chromatin, demonstrated the existence of a positional nucleosome between the ERE and the promoter. Deletion of the region where the nucleosome is bound or an alteration in its position (i.e., packaging into nucleosomes) leads to a 10-fold increase in estrogen-dependent transcription of the B1 gene.

There are many other reports in the literature of ER and other regulatory proteins, such as GR, HSP 26, and yeast PHO5, altering the chromatin structure of their target genes.[99-101] It thus appears that chromatin alteration is a common mechanism for the regulation of certain genes. What remains unclear is how the ER induces these chromatin alterations and how these changes lead to transcription regulation. It is possible that the ER's effect on chromatin

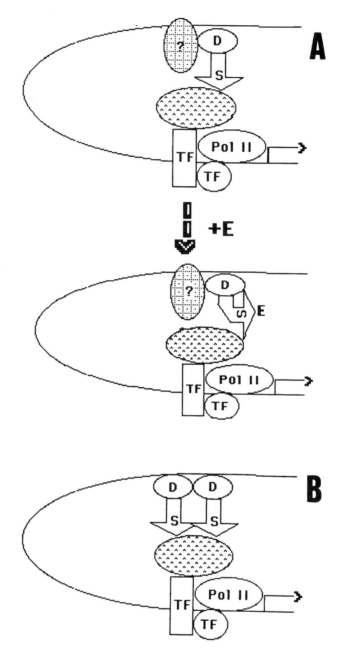

FIGURE 4. Models of estrogen and ER action. (**A**) New model. D, DNA binding domain of the ER; S, steroid binding domain of the ER; E, estrogen; Pol II, RNA polymerase II; TF, transcription factors; arrow, site of initiation. (**B**) Old model. (From Gorski et al., *Biol. Reprod.*, 48, 8, 1993. With permissionp.)

involves both local and global phenomena. When the ER binds the DNA, it causes a local bending of the DNA.[78,102] Such bending may, although there is no direct evidence, contribute to more global changes in the chromatin. Once the chromatin is "open," it then may become more accessible to other transcription factors or other proteins involved in transcription. Thus, ER and other steroid receptors induce alterations in chromatin structure, which lead to an increase in transcription by allowing a critical interaction of the receptor and some component of the transcriptional machinery.

ESTROGEN RECEPTOR PROTEIN-PROTEIN INTERACTIONS

It is generally agreed that chromatin alteration (looping and/or bending) results in a positioning of factors that are in close proximity to each other.[101] In this position, the ER and other steroid receptors are able to communicate with the general transcriptional machinery through protein-protein interactions by binding with other transcription factors. Identification of these factors, or so-called "coactivators," has been the subject of extensive investigation. In many cases, these factors are both tissue and gene specific. These proteins may be associated with the receptor prior to activation of transcription or form complexes with the receptor during activation. Which proteins or transactivators are associated with the ER during transcription? Are they common to all ER-responsive genes? Do all ER-responsive genes use the same bridging proteins?

In an attempt to answer these questions, investigators have begun to identify proteins that are associated (or function in conjunction) with the steroid receptors. It is generally accepted that only the hormone receptor and its DNA binding site (HRE) are required for transcription. However, *in vitro* transcription assays have indicated that for maximum transcription to occur, components other than the receptor are involved. One cellular component associated with steroid receptors is the group stress proteins, referred to as heat shock proteins (hsp). All the steroid receptors have been reported to be associated with one form of hsp.[103,104] In the absence of ligand and under low ionic conditions, the ER (PR and GR as well) is found in a complex with an hsp90 protein and is unable to bind DNA. The role of hsp in ER function is not clear. It appears that hsp associates with steroid receptors in the absence of ligand *in vitro*. This association results in an inactive receptor that is incapable of binding to DNA. The binding of ligand to the ER results in dissociation of hsp90 and the conversion of the receptor to an active state.[105] This view, however, is inconsistent with much of the current literature.

If the role of hsp90 is to block the ER's ability to bind DNA until ligand is bound, it follows that the ER would bind to DNA only in the presence of ligand. However, this is not the case. As mentioned earlier, it has been demonstrated that the ER is capable of binding DNA in the presence or absence of ligand under both *in vitro* and *in vivo* conditions.[63] Likewise, there have been no reports of an hsp90-ER-DNA complex or of hsp found in the nucleus of an estrogen-responsive cell. Recently, immunocytochemical data indicated that although the PR is localized primarily in the nucleus, anti-hsp90-reactive antigens are localized exclusively in the cytosol. Thus, it appears unlikely that the association of the steroid receptor and the hsp is to modulate DNA binding.

Most reports in the literature have assessed an inhibitory role to the steroid-heat shock protein interaction. Picard et al.[103] used an *in vivo* yeast system to determine the functional relevance of the steroid-heat shock protein interaction. When the ER was expressed (GR as well) in a yeast strain in which the levels of hsp82 (the yeast homologue of hsp90) could be regulated, this group found no enhancement of transcription when ER and GR were free of hsp. Transcription was enhanced to a small degree upon addition of hormone. Furthermore, the hormonal activation by the ER and GR depended on hsp82 expression levels. This experiment demonstrated that hsp is not essential for suppression of transcription when hormone is absent. These results suggest an alternative role for hsp in steroid action.

Thus, the findings of Picard et al.[103] suggest a possible physiological role for the heat shock protein family. An alternative role for hsp is supported by the fact that the ER makes several different contacts with hsp90, indicating that the ER may still be able bind to DNA and/or hormone in the presence of hsp90.[106] Based on the available data, it seems likely that hsp90 does interact with the ER, but a direct role in ER activation appears unlikely. Hsp90 has been shown to function as a chaperone. Therefore, one possible physiological function of the hsp90-ER association and other steroid hormone receptors could be to stabilize the receptor or to maintain it in an active conformation. Alternatively, heat shock protein function may be to shuttle newly synthesized receptor into the nucleus and then to maintain this equilibrium.

In addition to hsp, other proteins are reported to be associated with the ER.[107,108] Halacchmi et al.[109] isolated a 160-kDa ER-associated protein (ERAP160) from MCF-7 cells. Using an *in vitro* protein affinity assay, they were able to demonstrate the association of this protein with the ER. Moreover, this interaction was dependent upon E_2. The association occurred specifically when estrogen was added to the cells. The antiestrogen tamoxifen was unable to promote the association. It was proposed that the ERAP160 may be involved in E_2-dependent transactivation by the ER. The presence of an ER-associated protein is consistent with the hypothesis that other proteins (coactivators) are involved in ER modulation of transcription. However, the effect of this protein (ERAP160) on ER-dependent transcription was not examined. Therefore, a determination of ERAP160 function (if any) awaits further analysis.

That the steroid receptors interact with other proteins to promote their activity is further supported by analysis of partially purified receptors. Some steroid receptors lose their ability to form complexes with DNA when they are purified. This observation led to the identification of a DNA binding stimulatory factor (DBSF) in both mammalian and yeast nuclear extracts.[14,110] This DBSF associates with the ER and has been purified from yeast.[110] It is a 40-kDa single-stranded DBP that increases (~8- to 10-fold) binding of the purified ER to DNA.[110] The ability of DBSF to stimulate ER-DNA binding may in some way result in transactivation of the receptor. Although ER-DBSF is present in both yeast and mammalian cells, its involvement in transcription has not been determined. In light of the known ER-DBSF stimulatory effect, it is possible that the ER-DBSF is a coactivator for ER transcription.

The tissue-specific pituitary factor 1 (Pit-1) appears to be a coactivator (bridging factor) for the ER on the PRL gene. The distal enhancer region (HSII site) of the PRL gene contains two EREs that can confer estrogen regulation of this gene.[111] This enhancer region also contains four binding sites for Pit-1, as well as sites for two or three other unidentified proteins. Induction of PRL transcription by estrogen requires both the ER and Pit-1.[112] Estrogen induction of PRL gene transcription is reduced to below basal level either by elimination of the Pit-1 binding site or the destruction of Pit-1 by mutation. This implies that both the ER and Pit-1 proteins are required to increase PRL gene transcription. Although a direct interaction of Pit-1 and ER has not been detected, it is clear that both proteins are needed for estrogen-dependent PRL gene transcription.[112,113] Cullen et al.[114] used a recyclization assay to demonstrate that the distal enhancer region of the endogenous PRL gene is in contact with the promoter region, presumably by alteration of the chromatin structure. The recyclization assay requires that two ends of DNA are close enough together to be enzymatically joined by DNA ligase. This cyclization of DNA is a function of protein binding. When Seyfred et al.[97] applied this assay to the PRL gene, they were able to show that ER bound at the distal enhancer induces a change in the DNA that decreases the distance between the promoter and the distal enhancer, allowing DNA ligase to join the two regions of DNA. The decreased distance between the ERE and the promoter is presumed to occur via protein-protein interactions between these two regions.

The search for these bridging proteins has led investigators to the general TF. Both TF IID and TF IIB have been reported to be putative coactivators of ER-mediated transcription. The ER is able to associate with the TF IIB in *in vitro* assays.[115] This binding was restricted to the transcriptional activation function, AF 1, in the A/B domain of the ER. *In vitro* experiments have demonstrated that in addition to ER, TF IIB interacts with the TR, orphan receptor COUP-TF, the glutamine-rich activation domain of the fushi tarazu (Ftz) gene product, and C-Rel protein.[116] The association of TR with TF IIB is ligand dependent and has been proposed to be the mechanism responsible for transcriptional silencing by the receptor (see review in Ref. 117). Nevertheless, the functional relevance of the association of these hormone receptors with TF IIB is unknown.

Several laboratories have reported an association of steroid/thyroid hormone receptors with other transcription factors. Keaveney et al.[118] demonstrated that activation of gene transcription by the retinoic acid receptor is mediated through the interaction of a cell-specific,

E1A-like activity and the TATA-binding protein, a component of TF IID.[115,119] TF IID has been proposed to be a transactivator/coactivator because it interacts with the acidic activation domain of several viral enhancer proteins.[120]

The ability of the steroid/thyroid hormone receptors to interact with cellular proteins and members of the basal transcription factors indicates that direct protein-protein interactions may be responsible for the increased transcription rate. It is not known whether the binding of ER and other enhancer proteins to TF IIB or TF IID causes the TATA-binding protein to induce bending and unwinding of the promoter, thus leading to the initiation of transcription.[120] It is apparent that the different steroid receptor-coactivator protein complexes that form at the promoter are partially responsible for the differential regulation of transcription by the ER and other steroid receptors.

PHOSPHORYLATION OF THE ESTROGEN RECEPTOR

The ER, like the other steroid/thyroid hormone receptors, exists in cells as a phosphoprotein.[121] And, like the other steroid receptors, phosphorylation levels change upon ligand binding. Most of these receptors have been shown to be phosphorylated principally on serine residues (reviewed in Refs. 121 and 122). Somewhat surprisingly, however, early studies on the phosphorylation of the ER from calf uterine cytosols showed that the ER was phosphorylated exclusively on tyrosine residues.[121-124] Moreover, it was demonstrated that dephosphorylation of phosphotyrosine(s) inhibited the receptor's ability to bind estrogen, and if it was rephosphorylated with a cytosolic tyrosine kinase, ligand binding was restored.[125] A calf uterine tyrosine kinase was recently purified.[126] This kinase phosphorylated the phosphatase-treated ER in the HBD and activated its hormone binding. The activity of the kinase requires purified ER complex and Ca^{2+} calmodulin. Site-directed mutagenesis of the receptor demonstrated that tyr-537 in the ligand binding domain is a site of phosphorylation by this kinase, and substitution of the tyrosine with alanine inhibits both phosphorylation and hormone binding.

In sharp contrast to these findings are those from several other groups who do not detect phosphotyrosine, but rather phosphoserine in the ER.[127-130] In each of these studies the receptor was shown to have a basal level of phosphorylation that increased about fourfold upon estrogen treatment. The antiestrogens transhydroxytamoxifen (TOT) and ICI also increase the level of phosphorylation to the same extent. Although the results from each of these studies are similar in the overall increase in receptor phosphorylation, they differ regarding the number and location of the phosphorylation sites. Denton et al.[128] found only one major and two minor phosphopeptides upon tryptic digest of the receptor. Ali et al.[127] found several hormone-dependent phosphorylation sites in the A/B, D, and E regions of the ER. Finally, Le Goff et al.[129] demonstrated several phosphorylation sites in the A/B domain that were increased in phosphorylation when treated with hormone. They were also able to demonstrate that the increase in phosphorylation occurred at all of the major sites that were basally phosphorylated and that no new major phosphorylation sites appeared upon estrogen treatment. They used site-directed mutagenesis to show that ser-104 and/or ser-106 and ser-118 were major sites of phosphorylation in the A/B domain when treated with estrogen, TOT, and ICI. Interestingly, Ali et al.[127] also used site-directed mutagenesis and similarly showed that ser-118 was the major phosphoamino acid in the A/B domain. However, they did not find phosphorylation of either ser-104 or ser-106. In the PR, ser-530 was shown to be phosphorylated in a progesterone-dependent manner.[131] However, ser-294, the corresponding amino acid in the ER, was not found to be phosphorylated.[129] All the above sites have the sequence X-S-P-X, the preferred sequence motif of the proline-directed protein kinases. Similar sequences are found around the hormone-inducible phosphorylation sites in the PR[132] and in the GR, where four of seven phosphorylation sites show this sequence motif.[133] This suggests that the proline-directed protein kinase may be involved in regulating the activities of these receptors. Although progress is being made in this area, it is clear that there is no consensus regarding the location of specific phosphorylation sites in the ER.

Phosphorylation is one of the mechanisms by which cells control protein activity. The role of phosphorylation in controlling steroid receptor function remains unclear. Some evidence suggests that phosphorylation of tyrosine residues in the ligand binding domain of the ER is required for ligand binding, as mentioned above.[123-125] Other analyses suggest a role for phosphorylation in transcriptional activation by the receptor.[127-129] Phosphorylation of specific serine residues in the PR has been shown to control transcriptional activation.[132] Similar results have been obtained for the ER. Le Goff et al.[129] demonstrated that an ER mutant containing ala-104, -106, and -118 in place of serine showed a 60% reduction in transcriptional activation from an estrogen-responsive reporter gene in transient transfections. However, single mutations of ser-104, -106, or -118 to alanine caused only a 15% reduction of transcription in each case. Results from similar studies by Ali et al.[127] demonstrated that the transcriptional activation of three different estrogen-responsive reporter gene constructs in two different cell lines was reduced to 25–60% of the wild-type levels. This suggests that phosphorylation of ser-118 affects transcription in a promoter- and cell-specific manner, which is characteristic of TAF 1. Therefore, one factor that may be contributing to TAF 1 function might be whether ser-118 is phosphorylated. Again, additional research in this area will be required to fully understand the role of phosphorylation in steroid hormone receptor function.

LIGAND-INDEPENDENT TRANSCRIPTIONAL ACTIVATION

One of the most strongly held beliefs in the field of steroid hormone research has been that ligand is required for transcriptional activation. However, this idea was recently challenged. As mentioned earlier, the activity of steroid receptors may be controlled by their phosphorylation state. To this end, it was recently shown that compounds that increase protein kinase activity, such as cAMP, phorbol esters, or growth factors, can activate steroid receptor-mediated transcription when their specific ligand is absent.[134-136] This activation of transcriptional activity is accompanied by an increase in receptor phosphorylation.[132,137] Katzenellenbogen and Norman[134] reported that transcription of the PR gene, an estrogen-responsive gene, was activated by serum, insulin-like growth factor I, or cAMP when the cells were grown in E_2-free medium. Moreover, the antiestrogen ICI blocked this activation, suggesting direct involvement of the ER. They have extended these studies to show that the ER is phosphorylated upon the addition of these compounds and that protein kinase inhibitors block phosphorylation and activation.[137] These compounds, cAMP, or phorbol esters, increase the ER phosphorylation about fourfold, which is the same as that for E_2. However, in the case of cAMP, the major site of phosphorylation differs from those induced by estrogen, antiestrogen, or the phorbol ester 12-*O*-tetradecanoylphorbol-13-acetate (TPA).[129] In addition, there are synergistic effects of these compounds when combined with estrogen that increase the transcriptional activity of the ER to levels higher than with estrogen alone.[138,139] These effects do, however, show cell-type specificity.[138]

The main question raised in regard to ligand-independent activation of the ER (or other steroid receptors) is what is its physiological role? The range of compounds that can stimulate ER transcriptional activity include, in addition to estrogen, compounds that activate protein kinase A and protein kinase C, and growth factor receptors that have intrinsic tyrosine kinase activities; i.e., essentially every signaling pathway. That such a broad range of compounds can activate the receptor brings into question the specificity and physiological significance of the effects. With the exception of the work on the endogenous PR gene, all the other studies used artificial reporter gene constructs transiently transfected into established cell lines or primary cell cultures. Although informative, such studies must be interpreted cautiously due to the inherent problems associated with this type of analysis. However, in the case of the PR, a physiological response was recently reported. Mani et al.[140] demonstrated that a mating response, lordosis, in mice normally controlled by progestrone, could be induced by intracerebroventricular administration of dopamine D1 receptor agonists. This response was specific for dopamine D1 receptor agonists and was blocked by the administration of the antiprogestin RU 38486. These results suggest that the PR is mediating this response. This report was the first demonstration of a physiological response that may function through this cross-talk mechanism. Another physiological response that may provide indirect evidence that such cross-talk functions in cells can be seen in breast cancer. There are many breast carcinomas and breast cancer cell lines that become estrogen independent for tumorigenic growth. That is, they exhibit a high growth rate even when estrogens are not present. The growth of some of these tumors can be blocked by antiestrogens, suggesting that the ER is being activated by some mechanism other than ligand binding. Additional research is needed to establish if this mechanism of activation of steroid receptors has physiological significance.

ESTROGEN RECEPTOR INVOLVEMENT IN BREAST CANCER

Estrogen exerts control over many cellular events, including cell proliferation in specific target tissues such as mammary and uterus. Therefore, proper control of such hormonal signals must be maintained for normal growth, development, and function. Alterations of such signals can lead to such diseases as breast and uterine cancer, endometriosis, and others.[141] Many breast tumors are dependent on estrogen for growth. Therefore, the clinical relevence of estrogen and the ER has been realized for quite some time.[142] One of the most common treatments for breast cancers is the use of antiestrogens to block the proliferative activation in these cells caused by the ER. The presence or absence of ER, and also the PR, in breast cancer cells is a good indicator of therapeutic effectiveness, probability of relapse, and patient survival.[143] Patients that are ER+/PR+ have the highest response rate to hormone therapy, about 75%. Receptor levels are typically measured by ligand binding assays. Therefore, the presence of PR, in addition to ER, is believed to indicate that the ER can both bind estrogen and activate transcription as well. Patients who are ER+/PR– have an intermediate response to antiestrogen therapy, about 50%, whereas those who are ER– have only about a 10% response rate to such treatments. In most cases, after long-term treatment with antiestrogens, there is a loss of hormone sensitivity and the therapeutic effectiveness is lost. The molecular mechanism of this change to hormone resistance is poorly understood and is an area of very active research. One possible mechanism that could explain the change in many cases is mutations in the ER. In fact, such mutants have been found in both breast cancer tissues and cell lines (recently reviewed in Refs. 144 and 145).

Many of the mutants described to date are deletion mutants that occur specifically at exon-intron junctions. One such mutant lacks exon 7 in the ligand binding domain.[146] The cDNA for this exon 7 deletion mutant receptor (Δ7ER) was isolated from primary breast tumors and shown to have a dominant-negative effect on the transcriptional activity of the wild-type ER (wtER). When the Δ7ER receptor cDNA was expressed in yeast and assayed for transcriptional activity, it was inactive. However, when the wtER was coexpressed in cells with the Δ7ER, the transcriptional activity of the wtER was reduced by about 60%, demonstrating the dominant negative inhibition of ER function. An exon 7 deletion mutant has also been described in the T47D breast cancer cell line.[147] However, this mutant did not inhibit the transcriptional activity of the wtER when expressed in HeLa cells. The differences detected between these two exon 7 deletion mutants may be due to the different systems used to analyze ER activity.

Other studies have demonstrated truncated forms of the ER that have some or all of the ligand binding domain removed.[148] In most cases their role in tumorigenesis or tumor progression, if any, remains unknown. It has been postulated that some truncated mutants may be constitutive activators of transcription because TAF 1, the constitutive transactivation function in the A/B domain, remains intact. One such receptor mutant has been described.

This mutant has exon 5 completely and precisely deleted, causing a frameshift mutation and a truncated protein.[149] The cDNA for this clone was isolated from ER–/PR+ breast tumors. When the cDNA of this mutant ER was expressed in yeast cells, it constitutively activated the transcription from an estrogen-dependent reporter gene. Interestingly, when overexpressed in MCF-7 cells, which have high levels of ER, these cells were no longer sensitive to the growth inhibitory effects of antiestrogens. This may indicate that such mutants are important for hormone resistance.[145] It is interesting that wtER is present in many carcinomas where the ER mutants have been identified.[145]

Other interesting deletions have been found in the DBD.[145,147] Yang and Miksicek[147] isolated both exon 2 and exon 3 deletions. Both mutants were transcriptionally inactive, but Δ3ER was able the block the transcriptional activity of the wtER in transient transfection assays in HeLa cells. The mechanism of this inhibition remains unclear but probably involves protein-protein interactions of the mutant and wtER or interactions of the mutant ER with other protein factors that in turn form inactive complexes and limit the available factors with which the wtER can interact. Many other ER mutants have been found in breast tumors and cell lines. For a more detailed analysis of this subject, see reviews (Refs. 144 and 145). There is obviously a great deal more research needed in order to understand the role of the ER and mutant forms of the receptor on tumor formation and progression.

ESTROGEN RECEPTOR "KNOCK OUT" MICE

As mentioned earlier, it has long been known that estrogens are involved in the development of secondary female sex characteristics, female reproductive function, and fetal development. To date there are no known naturally occurring ER mutants.[150] This contrasts sharply to the androgen receptor, for which many receptor mutations have been described.[151,152] On the basis of these observations it was believed that estrogen and its receptor were required for fetal development and that mutations that blocked or significantly interfered with this normal signaling pathway were lethal. However, the first genetically engineered strain of ER knock out mice was recently developed.[153] These mice did develop to adulthood and their gross external anatomy appeared normal. However, the females were sterile and the males exhibited greatly reduced fertility, probably due to reduced sperm counts (about 10% of normal levels). The uteri of the females were hypoplastic and did not respond to 3 days of estrogen administration. Their ovaries were hyperemic with no apparent corpora lutea. Extracts prepared from the uteri of these knock out mice retained about 5% of the wild-type level of estrogen binding. Moreover, enzyme-linked immunosorbent assays also showed low levels of a protein that was reactive with an anti-ER monoclonal antibody. Therefore, it cannot be ruled out that these low levels of ER and estrogen binding may be enough to facilitate proper development. Additional analyses of these mice are needed to fully understand the role of the ER and estrogen in development. However, there is little doubt that these mice will provide one of the most interesting systems for studying the ER in coming years. For a detailed analysis of the role of the ER in development see Chapter 9.

TYPES OF ESTROGEN RECEPTORS

During the 1980s steroid binding analyses demonstrated that there are two E_2 binding macromolecules present in target tissue that have different affinities for E_2.[154-156] These macromolecules are referred to as the high-affinity ER (type I ER), with an affinity constant (Kd) of 0.1–1.0 nM, and the low-affinity estrogen binding site (type II ER, or low-affinity E_2 binding site, EBS), with a Kd of 20–30 nM. Type I ER is the classical ER and has been the focus of this chapter.

The structure and function of type I ERs have been studied extensively. However, little or no attention has been given to type II ER partly because of its low affinity for E_2. Eriksson et al.[157] were the first to demonstrate the presence of type II ER. Rats injected with E_2 show elevated concentrations of type II ER after 96 h, while type I ER decrease to less than 50% of its initial concentration within 4 h. The type II ER displays cooperative binding of estrogen.[158,159] It has a 400-fold lower affinity for estrogen than the type I receptor and is sensitive to sulfhydryl group reducing reagents.[158,160] Moreover, type II ER has been shown to bind bioflavonoids with an apparent Kd of 5 μM. These bioflavonoids have been proposed to be high-affinity endogenous inhibitors of the type II ER.[161] The type II ER was purified from uteri of pregnant rats and found to have many of the same characteristics as those reported for the crude protein.[162] The purified sample contains two major protein bands (73- and 67-kDa) as detected by silver staining on a sodium dodecyl sulfate-polyacrylamide agarose gel, electrophoresis, with the 73 kDa co-migrating with the type II ER. The 67-kDa protein is similar in size to the type I ER but is clearly distinct, because antibody to the type I ER does not cross-react with either it or the 73-kDa protein. Furthermore, neither of the proteins in the final preparation were able to bind to the vitellogenin ERE.

Recently, uteri from pregnant rats were identified as a rich source for the type II ER. Gray et al.[162] showed that on days 19–20 of gestation, levels of type II ER were 85-fold higher in the uteri of pregnant rats as compared with nonpregnant rats and 100 times greater than levels found in chickens or rats that had been treated with E_2.[163] Estrogen and progesterone are known to be involved in fetal maintenance; thus, high levels of type II ER combined with higher concentrations of E_2 may play a significant role in fetal growth and development.[164] However, whether the type II ER is involved in pregnancy was not addressed.

Despite these advancements in the biochemical characterization of the type II ER, very little progress has been made in elucidating the function of the protein. The limited physiochemical information that is available about type II ER has been used as a guide to assess the function of this protein. Type II ER has since been identified in a variety of tissues and cell lines.[156,165,166] This receptor has been implicated in mediating the effects of antitumor agents in certain cell lines via its ability to bind bioflavonoids. Type II ER levels have been shown to be high in estrogen-dependent mouse mammary tumors, human breast cancer, and certain cell lines, suggesting a possible role in these tumors. However, its apparent presence in normal tissue, such as the rat uterus, is observed only with exogenous administration of E_2. The administration of E_2 to rat results in stimulated uterine growth as well as type II ER levels. Thus, type II ER may be involved in uterine growth and perhaps uterine cell proliferation during gestation. Furthermore, its presence in endometrial cancer and different cancer cell lines has led to the hypothesis that the type II ER may play a crucial regulatory role in estrogen-stimulated pathways. Cloning of the gene encoding the type II ER would aid in determining the role of this receptor in regulating cellular activities.

CONCLUSION

Great strides have been made in the area of ER structure and function since the 1960s. We now have a good understanding of the basic mechanism of how estrogens function to alter cellular physiology. However, we have a long way before we fully understand the mechanism of steroid hormone function at the molecular level. There are still many areas of contention that will undoubtedly facilitate the advancement of research in this area and continually challenge us to reevaluate the model of estrogen action as new data are generated. Much more research is needed in all aspects of receptor biology. From basic research, such as receptor-associated proteins, to clinical aspects, such as the therapeutic possibilities associated with the receptor, this is and should remain a very exciting and active area of investigation that will continue to develop at a rapid pace, as it has over the last few decades.

REFERENCES

1. **Mueller, G.C., Herranen, A.M., and Jervell, K.,** Studies on the mechanisms of action of estrogens, *Recent Prog. Horm. Res.,* 14, 95, 1958.
2. **Beerman, W.,** Nuclear differentiation and functional morphology of chromosomes, *Cold Spring Harbor Symp. Quant. Biol.,* 21, 217, 1956.
3. **Clever, U. and Karlson, P.,** Induction of puff changes in salivary gland chromosomes of Chironomus tentans by ecdysone, *Exp. Cell Res.,* 20, 623, 1960.
4. **Ashburner, M.,** Patterns of puffing activity in the salivary gland chromosomes of *Drosophila*. VI. Induction by ecdysone in salivary glands of *D. melanogaster* cultured *in vitro*, *Chromosoma*, 38, 255, 1972.
5. **Landers, J.P. and Spelsberg, T.C.,** New concepts in steroid hormone action: transcription factors, proto-oncogenes, and the cascade model for steroid regulation of gene expression, *Crit. Rev. Eukaryotic Gene Expression*, 2, 19, 1992.
6. **Jensen, E.V. and Jacobson, H.I.,** Fate of steroid estrogens in target tissues, in *Biological Activities of Steroids in Relation to Cancer,* Pincus, G. and Vollmer, E.P., Eds., Academic Press, New York, 1960, 161.
7. **Toft, D. and Gorski, J.,** A receptor molecule for estrogens: isolation from the rat uterus and preliminary characterization, *Proc. Natl. Acad. Sci. U.S.A.,* 55, 1574, 1966.
8. **Toft, D., Shyamala, G., and Gorski, J.,** A receptor molecule for estrogens: studies using a cell-free system, *Proc. Natl. Acad. Sci. U.S.A.,* 57, 1740, 1967.
9. **Gorski, J., Toft, D., Shyamala, G., Smith, D., and Notides, A.,** Hormone receptors: studies on the interaction of estrogen with the uterus, *Recent Prog. Horm. Res.,* 24, 45, 1968.
10. **Jensen, E.V., Suzuki, T., Kawashima, T., Stumpf, W.E., Jungblut, P.W., and DeSombre, E.R.,** A two-step mechanism for the interaction of estradiol with rat uterus, *Proc. Natl. Acad. Sci. U.S.A.,* 59, 622, 1968.
11. **Gorski, J., Furlow, J.D., Murdoch, F.E., Fritsch, M., Kaneko, K., Ying, C., and Malayer, J.R.,** Perturbations in the model of estrogen receptor regulation of gene expression, *Biol. Reprod.,* 48, 8, 1993.
12. **Carson-Jurica, M.A., Schrader, W.T., and O'Malley, B.W.,** Steroid receptor family: structure and functions, *Endocr. Rev.,* 11, 201, 1990.
13. **Evans, R.M.,** The steroid and thyroid hormone receptor superfamily, *Science*, 240, 889, 1988.
14. **Gronemeyer, H.,** Transcription activation by estrogen and progesterone receptors, *Annu. Rev. Genet.,* 25, 89, 1991.
15. **Malayer, J.R. and Gorski, J.,** An integrated model of estrogen receptor action, *Domest. Anim. Endocrinol.,* 10, 159, 1993.
16. **Wahli, W. and Martinez, E.,** Superfamily of steroid nuclear receptors: positive and negative regulators of gene expression, *FASEB J.,* 5, 2243, 1991.
17. **Petkovich, M., Brand, N.J., Krust, A., and Chambon, P.,** A human retinoic acid receptor which belongs to the family of nuclear receptors, *Nature (London)*, 330, 444, 1987.
18. **Weinberger, C., Thompson, C.C., Ong, E.S., Lebo, R., Gruol, D.J., and Evans, R.M.,** The c-*erb*-A gene encodes a thyroid hormone receptor, *Nature (London)*, 324, 641, 1986.
19. **O'Malley, B.W. and Conneely, O.M.,** Orphan receptors: in search of a unifying hypothesis for activation, *Mol. Endocrinol.,* 6, 1359, 1992.
20. **Conneely, O.M., Sullivan, W.P., Toft, D.O., Birnbaumer, M., Cook, R.G., Maxwell, B.L., Zarucki-Schulz, T., Green, G.L., Schrader, W.T., and O'Malley, B.W.,** Molecular cloning of the chicken progesterone receptor, *Science*, 233, 767, 1986.
21. **Encio, I. and Detera-Wadleigh, S.D.,** The genomic structure of the human glucocorticoid receptor, *J. Biol. Chem.,* 266, 7182, 1991.
22. **Huckaby, C.S., Conneely, O.M., Beattie, W.G., Dobson, A.D.W., Tsai, M.-J., and O'Malley, B.W.,** Structure of the chromosomal chicken progesterone receptor gene, *Proc. Natl. Acad. Sci. U.S.A.,* 84, 8380, 1987.
23. **Lehmann, J.M., Hoffmann, B., and Pfahl, M.,** Genomic organization of the retinoic acid receptor gamma gene, *Nucleic Acids Res.,* 19, 573, 1991.
24. **Ponglikitmongkol, M., Green, S., and Chambon, P.,** Genomic organization of the human oestrogen receptor gene, *EMBO J.,* 7, 3385, 1988.
25. **Kumar, V., Green, S., Stack, G., Berry, M., Jin, J.-R., and Chambon, P.,** Functional domains of the human estrogen receptor, *Cell*, 51, 941, 1987.
26. **Lees, J.A., Fawell, S.E., and Parker, M.G.,** Identification of constitutive and steroid-dependent transactivation domains in the mouse oestrogen receptor, *J. Steroid Biochem.,* 34, 33, 1989.
27. **Tora, L., White, J., Brou, C., Tasset, D., Webster, N., Scheer, E., and Chambon, P.,** The human estrogen receptor has two independent nonacidic transcriptional activation functions, *Cell*, 59, 477, 1989.
28. **Tzukerman, M.T., Esty, A., Santiso-Mere, D., Danielian, P., Parker, M.G., Stein, R.B., Pike, J.W., and McDonnell, D.P.,** Human estrogen receptor transactivational capacity is determined by both cellular and promoter context and mediated by two functionally distinct intramolecular regions, *Mol. Endocrinol.,* 8, 21, 1994.

29. **Truss, M. and Beato, M.,** Steroid hormone receptors: interaction with deoxyribonucleic acid and transcription factors, *Endocr. Rev.*, 14, 459, 1993.

30. **Klein-Hitpass, L., Ryffel, G.U., Heitlinger, E., and Cato, A.C.B.,** A 13 bp palindrome is a functional estrogen responsive element and interacts specifically with estrogen receptor, *Nucleic Acids Res.*, 16, 647, 1988.

31. **Schwabe, J.W.R., Chapman, L., Finch, J.T., and Rhodes, D.,** The crystal structure of the estrogen receptor DNA-binding domain bound to DNA: how receptors discriminate between their response elements, *Cell*, 75, 567, 1993.

32. **Darwish, H., Krisinger, J., Furlow, J.D., Smith, C., Murdoch, F.E., and DeLulca, H.F.,** An estrogen-responsive element mediates the transcriptional regulation of calbindin D-9K gene in rat uterus, *J. Biol. Chem.*, 266, 551, 1991.

33. **Kato, S., Tora, L., Yamauchi, J., Masushige, S., and Chambon, P.,** A far upstream estrogen response element of the ovalbumin gene contains several half-palindromic 5′-TGACC-3′ motifs acting synergistically, *Cell*, 68, 731, 1992.

34. **Martinez, E. and Wahli, W.,** Cooperative binding of estrogen receptor to imperfect estrogen-responsive DNA elements correlates with their synergistic hormone-dependent enhancer activity, *EMBO J.*, 8, 3781, 1989.

35. **Schwabe, J.W.R., Neuhaus, D., and Rhodes, D.,** Solution structure of the DNA-binding domain of the oestrogen receptor, *Nature (London)*, 348, 458, 1990.

36. **Mader, S., Kumar, V., de Verneuil, H., and Chambon, P.,** Three amino acids of the oestrogen receptor are essential to its ability to distinguish an oestrogen from a glucocorticoid responsive element, *Nature (London)*, 338, 271, 1989.

37. **Hard, T., Kellenbach, E., Boelens, R., Kaptein, R., Dahlman, K., Carlstedt-Duke, J., Freedman, L.P., Maler, B.A., Hyde, E.I., Gustafsson, J.-A., and Yamamoto, K.R.,** 1H NMR studies of the glucocorticoid receptor DNA-binding domain: sequential assignments and identification of secondary structure elements, *Biochemistry*, 29, 9015, 1990.

38. **Luisi, B.F., Xu, W.X., Otwinowski, Z., Freedman, L.P., Yamamoto, K.R., and Sigler, P.B.,** Crystallographic analysis of the interaction of the glucocorticoid receptor with DNA, *Nature (London)*, 352, 497, 1991.

39. **Picard, D. and Yamamoto, K.R.,** Two signals mediate hormone-dependent nuclear localization of the glucocorticoid receptor, *EMBO J.*, 6, 3333, 1987.

40. **Picard, D., Kumar, V., Chambon, P., and Yamamoto, K.,** Signal transduction by steroid hormones: nuclear localization is differentially regulated in estrogen and glucocorticoid receptor, *Cell Regulation*, 1, 291, 1990.

41. **Ylikomi, T., Bocquel, M.T., Berry, M., Gronemeyer, H., and Chambon, P.,** Cooperation of proto-signals for nuclear accumulation of estrogen and progesterone receptors, *EMBO J.*, 11, 3681, 1992.

42. **Harlow, K.W., Smith, D.N., Katzenellenbogen, J.A., Greene, G.L., and Katzenellenbogen, B.S.,** Identification of cysteine 530 as the covalent attachment site of an affinity-labeling estrogen (ketononestrol aziridine) and antiestrogen (tamoxifen aziridine) in the human estrogen receptor, *J. Biol. Chem.*, 264, 17476, 1989.

43. **Pakdel, F. and Katzenellenbogan, B.S.,** Human estrogen receptor mutants with altered estrogen and antiestrogen ligand discrimination, *J. Biol. Chem.*, 267, 3429, 1992.

44. **Danielian, P.S., White, R., Hoarse, S.A., Fawell, S.E., and Parker, M.G.,** Identification of residues in the estrogen receptor that confer differential sensitivity to estrogen and hydroxytamoxifen, *Mol. Endocrinol.*, 7, 232, 1993.

45. **Wrenn, C.K. and Katzenellenbogen, B.S.,** Structure-function analysis of the hormone binding domain of the human estrogen receptor by region-specific mutagenesis and phenotypic screening in yeast, *J. Biol. Chem.*, 268, 24089, 1993.

46. **Danielian, P.S., White, R., Lees, J.A., and Parker, M.,** Identification of a conserved region required for hormone dependent transcriptional activation by steroid hormone receptors, *EMBO J.*, 11, 1025, 1992.

47. **Webster, N.J., Green, S., Jin, J.R., and Chambon, P.,** The hormone-binding domains of the estrogen and glucocorticoid receptors contain an inducible transcription activation function, *Cell*, 54, 199, 1988.

48. **Metzger, D., Lossen, R., Bornet, J.-M., Lemoine, J., and Chambon, P.,** Promotor specificity of the two transcriptional activation functions on the human estrogen receptor in yeast, *Nucleic Acids Res.*, 20, 2813, 1992.

49. **Pierrat, B., Henry, D.M., Chambon, P., and Losson, R.,** A highly conserved region in the hormone-binding domain of the human estrogen receptor functions as an efficient transactivation domain in yeast, *Gene*, 143, 193, 1994.

50. **Hollenberg, S.M. and Evans, R.M.,** Multiple and cooperative *trans*-activation domains of the human glucocorticoid receptor, *Cell*, 55, 899, 1988.

51. **Fawell, S.E., Lees, J.A., White, R., and Parker, M.G.,** Characterization and colocalization of steroid binding and dimerization activities in the mouse estrogen receptor, *Cell*, 60, 953, 1990.

52. **Fuxe, K., Wikstrom, A.-C., Okret, S., Agnati, L.F., Harfstrand, A., Yu, Z.-Y., Granholm, L., Zoli, M., Vale, W., and Gustafsson, J.A.,** Mapping of glucocorticoid receptor immunoreactive neurons in the rat tel- and diencephalon using a monoclonal antibody against rat liver glucocorticoid receptor, *Endocrinology*, 117, 1803, 1985.

53. **Wikstrom, A.-C., Bakke, O., Okret, S., Bronnegard, M., and Gustafsson, J.-A.,** Intracellular localization of the glucocorticoid receptor: evidence for cytoplasmic and nuclear localization, *Endocrinology*, 120, 1232, 1987.

54. **Brink, M., Humbel, B.M., De Kloet, E.R., and Van Driel, R.,** The unliganded glucocorticoid receptor is localized in the nucleus, not in the cytoplasm, *Endocrinology*, 130, 3575, 1992.

55. **Welshons, W.V., Krummel, B.M., and Gorski, J.,** Nuclear localization of unoccupied receptors for gluco- corticoids, estrogens, and progesterone in GH_3 cells, *Endocrinology*, 117, 2140, 1985.

56. **Welshons, W.V. and Gorski, J.,** Nuclear location of estrogen receptors, *Receptors*, 4, 97, 1986.

57. **Gorski, J., Malayer, J.R., Gregg, D.W., and Lundeen, S.G.,** Just where are the steroid hormone receptors anyway? *Endocrine J.*, 2, 99, 1994.

58. **Gorski, J. and Gannon, F.,** Current models of steroid hormone action: a critique, *Annu. Rev. Physiol.*, 38, 425, 1976.

59. **Welshons, W.V., Lieberman, M.E., and Gorski, J.,** Nuclear location of unoccupied estrogen receptor, *Nature (London)*, 307, 747, 1984.

60. **King, W.J. and Greene, G.L.,** Monoclonal antibodies localize oestrogen receptor in the nuclei of target cells, *Nature (London)*, 307, 745, 1984.

61. **McClellan, M.C., West, N.B., Tacha, D.E., Greene, G.L., and Brenner, R.M.,** Immunocytochemical localization of estrogen receptors in the Macaque reproductive tract with monoclonal antiestrophilins, *En- docrinology*, 114, 2002, 1984.

62. **Roberts, B.,** Nuclear location signal-mediated protein transport, *Biochim. Biophys. Acta*, 1008, 263, 1989.

63. **Murdoch, F.E., Grunwald, K.A.A., and Gorski, J.,** Marked effects of salt on estrogen receptor binding to DNA: biologically relevant discrimination between DNA sequences, *Biochemistry*, 30, 10838, 1991.

64. **Pekki, A., Ylikomi, T., Syvala, H., and Tuohimaa, P.,** Progesterone receptor and hsp90 are not complexed in intact nuclei, *J. Steroid Biochem. Mol. Biol.*, 48, 475, 1994.

65. **Tuohimaa, P., Pekki, A., Bläuer, M., Joensuu, T., Vilja, P., and Ylikomi, T.,** Nuclear progesterone receptor is mainly heat shock protein 90-free *in vivo, Proc. Natl. Acad. Sci. U.S.A.*, 90, 5848, 1993.

66. **Reese, J.C. and Katzenellenbogen, B. S.,** Examination of the DNA-binding ability of estrogen receptor in whole cells: implications for hormone-independent transactivation and the actions of antiestrogens, *Mol. Cell. Biol.*, 12, 4531, 1992.

67. **McDonnell, D.P., Nawaz, Z., and O'Malley, B.W.,** In situ distinction between steroid receptor binding and transactivation at a target gene, *Mol. Cell. Biol.*, 11, 4350, 1991.

68. **Wrenn, C.K. and Katzenellenbogen, B.S.,** Cross-linking of estrogen receptor to chromatin in intact MCF- 7 human breast cancer cells: optimization and effect of ligand, *Mol. Endocrinol.*, 4, 1647, 1990.

69. **Nelson, K., van Nagell, J.R., Gallion, H., Donaldson, E.S., and Pavlik, E.J.,** Estrogens and antiestrogens mediate contrasting transitions in estrogen receptor conformation which determine chromatin access: a review and synthesis of recent observations, in *Hormones, Cell Biology, and Cancer: Perspectives and Potentials*, Hankins, W.D. and Puett, D., Eds., Alan R. Liss, New York, 1988, 85.

70. **Hansen, J.C.,** Analysis of structural changes in steroid receptor proteins by partitioning, in *Aqueous Two- Phase Systems*, Walter, H. and Johansson, G., Eds., Academic Press, San Diego, CA, 1994, 276.

71. **Hansen, J.C. and Gorski, J.,** Conformational transitions of the estrogen receptor monomer: effects of estrogens, antiestrogen, and temperature, *J. Biol. Chem.*, 261, 13990, 1986.

72. **Fritsch, M., Leary, C., Furlow, J.D., Ahrens, H., Schuh, T., Mueller, G., and Gorski, J.,** The ligand induced decrease in surface hydrophobicity of the estrogen receptor is localized in the steroid binding domain, *Biochemistry*, 31, 5303, 1992.

73. **Beekman, J.M., Allan, G.F., Tsai, S.Y., Tsai, M.-J., and O'Malley, B.W.,** Transcriptional activation by the estrogen receptor requires a conformational change in the ligand binding domain, *Mol. Endocrinol.*, 7, 1266, 1993.

74. **Brown, M. and Sharp, P.A.,** Human estrogen receptor forms multiple protein-DNA complexes, *J. Biol. Chem.*, 265, 11238, 1990.

75. **Kumar, V. and Chambon, P.,** The estrogen receptor binds tightly to its responsive element as a ligand- induced homodimer, *Cell*, 55, 145, 1988.

76. **Sabbah, M., Gouilleux, F., Sola, B., Redeuilh, G., and Baulieu, E.-E.,** Structural differences between the hormone and antihormone estrogen receptor complexes bound to the hormone response element, *Proc. Natl. Acad. Sci. U.S.A.*, 88, 390, 1991.

77. **Borgna, J.-L. and Scali, J.,** Differential interactions of estrogens and antiestrogens at the 17β-hydroxy or counterpart function with the estrogen receptor, *Eur. J. Biochem.*, 199, 575, 1991.

78. **Nardulli, A.M. and Shapiro, D.J.,** Binding of the estrogen receptor DNA-binding domain to the estrogen response element induces DNA bending, *Mol. Cell. Biol.*, 12, 2037, 1992.

79. **Nardulli, A.M., Greene, G.L., and Shapiro, D.J.,** Human estrogen receptor bound to an estrogen response element bends DNA, *Mol. Endocrinol.*, 7, 331, 1993.

80. **Fritsch, M., Welch, R.D., Murdoch, F.E., Anderson, I., and Gorski, J.,** DNA allosterically modulates the steroid binding domain of the estrogen receptor, *J. Biol. Chem.*, 267, 1823, 1992.

81. **Klein-Hitpass, L., Tsai, S.Y., Greene, G.L., Clark, J.H., Tsai, M.-J., and O'Malley, B.W.,** Specific binding of estrogen receptor to the estrogen response element, *Mol. Cell. Biol.*, 9, 43, 1989.

82. **Ince, B.A., Zhuang, Y., Wrenn, C.K., Shapiro, D.J., and Katzenellenbogen, B.S.,** Powerful dominant negative mutants of the human estrogen receptor, *J. Biol. Chem.*, 268, 14026, 1993.

83. **Mader, S., Chambon, P., and White, J.H.,** Defining a minimal estrogen receptor DNA binding domain, *Nucleic Acids Res.*, 21, 1125, 1993.

84. **Furlow, J.D., Murdoch, F.E., and Gorski, J.,** High affinity binding of the estrogen receptor to a DNA response element does not require homodimer formation or estrogen, *J. Biol. Chem.*, 268, 12519, 1993.

85. **Slater, E.P., Redeuilh, G., Theis, K., Suske, G., and Beato, M.,** The uteroglobin promoter contains a noncanonical estrogen responsive element, *Mol. Endocrinol.*, 4, 604, 1990.

86. **Augerau, P., Miralles, F., Cavaillès, V., Gaudelet, C., Parker, M., and Rochefort, H.,** Characterization of the proximal estrogen-responsive element of human cathepsin D gene, *Mol. Endocrinol.*, 8, 693, 1994.

87. **Cohen-Solal, K., Bailly, A., Rauch, C., Quesne, M., and Milgrom, E.,** Specific binding of progesterone receptor to progesterone-responsive elements does not require prior dimerization, *Eur. J. Biochem.*, 214, 189, 1993.

88. **Hard, T., Dahlman, K., Carlstedt-Duke, J., Gustafsson, J.-Å., and Rigler, R.,** Cooperativity and specificity in the interactions between DNA and the glucocorticoid receptor DNA-binding domain, *Biochemistry*, 29, 5358, 1990.

89. **Notides, A.C., Lerner, N., and Hamilton, D.E.,** Positive cooperativity of the estrogen receptor, *Proc. Natl. Acad. Sci. U.S.A.*, 78, 4926, 1981.

90. **Sabbah, M., Redeuilh, G., and Baulieu, E.-E.,** Subunit composition of the estrogen receptor: involvement of the hormone-binding domain in the dimeric state, *J. Biol. Chem.*, 264, 2397, 1989.

91. **Tora, L., Mullick, A., Metzger, D., Ponglikitmongkol, M., Park, I., and Chambon, P.,** The cloned human oestrogen receptor contains a mutation which alters its hormone binding properties, *EMBO J.*, 8, 1981, 1989.

92. **Murdoch, F.E. and Gorski, J.,** The role of ligand in estrogen receptor regulation of gene expression, *Mol. Cell. Endocrinol.*, 78, C103, 1991.

93. **Buratowski, S.,** The basics of basal transcription by RNA polymerase II, *Cell*, 77, 1, 1994.

94. **Malik, S., Kun Lee, D., and Roeder, R.G.,** Potential RNA polymerase II-induced interactions of transcription factor TFIIB, *Mol. Cell. Biol.*, 13, 6253, 1993.

95. **Gilbert, D.M., Losson, R., and Chambone, P.,** Ligand dependence of estrogen receptor induced changes in chromatin structure, *Nucleic Acids Res.*, 20, 4525, 1992.

96. **Pham, T.A., Hwung, Y.-P., McDonnell, D.P., and O'Malley, B.,** Transactivation functions facilitate the disruption of chromatin structure by estrogen receptor derivatives *in vivo*, *J. Biol. Chem.*, 266, 18179, 1991.

97. **Seyfred, M.A., Kladde, M.P., and Gorski, J.,** Transcriptional regulation by estrogen of episomal prolactin gene regulatory elements, *Mol. Endocrinol.*, 3, 305, 1989.

98. **Schild, C., Claret, F.-X., Whali, W., and Wolffe, A.P.,** A nucleosome-dependent static loop potentiates estrogen-regulated transcription from the Xenopus vitellogenin B1 promoter *in vitro*, *EMBO J.*, 12, 423, 1993.

99. **Qin, L., Wallrath, L.L., Granok, H., and Elgin, S.C.R.,** $(CT)_n.(GA)_n$ repeats and heat shock elements have distinct roles in chromatin structure and transcriptional activation of the *Drosophila* hsp 26 gene, *Mol. Cell. Biol.*, 13, 2802, 1993.

100. **Stroka, C. and Wolfram, A.H.,** A functional role for nucleosomes in the repression of a yeast promoter, *EMBO J.*, 10, 361, 1991.

101. **Wolffe, A.P.,** Nucleosome positioning and modification: chromatin structures that potentiate transcription, *TIBS*, 19, 240, 1994.

102. **Sabbah, M., Le Ricousse, S., Redeuilh, G., and Baulieu, E.-E.,** Estrogen receptor-induced bending of the Xenopus vitellogenin A2 gene hormone responsive element, *Biochem. Biophys. Res. Commun.*, 185, 944, 1992.

103. **Picard, D., Khuresheed, B., Garabedian, M.J., Fortin, M.G., Lindquist, S., and Yamamoto, K.R.,** Reduced levels of hsp90 compromise steroid receptor action *in vivo*, *Nature (London)*, 348, 166, 1990.

104. **Veldscholte, J., Berrevoets, C.A., Zegers, N.D., Van-Der-Kwast, T.H., Grootegoed, J.A., and Mulder, E.,** Hormone-induced dissociation of the androgen receptor heat-shock protein complex: use of a new monoclonal antibody to distinguish transformed from nontransformed receptors, *Biochemistry*, 31, 7422, 1992.

105. **Bagchi, M.K., Tsai, M.-J., O'Malley, B.W., and Tsai, S.Y.,** Analysis of the mechanism of steroid hormone receptor-dependent gene activation in cell-free systems, *Endocr. Rev.*, 13, 525, 1992.

106. **Chambraud, B., Berry, M., Redveilh, G., and Chambon, P.,** Several regions of human estrogen receptor are involved in the formation of receptor-heat shock protein 90 complexes, *J. Biol. Chem.*, 265, 20686, 1990.

107. **Cavailles, V., Dauvois, S., Danielian, P.S., and Parker, M.G.,** Interaction of proteins with transcriptionally active estrogen receptors, *Proc. Natl. Acad. Sci. U.S.A.,* 91, 10009, 1994.

108. **Jacq, X., Brou, C., Lutz, Y., Davidson, I., and Chambon, P.,** Human TAFII 30 is present in a distinct TF IID complex and is required for transcriptional activation by the estrogen receptor, *Cell,* 79, 107, 1994.

109. **Halacchmi, S., Marden, E., Martin, G., MacKay, H., Addondanza, C., and Brown, M.,** Estrogen receptor-associated proteins: possible mediators of hormone-induced transcription, *Science,* 264, 1455, 1994.

110. **Mukherjee, R. and Chambone, P.,** A single stranded DNA-binding protein promotes the binding of the purified oestrogen receptor to its responsive element, *Nucleic Acids Res.,* 18, 5713, 1990.

111. **Somasekhar, M. and Gorski, J.,** Two elements of the rat prolactin 5' flanking region are required for its regulation by estrogen and glucocorticoids, *Gene,* 69, 13, 1988.

112. **Day, R., Koike, S., Sakai, M., Muramatsu, M., and Maurer, R.,** Both Pit-1 and the estrogen receptor are required for estrogen responsiveness of the rat prolactin gene, *Mol. Cell. Endocrinol.,* 4, 1964, 1990.

113. **Kaneko, K.J., Gélinas, C., and Gorski, J.,** Activation of the silent progesterone receptor gene by ectopic expression of estrogen receptors in a rat fibroblast cell line, *Biochemistry,* 32, 8348, 1993.

114. **Cullen, K.E., Kladde, M.P., and Seyfred, M.A.,** Interaction between transcription regulatory regions of prolactin chromatin, *Science,* 261, 203, 1993.

115. **Ing, N., Beekman, J., Tsai, S., Tsai, M.-J., and O'Malley, B.,** Members of the steroid hormone receptor superfamily interact with TFIIB (S300-II), *J. Biol. Chem.,* 267, 17617, 1992.

116. **Colgan, J., Wampler, S., and Manlet, J.L.,** Interaction between a transcriptional activator and transcription factor IIB *in vivo, Nature (London),* 362, 549, 1993.

117. **Tsai, M.-J. and O'Malley, B.W.,** Molecular mechanisms of action of steroid/thyroid receptor superfamily members, *Annu. Rev. Biochem.,* 63, 451, 1994.

118. **Keaveney, M., Berkenstam, A., Feigenbutz, M., Vriend, G., and Stunnenberg, H.,** Residues in the TATA-binding protein required to mediate a transcriptional response to retinoic acid in EC cells, *Nature (London),* 365, 562, 1993.

119. **Baniahmad, A., Ha, I., Reinberg, D., Tsai, S., Tsai, M.-J., and O'Malley, B.,** Interaction of human thyroid hormone receptor β with transcription factor TFIIB may mediate target gene depression and activation by thyroid hormone, *Proc. Natl. Acad. Sci. U.S.A.,* 90, 8832, 1993.

120. **Kerr, L., Ransone, L., Wamsley, P., Schmitt, M., Boyer, T., Zhou, Q., Berk, A., and Verma, I.,** Association between proto-oncoprotein Rel and TATA-binding protein mediates transcriptional activation by NF-*k*B, *Nature (London),* 365, 412, 1993.

121. **Orti, E., Bodwell, J.E., and Munck, A.,** Phosphorylation of steroid hormone receptors, *Endocr. Rev.,* 13, 105, 1992.

122. **Moudgil, V.K.,** Phosphorylation of steroid hormone receptors, *Biochim. Biophys. Acta,* 1055, 243, 1990.

123. **Migliaccio, A., Rotondi, A., and Auricchio, F.,** Calmodulin-stimulated phosphorylation of 17β-estradiol receptor on tyrosine, *Proc. Natl. Acad. Sci. U.S.A.,* 81, 5921, 1984.

124. **Migliaccio, A., Rotondi, A., and Auricchio, F.,** Estradiol receptor: phosphorylation on tyrosine in uterus and interaction with antiphosphotyrosine antibody, *EMBO J.,* 5, 2867, 1984.

125. **Auricchio, F., Migliaccio, A., Castoria, G., Rotondi, A., and Lastoria, S.,** Direct evidence of *in vitro* phosphorylation-dephosphorylation of the estradiol-17β receptor, Role of Ca²⁺-calmodulin in the activation of hormone binding sites, *J. Steroid Biochem.,* 20, 31, 1984.

126. **Castoria, G., Migliaccio, A., Green, S., Di Domenico, M., Chambon, P., and Auricchio, F.,** Properties of a purified estradiol-dependent calf uterus tyrosine kinase, *Biochemistry,* 32, 1740, 1993.

127. **Ali, S., Metzger, D., Bornert, J.M., and Chambon, P.,** Modulation of transcriptional activation by ligand dependent phosphorylation of the human oestrogen receptor A/B domain, *EMBO J.,* 12, 1153, 1993.

128. **Denton, R.R., Koszewski, N.J., and Notides, A.C.,** Estrogen receptor phosphorylation, *J. Biol. Chem.,* 267, 7263, 1992.

129. **Le Goff, P., Montano, M.M., Schodin, D.J., and Katzenellenbogen, B.S.,** Phosphorylation of the human estrogen receptor, *J. Biol. Chem.,* 269, 4458, 1994.

130. **Washburn, T., Hocutt, A., Brautigan, D.L., and Korach, K.S.,** Uterine estrogen receptor *in vivo*: phosphorylation of nuclear specific forms on serine residues, *Mol. Endocrinol.,* 5, 235, 1991.

131. **Denner, L.A., Weigel, N.L., Maxwell, B.L., Schrader, W.T., and O'Malley, B.W.,** Regulation of progesterone receptor-mediated transcription of phosphorylation, *Science,* 250, 1740, 1990.

132. **Denner, L.A., Schrader, W.T., O'Malley, B.W., and Weigel, N.L.,** Hormonal regulation and identification of chicken progesterone receptor phosphorylation sites, *J. Biol. Chem.,* 265, 513, 1990.

133. **Bodwell, J.E., Orti, E., Coull, J.M., Pappin, D.J.C., Smith, L.I., and Swift, F.,** Identification of phosphorylated sites in the mouse glucocorticoid receptor, *J. Biol. Chem.,* 266, 7549, 1991.

134. **Katzenellenbogen, B.S. and Norman, M.J.,** Multihormonal regulation of the progesterone receptor in MCF-7 human breast cancer cells: interrelationships among insulin/insulin-like growth factor-1, serum, and estrogen, *Endocrinology,* 126, 891, 1990.

135. **Power, R.F., Mani, S.K., Codina, J., Conneely, O.M., and O'Malley, B.W.,** Dopaminergic and ligand-independent activation of steroid hormone receptors, *Science,* 254, 1636, 1991.

136. **Zhang, Y., Bai, W., Allgood, V.E., and Weigel, N.L.,** Multiple signaling pathways activate the chicken progesterone receptor, *Mol. Endocrinol.,* 8, 577, 1994.

137. **Aronica, S.M. and Katzenellenbogen, B.S.,** Stimulation of estrogen receptor-mediated transcription and alteration in the phosphorylation state of the rat uterine estrogen receptor by estrogen, cyclic adenosine monophosphate, and insulin-like growth factor-I, *Mol. Endocrinol.,* 7, 743, 1993.

138. **Cho, H. and Katzenellenbogen, B.S.,** Synergistic activation of estrogen receptor-mediated transcription by estradiol and protein kinase activators, *Mol. Endocrinol.,* 7, 441, 1993.

139. **Fujimoto, N. and Katzenellenbogen, B.S.,** Alteration in the agonist/antagonist balance of antiestrogens by activation of protein kinase A signaling pathways in breast cancer cells: antiestrogen selectivity and promoter dependence, *Mol. Endocrinol.,* 8, 296, 1994.

140. **Mani, S.K., Allen, J.M.C., Clark, J.H., Blaustein, J.D., and O'Malley, B.W.,** Convergent pathways for steroid hormone- and neurotransmitter-induced rat sexual behavior, *Science,* 265, 1246, 1994.

141. **Lippman, M.E. and Dickson, R.B.,** Regulation of normal and malignant breast epithelial proliferation, in *Growth Regulation in Cancer II,* Dickson, M.L. and Dickson, R., Eds., Alan R. Liss, New York, 1990, 127.

142. **Clark, G.M. and McGuire, W.L.,** Steroid receptors and other prognostic factors in primary breast cancer, *Semin. Oncol.,* 15, 20, 1988.

143. **Klijn, J.G.M., Berns, E.M.J.J., and Foekens, J.A.,** Prognostic factors and response to therapy in breast cancer, in *Breast Cancer,* Fentiman, I.S. and Taylor-Papadimitriou, J., Eds., Cold Spring Harbor Laboratory Press, Plainview, NY, 1993, 165.

144. **Encarnacion, C.A. and Fuqua, S.A.W.,** Estrogen receptor variants in breast cancer, in *Steroid Hormone Receptors: Basic and Clinical Aspects,* Moudgil, V.K., Ed., Birkhauser, Boston, 1994, 427.

145. **Fuqua, S.A.W., Chamness, G.C., and McGuire, W.L.,** Estrogen receptor mutations in breast cancer, *J. Cell. Biochem.,* 51, 135, 1993.

146. **Fuqua, S.A.W., Fitzgerald, S.D., Allred, D.C., Elledge, R.M., Nawaz, Z., McDonnell, D.P., O'Malley, B.W., Greene, G.L., and McGuire, W.L.,** Inhibition of estrogen receptor action by a naturally occurring variant in human breast tumors, *Cancer Res.,* 52, 483, 1992.

147. **Yang, Y. and Miksicek, R.J.,** Identification of a dominant negative form of the human estrogen receptor, *Mol. Endocrinol.,* 5, 1707, 1991.

148. **Murphy, L.C. and Dotzlaw, H.,** Variant estrogen receptor mRNA species detected in human breast cancer biopsy samples, *Mol. Endocrinol.,* 3, 687, 1989.

149. **Fuqua, S.A.W., Fitzgerald, S.D., Chamness, G.C., Tandon, A.K., McDonnell, D.P., Nawaz, Z., O'Malley, B.W., and McGuire, W.L.,** Variant human breast tumor estrogen receptor with constitutive transcriptional activity, *Cancer Res.,* 51, 105, 1991.

150. **George, F.W. and Wilson, J.D.,** Sex determination and differentiation, in *The Physiology of Reproduction,* Knobil, E., Neill, J.D., Ewing, L.L., Greenwald, G.S., Markert, C.L., and Pfaff, D.W., Eds., Raven Press, New York, 1988, 3.

151. **Brown, T.R. and Migeon, C.J.,** Androgen insensitivity syndromes: paradox of phenotypic feminization with male genotype and normal testicular androgen secretion, in *Hormone Resistance and Other Endocrine Paradoxes,* Cohen, M.P. and Foa, P.P., Eds., Springer, New York, 1987, 157.

152. **Lubahn, D.B., Brown, T.R., Simental, J.A., Higgs, H.N., Migeon, C.J., Wilson, E.M., and French, F.S.,** Sequence of the intron/exon junction of the coding region of the human androgen receptor gene and identification of a point mutation in a family with complete androgen insensitivity, *Proc. Natl. Acad. Sci. U.S.A.,* 86, 9534, 1989.

153. **Lubahn, D.B., Moyer, J.S., Golding, T.S., Couse, J.S., Korach, K.S., and Smithies, O.,** Alteration of reproductive function but not prenatal sexual development after insertional disruption of the mouse estrogen receptor gene, *Proc. Natl. Acad. Sci. U.S.A.,* 90, 11162, 1993.

154. **Clark, J.H., Hardin, J.W., Upchurch, S., and Eriksson, H.,** Heterogeneity of estrogen binding sites in the cytosol of the rat uterus, *J. Biol. Chem.,* 253, 7630, l978.

155. **Markaverich, B.M., Williams, M., Upchurch, S., and Clark, J.H.,** Heterogeneity of nuclear estrogen-binding site in the rat uterus: a simple method for the quantitation of type I and type II sites by [³H] estradiol exchange, *Endocrinology,* 109, 62, 1981.

156. **Marsigliante, S., Biscozzo, L., Puddefoot, J.R., Vinson, G.P., and Steorelli, C.,** Type II oestrogen binding site is associated with the major 4S oestrogen receptor isoform in breast tumors, *J. Steroid Biochem. Mol. Biol.,* 42, 777, 1992.

157. **Eriksson, H., Upchurch, S., Hardin, J.W., Peck, E.J., and Clark, J.H.,** Heterogeneity of estrogen receptors in the cytosol and nuclear fractions of the rat uterus, *Biochem. Biophys. Res. Commun.,* 81, 1, 1978.

158. **Densmore, C.L., Markaverich, B.M., O'Malley, B.W., and Clark, J.H.,** Characterization and purification of an estrogen type II binding site in chick oviduct cytosol, *Biochemistry,* 28, 7788, 1989.

159. **Markaverich, M.B., Roberts, R.R., Finney, W.R., and Clark, H.J.,** Preliminary characterization of an endogenous inhibitor of [³H]estradiol binding in rat uterine nuclei, *J. Biol. Chem.,* 258, 11663, 1983.

160. **Markaverich, B.M. and Gregory, R.R.,** Preliminary characterization and partial purification of rat uterine nuclear type II binding sites, *Biochem. Biophys. Res. Commun.,* 177, 1283, 1991.

161. **Scambia, G., Ranelletti, F.O., Panici, P.B., Piantelli, M., Bonanno, G., De Vincenzo, R., Ferranadina, G., Pierelli, L., Capelli, A., and Mancuso, S.,** Quercetin inhibits the growth of a multidrug-resistant estrogen-receptor-negative MCF-7 human breast-cancer cell line expressing type II estrogen-binding sites, *Cancer Chemother. Pharmacol.*, 28, 248, 1991.

162. **Gray, W.G.N., Biswas, E.E., Bashirelahi, N.B., and Biswas, S.B.,** A low-affinity estrogen binding site in pregnant rat uteri: analysis and partial purification, *Proc. Natl. Acad. Sci. U.S.A.*, 91, 11502, 1994.

163. **Anderson, J.N., Clark, J.H., and Peck, E.J., Jr.,** The relationship between nuclear receptor-estrogen binding and uterotrophic responses, *Biochem. Biophys. Res. Commun.*, 48, 1460, 1972.

164. **Markaverich, M.B., Upchurch, S., and Clarj, J.H.,** Progesterone and dexamethasone antagonism of uterine growth: a role for a second nuclear binding site for estradiol in estrogen action, *J. Steroid Biochem.*, 14, 125, 1981.

165. **Poirot, M., Chailleux, C., Bayard, F., and Paye, J.,** Cytosolic type II estrogen binding site in rat uterus: specific photolabeling with estrone, *J. Receptor Res.*, 12, 217, 1992.

166. **Scambia, G., Ranelletti, O.F., Panici, B.P., and Mancuso, S.,** Type-II estrogen binding sites in a lymphoblastoid cell line and growth-inhibitory effect of estrogen, anti-estrogen and bioflavonoids, *Int. J. Cancer*, 46, 1112, 1990.

167. **Gorski, J. and Hansen, J.C.,** The "one and only" step model of estrogen action, *Steroids*, 49, 461, 1987.

168. **Seyfred, M.A. and Gorski, J.,** An interaction between 5′ flanking distal and proximal regulatory domains of the rat prolactin gene is required for transcriptional activation by estrogens, *Mol. Endocrinol.*, 4, 1226, 1990.

Chapter 9

ESTROGEN RECEPTORS IN EMBRYOGENESIS

Qunfang Hou, Tamara Greco, Theresa Duello, and Jack Gorski

CONTENTS

INTRODUCTION

Estrogens are the primary female sex hormones, which are mainly synthesized by the ovaries of mature animals. Estrogens circulate in the blood and promote RNA and protein synthesis and growth in a variety of target tissues.[1] It is well established that estrogen elicits its function by binding to a receptor protein, the estrogen receptor (ER). The ER belongs to a receptor superfamily that includes the receptors for progesterone, androgen, glucocorticoid, mineralocorticoid, vitamin D, thyroid hormone, retinoic acid, and a growing number of orphan receptors whose ligands are not yet known (for reviews, see Refs. 1–6). These receptors share similar structural organization and act in a similar fashion as ligand-modulated transcriptional factors. The ER regulates transcription by binding to a specific DNA sequence termed the estrogen response element, located on the target gene of the ER. The other members of the receptor superfamily bind to their own unique, but similar, sequences or response elements. Estrogens are able to diffuse into the cell freely because of their hydrophobicity. The binding of estrogen to its receptor induces conformational changes in the ER, which results in ER activation. The interaction of activated ER with the transcription machinery affects the assembly of the transcriptional initiation complex and results in changes in the rate of transcription of certain target genes. These changes eventually lead to changes in cellular function, such as a change in the growth rate or physiology of the cell. Clearly, the ER is the critical component that mediates estrogen's effects. Its presence will dictate whether a tissue or a population of cells is estrogen responsive. The primary targets of estrogen are the female sexual organs such as the fallopian tubes, uterus, vagina, and the breast.[7] Correspondingly, these sexual organs are also well-characterized, ER-containing tissues. However, the expression of ER is not restricted to the female sexual organs and the time of ER expression occurs prior to puberty. Estrogen is known to have effects that are not directly related to the development of sexual organs. For example, estrogen affects skeletal growth, skin texture, and general metabolism such as protein deposition, fat deposition, and electrolyte balance.[7] Recent findings that ER is present in low amounts in bone[8-10] and adipose tissue[11-13] correspond well to these tissues' responsiveness to estrogen. The observation that prenatal exposure to diethylstilbestrol (DES), a synthetic estrogen, has a deleterious effect on the offspring later in development prompted scientists to investigate the prenatal expression of ER. In this chapter, we will review what is known about ER expression during embryogenesis, primarily in the mouse. This will include the period from the day of conception to the day of birth. These findings will aid our understanding of the possible role of estrogen and ER in development.

THE EFFECT OF DIETHYLSTILBESTROL

HISTORY OF USE IN HUMANS

During the 1940s and 1950s, progesterone deficiency was assumed to result in abortion, miscarriage, and premature delivery. Because doctors believed that estrogen could enhance progesterone secretion, pregnant women who were considered to be at risk were given a synthetic estrogenic compound, DES, beginning as early as the sixth week of pregnancy to prevent miscarriage.[14] The practice was widespread in the late 1940s and early 1950s, and seemed to be effective.[14,15] However, in 1966–1969, the sudden appearance of an extremely rare form of cancer, vaginal adenocarcinoma, in young females led Herbst et al.[16] to associate tumor appearance with maternal DES therapy. It was estimated that only 5–10% of pregnant women received DES. However, a survey showed that among patients exhibiting adenocarcinoma of the vagina and cervix whose maternal history was available, those who had been exposed to DES *in utero* accounted for 65%.[17] Thus, a much higher percentage of the DES-exposed population developed cancer than the general population. The number of cancer cases peaked in the early 1970s when the DES-exposed population reached puberty.[17] In addition to the carcinoma, studies revealed benign changes that occurred more frequently, including vaginal adenosis, cervical erosion, and transverse vaginal and cervical ridges.[18,19] Lesions were also present in male offspring exposed to DES *in utero*. A higher incidence of epididymal cysts, hypotrophic testis, hypoplastic penis, and low sperm count was observed in DES-exposed offspring compared with unexposed controls.[19,20] It is worth noting that there were no noticeable abnormalities of these DES-exposed children at the time of birth. Development appeared normal until puberty.[19] Therefore, the effects of DES were manifest only many years after the initial exposure and appeared to depend on a subsequent exposure to estrogen.

THE MOUSE AS A MODEL

To study the effect of prenatal exposure to DES more thoroughly, McLachlan's lab investigated whether mice could be used as an animal model.[21-28] DES was injected into pregnant mice at different doses between gestation days 9 and 16, a period corresponding to the developmental stage during which humans were exposed. The exposed mice were examined when they reached adulthood. Lesions in the reproductive tract similar to those found in humans were also found in mice. In the female, the prevalence of histological abnormalities of the ovary, oviduct, vagina, cervix, and uterus was as high as 50–100% at the highest dose (100 µg/kg body weight) of DES tested, whereas controls exhibited these abnormalities at 0–10%. The changes included ovarian cysts, inflammation, and oophoritis in the ovary; oviductal malformation and oviductal hyperplasia; vaginal concretions, and excess keratinization; cervical enlargement; uterine squamous metaplasia and cystic endometrial hyperplasia. Also, a low incidence of vaginal, cervical, and/or uterine cancer was observed. In the male, lesions in the reproductive tract included intraabdominal or fibrotic testes, epididymal cysts, inflammation, cryptorchidism, and nodular masses in the seminal vesicles and/or prostate gland. An exceptionally rare adenocarcinoma of the rete testis was also observed in the prenatally DES-treated mice. In addition, both female and male mice exhibited dose-related decreased fertility. As in humans, some of the effects of DES on mice also appears to depend on subsequent exposure to estrogen, because DES-exposed neonatal mice that were ovariectomized before puberty did not exhibit squamous metaplasia or tumor in the uterus shown in the DES-exposed intact animals.[29,30]

TARGET TISSUES

McLachlan's group used radiolabeled DES to show that maternally administrated DES does pass the placenta, reach the fetus, and accumulate in the fetal reproductive tract.[25] The Mullerian duct seemed to be the primary target of DES in these cases. It was suggested that the adenocarcinoma were of Mullerian origin and vaginal adenosis resulted when the Mullerian anlage was not replaced completely by the upgrowing vaginal plate of squamous epithelium.[16,18] The data on mice support this idea. The persistence of Mullerian structures resembling portions of the mature female reproductive tract was observed in males in addition to well-defined Wolffian ducts.[27] When fetal Mullerian ducts from DES-exposed males were cultured *in vitro*, Mullerian duct regression was severely compromised.[31] Recombination experiments with Mullerian duct and testis from either control or exposed males demonstrated that the inhibitory effect on regression is primarily due to decreased responsiveness of the Mullerian duct itself. Modification of the development of Mullerian duct tissue appeared to represent a common response to DES in both the male and female fetus.[25,27] In addition to the Mullerian duct, the Wolffian duct was also stimulated *in utero* by DES.[28] Wolffian duct remnants were frequently observed in DES-treated females.[23,28] These remnants were often enlarged and incorporated in the oviductal stroma.[22] The developmental modification of the fetal genital tract may arise from stimulation of DES during a particular stage of cellular differentiation at a critical time of development. The ability of DES injected during pregnancy to modulate development of the offspring suggests that the responsive mechanism for estrogen, which includes the presence of ER, has developed at an early age.

ESTROGEN RECEPTOR DURING PREIMPLANTATION DEVELOPMENT

OVERVIEW OF PREIMPLANTATION DEVELOPMENT

After ovulation, the oocyte is fertilized in a swollen region of the oviduct called the ampulla. The fusion of the oocyte and the sperm results in a fertilized egg that has two pronuclei and thus two diploid chromosomes per cell. This fertilized egg marks the start of a new life; the one-cell embryo. From two cells to morula, the embryo travels down the oviduct and reaches the uterus 3–4 days postcoitum (d.p.c.). At that time, the embryo develops into a blastocyst. Mouse embryos remain as free identities until they implant in the uterus on 4–5 d.p.c. This is the preimplantation period (for reviews on preimplantation development, see Refs. 32 and 33).

First Cleavage

Development at the one-cell stage depends largely on proteins and RNAs synthesized during oogenesis. DNA replication begins at about 11–18 h postfertilization. The first cleavage occurs 17–20 h postfertilization.[32] The majority of transcription and translation of the zygotic genes does not begin until the two-cell stage of development.[34] Initiation of zygotic gene expression is governed by a "clock" that initiates transcription about 20 h postfertilization, regardless of whether the one-cell embryo has completed DNA replication or undergone mitosis.[35]

Based on the effect of a polyoma virus enhancer on gene expression in oocytes, one-cell, and two-cell embryos, it was proposed that the need for enhancers and, therefore, transcriptional activators in gene expression is acquired upon formation of a diploid nucleus.[36] The need for an enhancer was thought to result from the first appearance of negative regulatory elements at this stage. However, activation of promoters by other enhancers was observed in one-cell as well as two-cell embryos when appropriate transactivators were introduced into the embryo, suggesting that enhancers were capable of functioning before the two-cell stage.[37] Apparently, whether an enhancer will have an effect on gene expression depends on the particular enhancers used because their corresponding transactivators may be present at different times during this period. Thus, as in adult tissues, the context of transactivators/repressors is very important in affecting gene expression at this stage. There seems to be no aberrant expression of tissue-specific genes, at least by microinjection of reporter genes linked to tissue-specific promoters,[37] presumably because of the lack of an appropriate, specific combination of transcription factors or the presence of specific repressors. The enhancers and their regulators together play a role in transcriptional regulation and perhaps the specificity of gene expression during this period.

From Two-Cell Embryo to Blastocyst

The subsequent development of the embryo beyond the two-cell stage depends on the embryonic synthesis of RNA and protein. Inhibition of RNA synthesis at the two-cell stage will inhibit further cleavage. There is an extensive reprogramming in the pattern of protein synthesis at the two-cell stage.[34,35] The degradation of maternal RNA that starts during oocyte maturation continues.[38] In most strains of mouse, the embryos divide at intervals of about 20–26 h for the first two cleavages and at intervals of approximately 10 h for later cleavages to progress to the two-cell, four-cell, eight-cell, morula, and blastocyst stages.[39] During this period, total RNA increases about 10-fold. The size of the embryo, however, remains similar to the mature oocyte. The stage-specific expression of particular RNA was observed at each stage. Up to the eight-cell stage, the blastomeres of the embryo are equipotent.[32] The first indication of cell differentiation occurs at the eight-cell stage when the embryos undergo compaction. Cellular polarization early in compaction results in differentiation of different cell types later. Cell adhesiveness changes during compaction so that individual cells can no longer be distinguished. The compacted 8–16-cell embryo is called a morula, which looks like a solid ball of cells. Later, a fluid-filled cavity, the blastocoele, starts to form and the embryo becomes a blastocyst. Different cell types, i.e., the inner cell mass and the trophectoderm, are clearly distinguishable at the early blastocyst stage. The blastocyst continues to grow and expand and when fully expanded, has 64 cells, of which about 20 are inner mass cells.[32] The blastocyst resembles a hollow ball, with a layer of trophectoderm cells covering the blastocoele cavity and a blob of inner cell mass clinging to the outer layer. At about 4.5 days postfertilization, the blastocyst begins to elongate and loses its *zona pellucida*. This process is called hatching. The embryo is now ready to implant in the uterus. Change in protein synthesis has been observed in both the morula-to-blastocyst and the early-to-late blastocyst transition.[40,41] The metabolic rate rises sharply from the morula-to-blastocyst stage.[33]

POSSIBLE EFFECTS OF ESTROGEN ON THE DEVELOPMENT AND IMPLANTATION OF PREIMPLANTATION EMBRYOS

Both estrogen and progesterone are needed for the establishment and maintenance of pregnancy. Hypophysectomy of pregnant rats on day 1 of pregnancy resulted in expulsion of most embryos from the uterus, delayed entry of embryos into the uterus, and retarded development of embryos.[42] Expulsion of embryos was prevented with injections of progesterone, although there was no effect on embryonic development. Embryonic development was significantly improved with a combined injection of progesterone and estrone. Blastocyst dormancy and implantation delay was observed in ovariectomized pregnant animals treated only with progesterone.[43] An injection of estrogen could reactivate the blastocyst and resume implantation. Estrogen's effect was reflected by changes in both the uterus and the embryo.

The delayed blastocyst was shown to have a lower metabolism rate and lower transcriptional activity compared with the normal embryo. After estrogen treatment of the pregnant animal, metabolic rate and transcriptional activity increased.[44-46] It was observed that stage-specific synthesis of proteins by the embryo occurred around the time of implantation. The changes included cell surface proteins[47] that could be involved in blastocyst invasion as well as secreted proteins[48] that could act as local signals for the uterus. Delayed blastocysts failed to show such a change, but estradiol injection would induce such a change. Because estrogen was administered to the mother, it could not be determined whether estrogen could act directly on the embryo or if the effect of estrogen was mediated solely through the uterus. The use of *in vitro* cultured embryos permitted a better evaluation of the mechanism of estrogen action. It was demonstrated that estradiol treatment *in vitro* did not stimulate uptake or incorporation of amino acids into morulae, but an increase was evident in early blastocysts and the increase was significant in late blastocysts.[49] It was also shown that estradiol stimulated ^{3}H-uridine uptake and RNA synthesis in *in vitro* cultured blastocysts.[50] Estrogen also seemed to affect the development of the embryo. When four- to eight-cell mouse embryos were cultured *in vitro* in the presence of the antiestrogen CI-628, the development to blastocysts was severely blocked.[51] In the absence of the drug, between 84 and 98% of the embryos developed to blastocysts after 48 h in culture. At a concentration of 1 μg/ml of CI-628, the percentage dropped to 45%. At a concentration of 1.5 μg/ml, none of the embryos developed to blastocyst. If 1 μg/ml 17β-estradiol was added together with 1 μg/ml CI-628, the development rate was brought back to 78%. One possible reason for the incomplete reversal of CI-628's effect by estradiol might be competition between the two drugs. Excess estradiol might be needed for a complete reversal. However, it should be pointed out that the concentration of antiestrogen used was at the micromolar level. At such a high concentration, toxic effects on the embryo not related to antiestrogenic activity may be taking place. It is difficult to assess to what degree the role of toxicity of the compound played in inhibiting embryonic development. Similarly, if the estrogen synthesis inhibitor 1,4,6-androstatriene-3,17-dione was included in the incubation, an inhibition of development to the blastocyst stage also occurred.[52] In this case, only 17β-estradiol, but not 17α-estradiol, was able to counter the inhibitory effect, which is in agreement with the estrogenicity of the compound. When antiestrogen was given to pregnant mice, implantation was inhibited. Paradoxically, this could not be overcome by the administration of estradiol, even though administration of progesterone seemed to be helpful.[53] Perhaps the antiestrogen, given at a large dose, can also act as a weak estrogen, because an excess of estrogen inhibits implantation (see below).

A report about embryos treated with estrogen *in vitro* showed a higher implantation rate than nontreated controls when transferred to a progesterone-treated ovariectomized foster mother.[54] However, no effect of hormone on embryonic development or implantation was observed in another study when estrogen or progesterone at levels higher than those found in physiological plasma were added directly to media.[55] In the latter study, a hormonal effect was only observed when embryos were cultured in oviductal fluid from hormone-treated animals. It was shown that oviductal fluid from estrogen-dominated donors inhibited embryo development as well as implantation. A similar study, in which oviductal fluid was also used to culture embryos, concluded that an optimal ratio of estrogen and progesterone given to the donor animal is required.[56] A large elevation of the estrogen/progesterone ratio inhibited implantation. In any case, these results would imply that the estrogen effect was indirectly exerted on the embryo through the mother. A delicate balance of hormones may be needed to ensure an optimal environment of the uterine lumenal milieu where the embryos exist. There is evidence that the protein content of uterine secretion changes at the time of implantation and this change is regulated by estrogen, because similar changes occur when ovariectomized rats receive estrogen.[57,58] It was postulated that these proteins could be regulators of embryonic metabolism. Nonetheless, the possibility of a direct effect of estrogen on embryos cannot be excluded.

The direct response of an embryo to estrogen would require the presence of ER in the embryo. Binding of ^{3}H-estradiol (38.1 Ci/mmol) was attempted in mouse blastocysts.[54] However, there were less than 20 counts per minute (cpm) per 100 embryos and the specificity for ER was not verified. The low counts are not surprising given the following calculation. Assuming that each blastocyst has 64 cells, even with the specific activity of ^{3}H-estradiol currently available (100 Ci/mmol), only 20 cpm per 100 embryos would be expected for a receptor level of 20,000 per cell, which is comparable to the receptor level of the uterine cells. However, 20 cpm is too close to background radiation. In order to detect binding with confidence for receptor levels at or below 20,000 receptors per cell, several hundred or more embryos would be required. In rabbit blastocysts, binding of estradiol was observed, although excess of antiestrogen only inhibited binding by 50%.[59] In pig, uptake of ^{3}H-estradiol amounted to 134 cpm per 10 blastocysts.[60] This could be reduced by 68% in the presence of excess unlabeled estradiol. Progesterone could compete only 23%, indicating that the estrogen uptake was specific to a certain degree. However, the presence of ER could not be directly demonstrated.

EXPRESSION OF ESTROGEN RECEPTOR

The advance of polymerase chain reaction (PCR) technology makes it possible to analyze gene expression in limited amounts of material. Due to its high sensitivity, precautions must be taken to avoid contamination of ER-positive maternal tissues. The expression of ER in preimplantation mouse embryos was studied using embryos cultured *in vitro*.[61] Figure 1 summarizes the findings of this study. In this analysis, total RNA from embryos at different stages of development were isolated and reverse transcribed to cDNA. Using primers specific for ER, DNA fragments corresponding to the ER were amplified and visualized on an agarose gel. A similar expression pattern of ER mRNA was shown by two different primer sets (Figure 2, A and B). The specificity of the amplified DNA was confirmed by Southern blot analysis. The integrity of the RNA sample was checked by analyzing the expression of ribosomal protein L-19, which should be present at every stage. ER mRNA was detected in unfertilized oocytes as well as in fertilized eggs. The detection of ER mRNA in oocytes and one-cell embryos by reverse transcriptase (RT)-PCR was also reported by Wu et al.[62] The reason for the presence of ER in the oocyte is not clear. It is probably related to oocyte growth and maturation because follicular growth is stimulated by estrogen.[63] Estrogen may have a direct effect on the oocyte as well. As the embryos went through a series of cell divisions, the level of ER mRNA declined from the two-cell to the five- to eight-cell stage. At the morula stage, ER mRNA was undetectable. The ER mRNA detected during this period was probably of maternal origin because the ER mRNA level was highest in the egg and the decrease is in agreement with the general degradation of maternal RNA. Because equal numbers of embryos at each stage were analyzed, the decrease in ER mRNA did not result from the dilution of existing ER mRNA because of the embryo's growth. The most interesting observation from this study is the reappearance of ER mRNA at the blastocyst stage. The

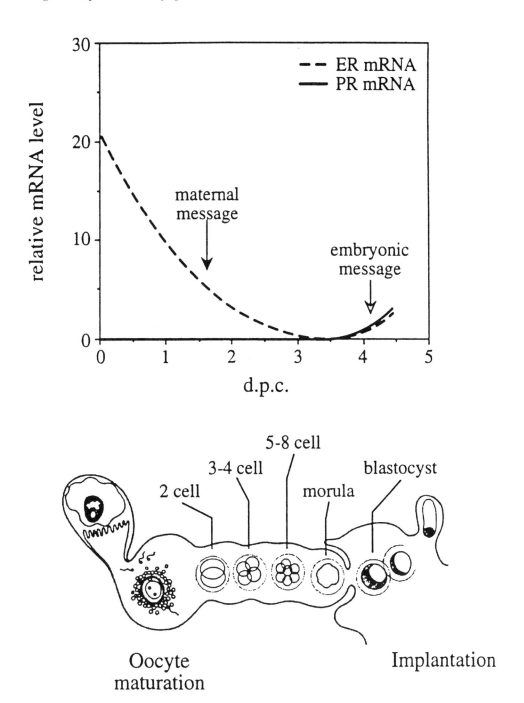

FIGURE 1. Summary of mRNA levels of estrogen receptor (ER) and progesterone receptor (PR) in mouse preimplantation embryos. The ER and PR mRNA levels per embryo are shown in relationship to the age of the embryos. The scale is arbitrary. The corresponding developmental stages are depicted. d.p.c., days postcoitum. The drawing of the embryo at various stages of development was adapted from Hogan et al.[32] with permission (Cold Spring Harbor Laboratory Press, copyright 1986). The origin of the mRNA and its possible function are also indicated. (From Hou, Q. and Gorski, J., *Proc. Natl. Acad. Sci. U.S.A.*, 90, 9460, 1993. With permission.)

mRNA detected at this stage must be synthesized by the embryo itself. Using RT-PCR, Wu et al.[62] was not able to detect ER mRNA in the blastocyst. This discrepancy could be caused by the different reaction conditions used and thus different sensitivity of the PCR.

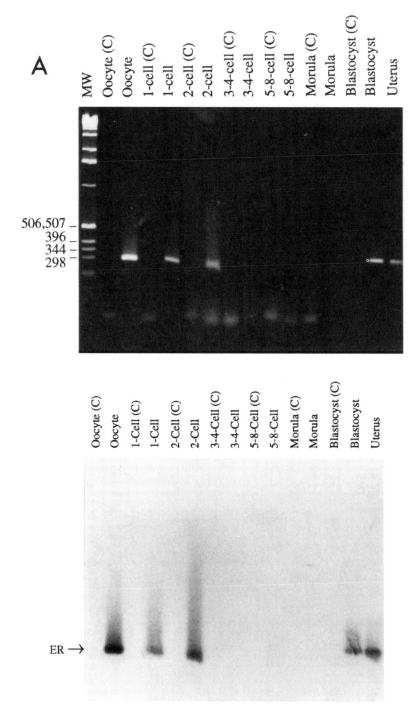

FIGURE 2. Expression of the ER gene. **(A; top panel)** Agarose gel showing the polymerase chain reaction (PCR) product amplified with primers mERo and mERp. RNA from 1.8 embryos was included in each sample. Lanes marked **(C)** are wash controls. Uterine RNA (50 pg) was used as a positive control. The annealing temperature for PCR was 65°C, and 17 plus 33 cycles were run. **(A; bottom panel)** Autoradiogram of Southern blot for the gel shown at top. **(B)** Southern blot analysis of the PCR product amplified with primers mERa and mERb. RNA from 3.6 embryos was included in each sample. Lanes marked **(C)** are as in **A.** Uterine RNA (100 pg) was used as a positive control. The annealing temperature for PCR was 62°C, and 20 plus 35 cycles were run. Lane M, molecular size markers (lengths at left in nucleotides). (From Hou, Q. and Gorski, J., *Proc. Natl. Acad. Sci. U.S.A.,* 90, 9460, 1993. With permission.)

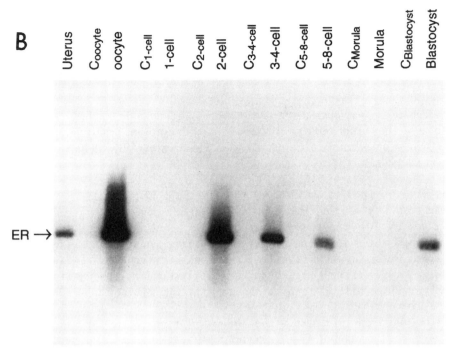

FIGURE 2B.

Mouse embryos implant at the late blastocyst stage. The embryonic expression of ER mRNA suggests a possible functional role for ER at this stage. Because it is the protein that executes function, and RT-PCR assays only for mRNA, it is desirable to determine if this mRNA is indeed translated into protein. Immunocytochemistry was performed on the blastocyst using an antibody developed in rabbit against a synthetic peptide corresponding to a region of the ER.[64] Nuclear staining was observed in all the cells of the blastocyst.[65] The specificity of the staining was validated by including the following controls in parallel samples. No staining or much reduced staining was observed when the antibody was pre-absorbed with an excess of the antigen peptide, or when normal rabbit IgG was substituted for the ER antibody, or when ER antibody was omitted in the incubation. The cellular location of the staining agrees with the cellular location of ER, which is in the nucleus.[66,67] There are two cell types in the blastocyst, the inner cell mass and the trophoblast. The fact that every cell contains ER protein suggests that both cell types express ER. It is known that both estrogen and progesterone are needed for implantation. ER in the trophoblast may respond to estrogen and prepare the embryo for implantation. The fetus is derived from the inner cell mass. It is possible that ER has a general function in the early development of the fetus. Because the progesterone receptor (PR) is generally subject to estrogen regulation, its expression for the first time in preimplantation embryos at the blastocyst stage[61] may be a consequence of ER expression. Whether this expression of PR is indeed dependent upon ER is not yet known.

The presence of ER at such an early age is consistent with the observation that mutations of ER are rare, in contrast to the male sex hormone receptor, the androgen receptor, where numerous mutants have been found.[68] The presence of functional ER may be needed for embryo survival. However, the ER gene was disrupted recently by insertional mutation to create ER "knock out" mice, in which the production of a normal ER transcript was prevented.[69] Paradoxically, the mutant mice were viable, though both females and males were nonfertile. The female reproductive tract was also abnormal. Because there was still 5%

estrogen binding ability in the uterus of the female mice, corresponding to about 1000 receptors per cell, residual expression of ER may be sufficient for survival. Alternatively, redundant pathways might exist. It is conceivable that such redundancy has evolved for certain critical genes, increasing the chances for animal survival. In fact, many genes thought to be very important resulted in viable mice that exhibit only limited phenotype when "knocked out."[70–72] In some cases, a double "knock out" of two genes was needed to result in a phenotypic change.[72] Another possible reason for the early presence of ER is that ER has to be present early in development to help with the organization of the chromatin structure. This is probably required for subsequent responsiveness to estrogen. Later in development, ER expression becomes restricted. But those tissues that do express ER will have chromatin that ER can act upon.

PREIMPLANTATION EMBRYO AS A SOURCE OF ESTROGEN

The possibility that preimplantation embryos make estrogen was proposed on the basis of the possible existence of enzymes important for steroidogenesis in the embryo. Using histochemical studies, Dickmann and Dey[73] demonstrated the presence of 3β-hydroxysteroid dehydrogenase activity in day 4 to day 6 rat embryos. The activity of 17β-hydroxysteroid dehydrogenase, which catalyzes the interconversion of estrone and estradiol, was also detected in embryos of the same age from rat, mouse, rabbit, and hamster using similar methods.[74] Mouse and hamster blastocysts were shown to be able to metabolize progesterone in culture, suggesting that both 5α-reductase and 3α- and 5β-hydroxysteroid dehydrogenase were active.[75,76] The formation of ^{3}H-17β-estradiol from ^{3}H-testosterone was detected directly in rabbit embryos.[77,78] In a recent study, the ability of *in vitro* fertilized human embryos to secrete estrogen in the presence of precursor androgen was demonstrated.[79] The activity seemed to peak right around the time of implantation. The role of estrogen synthesized by embryos was postulated to be important for morula-to-blastocyst transformation, shedding and dissolution of the *zona pellucida*, and implantation of the blastocyst by exerting a local hormonal effect on the uterus.[74,80,81] However, Grube et al.[82] did not detect any secretion of estradiol and progesterone from mouse embryos in culture by radioimmunoassays. So whether preimplantation embryos actually synthesize estrogen normally remains to be seen. Because the embryo exists in a sea of maternal hormones, the role of embryonic-made hormone, if any, may only be supplemental.

ESTROGEN RECEPTOR DURING FETAL DEVELOPMENT

The trophectoderm of the blastocyst contributes only to the extraembryonic tissue. The embryo is derived from the inner cell mass. The inner cell mass forms two layers: the primitive endoderm, which also contributes to extraembryonic tissues, and the primitive ectoderm. The primitive ectoderm gives rise to three layers: the endoderm, the mesoderm, and the ectoderm. The ectoderm gives rise to skin and the nervous system. The endoderm gives rise to intestine, lungs, liver, etc. The mesoderm gives rise to vertebrae, dermis, and muscles as well as the genital ridges, kidney, etc. (for reviews of mouse development, see Refs. 32 and 83).

ESTROGEN RECEPTOR DETECTION USING LIGAND BINDING ASSAYS

The distribution of ER in fetal mouse was examined systematically by the collective efforts of Stumpf, Narbaitz, and Sar using autoradiography.[84–86] In these studies, ^{3}H-DES was injected into mice on the 16th day of pregnancy. The choice of DES as the labeled estrogen circumvents the interference of α-fetoprotein, which binds estradiol with a much higher affinity than DES.[87] Fetuses were collected 80 min to 6 h after injection and frozen sections were prepared. After 18 months of exposure, the distribution of silver grains was analyzed. Cells that showed some concentration of radioactivity in the nucleus were considered to be estrogen targets containing ER. A wide distribution of estrogen target cells was found, including certain hypothalamic and extrahypothalamic brain regions, the anterior pituitary, the larynx, the mesenchyme that surrounds the genital tracts, urogenital sinus, the rectum, the mammary glands, the gubernaculum testis, and the skin. In these studies no competition controls were included to prove specificity of the assay. Using a similar method, Holderegger and Keefer[88,89] extended the study to include fetuses at different gestation ages, namely, days 4, 7, 10, 13, 14, 15, and 17. They also included animals that were injected with a 10-fold higher dose of unlabeled estrogen prior to the injection of ^{3}H-DES at day 7 and day 15 to serve as controls. The earliest day that they could observe even a slight nuclear concentration of radioactivity in the mesenchyme around the genital ducts was day 13 of gestation. On subsequent days they were able to detect ER in certain mammary gland cells, connective tissues, perichondrium associated with specific developing bones, skin, interstitial tissue of the testis, and cells surrounding the colon and the urethra. ER in the brain was first detected on day 14. The number of labeled cells and the intensity of labeling increased during prenatal development. They were not able to detect ER at times earlier than day 13. Attempts to incubate embryos *in vitro* with labeled DES were unsuccessful due to high background.

The autoradiographic method has the advantage of being able to localize the ligand, thus indirectly providing evidence for the presence of ER. The limited sensitivity of this assay, however, requires prolonged exposure. There is also a high background associated with the method. Another disadvantage of this method is that localization of ligand binding does not distinguish high- and low-affinity binding and therefore does not definitely prove the existence of ER.

Ligand binding assays using tissue extracts, which require more material, have also been employed by other investigators. This type of assay provides quantitative information regarding binding affinity and the amount of receptor present. In the 18-day-old fetal mouse uterus, it was determined that the ER level was 140 fmol of ER per milligram of protein.[90] In the fetal mouse forebrain, 0.86 fmol ER/mg of protein on day 13 and 2.65 fmol ER/mg on day 18 was measured.[91] The dissociation constant was determined to be 0.14 nM at fetal day 15 and 0.18 nM at fetal day 18, which is similar to that found in adult tissues.

IMMUNODETECTION OF ESTROGEN RECEPTOR IN MALE AND FEMALE REPRODUCTIVE TRACTS
Development of the Fetal Reproductive System

The fetal development of the reproductive system includes both the gonads and their associated ducts (for reviews, see Refs. 92 and 93). The gonad develops from the genital ridge near the ventral area of the primitive kidney, the mesonephros. Germ cells derived from primordial cells migrate from the epithelium of the dorsal endoderm of the yolk sac outside the embryo proper to reach the area of the genital ridge.[32,92,93] By 11.5 d.p.c., the first indication of the gonadal primordium is seen. At this stage it is not possible to distinguish between the developing ovary or testis.[83] The undifferentiated gonad consists of mesenchymal cells and three other cell types: the germ cells, cells derived from mesonephros, and cells originated in the coelomic epithelium.[92,93] During gonadal sex differentiation in the male, cords develop in the testis that enclose the germ cells together with somatic cells. In the female, germ cells are not confined to cords and the ovary is compact. The supporting somatic cells of the gonad, granulosa cells and Sertoli cells, are thought to have a dual origin of both mesonephros and surface epithelium.[93] The steroid-producing Leydig cells may derive from mesenchymal cells or mesonephric cells. During fetal development, the gonads continue to increase in volume. Between about 13 and 13.5 d.p.c., there is a critical change in the cellular architecture and histological appearance of the gonads so that the ovary and testis can be distinguished.[83] By 14–14.5 d.p.c. the ovaries and testes no longer have a similar size and shape.

The male- and female-associated ducts are derived from the wolffian duct (mesonephric duct) and the Müllerian duct (paranephric duct), respectively.[92,93] At the undifferentiated stage, both ducts are present in both sexes. The Wolffian duct is the excretory duct of the mesonephros, which is formed well before gonad formation. The Müllerian duct develops later. It is hypothesized that the wolffian duct guides the early growth of the Müllerian duct.[93] Both ducts consist of epithelial cells and mesenchymal cells. The epithelial cells line the tube and the mesenchymal cells are arranged in concentric layers around the tube. At early stages of differentiation, both ducts are simple, straight tubes. During sex differentiation in the male, the Wolffian duct differentiates into the epididymis, vas deferens, and seminal vesicles. In the female, the Müllerian duct gives rise to oviducts, uterus, and part of the vagina.

It was demonstrated by Jost et al.[94] that removal of the gonads from the rabbit fetus results in a female phenotype. It is the hormones from the fetal testis that play a critical role in the determination of phenotypic sex. Testosterone synthesized by Leydig cells is responsible for the virilization of the Wolffian duct. Müllerian inhibitory hormone (MIH) secreted by the Sertoli cells causes the regression of the Müllerian duct. The role of female hormones in sexual determination is not clear. However, it seems that the female phenotype develops by default in the absence of the testes. The Wolffian duct regresses without androgen. The Müllerian duct differentiates into female-associated ducts in the absence of MIH.

Estrogen Receptor Expression

The abnormalities in the reproductive system observed in DES-exposed animals indicate that the developmental course of reproductive tissue is altered by an early estrogen stimulus, suggesting the existence of ER in the developing reproductive tissues at an early age. Autoradiographic studies were able to detect ligand binding in the mesenchyme surrounding the reproductive tract. The use of antibodies against ER permits the detection of ER protein independent of its ability to bind ligand, thus the endogenous estrogens will not interfere with the assay. Using a combination of immunoblotting and immunocytochemistry methods, Greco et al.[95–98] carefully examined the ontogeny of ER in the male and female reproductive tract during fetal development. The earliest stage examined by immunodetection was fetal day 10 in the mouse. When protein extracts of the whole embryo were separated on a sodium dodecyl sulfate-polyacrylamide gel and analyzed by immunoblotting, a protein band with the correct molecular weight of the ER, 66,000 Da, was detected. In a parallel experiment, the antibody was preabsorbed with an excess of antigen peptide, and the band could no longer be detected.[95] This proves that the 66-kDa band detected was indeed the ER. On day 10, the sex of the fetus cannot be discriminated morphologically; however, the consistent detection of ER in several single-embryo preparations argues that ER is present in both sexes. On day 13, it is possible to dissect the reproductive tract out of the fetus. When the protein extract of the reproductive tract was subject to immunoblotting, ER was detected. At this stage, the sex of the fetus still cannot be definitely determined by morphology. Beginning on day 15, sexual differentiation begins and the gender of the fetus becomes apparent, allowing males and females to be investigated separately. Extracts of female reproductive tracts on days 15, 17, and 19 were analyzed by immunoblotting (Figure 3), and ER was detected on all three days. The amount of ER increased with age. In the male, the gonad and the associated ducts were examined separately. Again, ER was detected at all ages in both tissues (Figure 3). In contrast to the female, in the male the intensity of the ER band actually decreased at the later stages of development and the overall ER level was much lower than that in the female.

Immunocytochemistry of frozen sections was used to determine the cellular localization and tissue distribution of ER in the reproductive tracts of the fetus. The validity of the method was assessed by including adjacent sections as controls. No staining could be observed if the antibody was preabsorbed with an excess of the antigenic peptide. Gonads and associated ducts were examined separately (Figures 4 and 5). On day 13, most tracts were ambisexual, but differentiation of the testis had occurred in some fetuses, so these fetuses could be identified as male and the rest were categorized as ambisexual. In the male reproductive tract, including the Wolffian duct and possibly the regressing Müllerian duct, ER staining was observed in both epithelial and mesenchymal cells. Gonadal cells also stained. In the

Immunoblot of fetal and neonatal mouse reproductive tracts

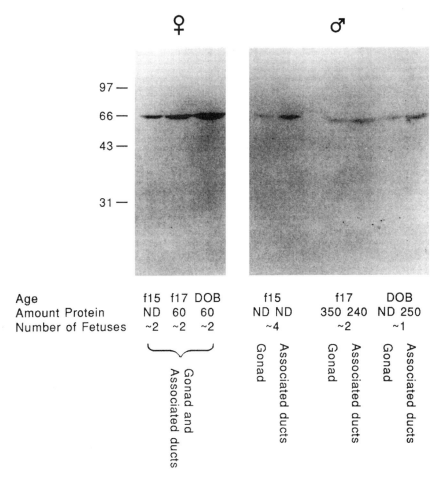

FIGURE 3. Immunoblots of extracts prepared from female and male reproductive tracts collected 15, 17, and 19 days after fertilization. For males, the testes were separated from the associated ducts of the reproductive tract and prepared separately for the immunoblots. Protein concentration (µg) and approximate number of fetuses pooled are listed below the photograph. ND, not determined. (From Greco, T. L., Duello, T. M., and Gorski, J., *Endocr. Rev.,* 14(1), 59, 1993. With permission.)

ambisexual individuals, staining was no different from the male. Later in development, male fetuses could be identified by the presence of seminiferous tubules in the testes and by the descended location of the testes. On fetal day 15, nuclear staining was observed in the cells within tubules and between tubules in the testes. Leydig cells represented most of the ER-positive cells. A smaller percentage of gonadal cells was found to contain ER on fetal day 17 and the day of birth. In the female, the ovary showed immunostaining on fetal day 15. The staining in the ovary was not consistent on fetal day 17. Little or no specific ER staining in the ovary was observed at later fetal stages.

In the associated tracts, ER was also detected in both sexes (Figure 5). On fetal day 15, nuclear staining for ER was observed in the Müllerian duct of the female and Wolffian duct of the male. Both epithelial cell types and mesenchymal cell types showed staining. On day 17, a primitive uterus is discernible in the female. Staining of the mesenchymal cells of the

Gonads

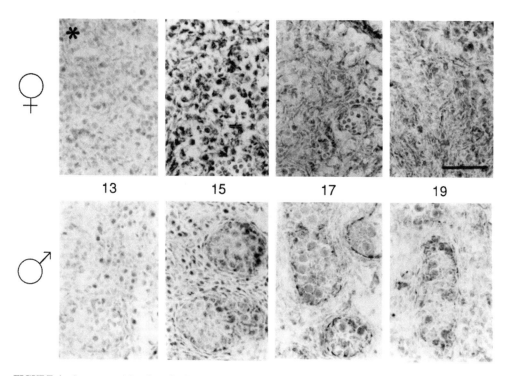

FIGURE 4. Immunocytochemistry for ER on frozen sections from fetal mouse gonads taken on days 13, 15, 17, and 19 postconception. An asterisk indicates that on day 13, gender was not apparent and the fetus could be either a female or a male before sexual differentiation. *Female*: Nuclear staining was observed only on day 15, and the intensity of staining varied between experiments. *Male*: Nuclear staining was observed on days 13 and 15; Leydig cells stained on fetal day 15. On days 17 and 19, peritubular cells of the testes for ER. Bar = 50 μm. (From Greco, T. L., Duello, T. M., and Gorski, J., *Endocr. Rev.,* 14(1), 59, 1993. With permission.)

uterus was observed. However, staining of the epithelial cells varied from very weak to positive staining. Compared with the connective tissue, staining in the epithelial cells was less intense. By the day of birth, day 19, there was no nuclear staining in the epithelium and the staining in the stromal cells was similar to that of the mesenchymal cells of day 17. In the male the intensity of staining and the number of cells stained in the associated ducts of the developing reproductive tract decreased during this period. Less staining was observed on day 17 in both epithelial and connective tissue. By the day of birth, epithelial cells of the epididymis persist in nuclear staining, but stromal cells are no longer ER positive.

The detection of ER in the mesenchymal cells of the reproductive tract agrees with the result of the autoradiographic studies. No ER was found in the epithelial cells in the autoradiographic studies, possibly due to a combination of the lower concentration of ER in these cells during fetal development and the limited sensitivity of the method. Immunocytochemistry, however, allowed the detection of ER in epithelial cells.

SUMMARY AND DISCUSSION

ER mRNA is present at the very beginning of embryogenesis in the fertilized egg.[61,62] Although the maternal messages are degraded, the embryo starts to express ER as early as the blastocyst stage.[61] At this time, the expression of ER is not restricted to any one cell type.[65] Little information is available about ER expression between days 5 and 9 of embryonic

Associated ducts

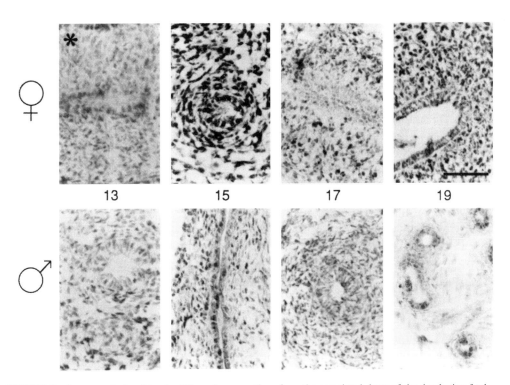

FIGURE 5. Immunocytochemistry for ER on frozen sections from the associated ducts of the developing fetal reproductive tracts taken on days 13, 15, 17, and 19 postconception. An asterisk indicates that the gender of the fetus could not be determined, but nuclear staining could be observed at this age. *Female*: Nuclei stain in mesenchymal and possibly epithelial cells in the Müllerian duct on fetal days 15, 17, and 19. *Male*: On day 13, a cross-section through the Wolffian duct is shown, and nuclei from epithelial and mesenchymal cells stain for ER. Similarly, nuclei are stained in epithelial and mesenchymal cells of the Wolffian duct on fetal day 15. Faint staining in epithelial and mesenchymal cells is noted on day 17; by day 19, epithelial cells, but not connective tissue cells, stain for ER in the epididymis. The section shown for day 15 was incubated with ER antibody ER 715 combined with an excess of Fos peptide to show that a nonrelated peptide would not compete for the antibody. Bar = 50 μm. (From Greco, T. L., Duello, T. M., and Gorski, J., *Endocr. Rev.*, 14(1), 59, 1993. With permission.)

development. Normal embryos cannot be cultured beyond day 5. The small size of the embryos during this period makes their dissection out of the maternal uterus very difficult and allows little confidence that they are free of maternal cell contamination for biochemical analysis. Nonetheless, it was reported that ER mRNA was detected on day 8 by RT-PCR.[62] The same authors also reported an increase in ER mRNA of the whole embryo from day 10 to day 18. On day 10, ER protein can be detected by immunoblotting.[95,98] From day 13 until the day of birth, ER is found in both male and female reproductive tracts as well as some other tissues.[84–86,88–91,95–98] Recently, ER has also been detected in the long bones of vertebrae of human fetuses by both immunocytochemistry and autoradiographic methods.[9] The early presence and wide distribution of ER during embryonic development suggests that ER may have a general role in development not restricted to the development of the female reproductive system.

It is paradoxical that ER mutant mice displayed only limited defects in the reproductive tract.[69] It is possible that the function of ER at an early stage requires only very low levels of receptor, thus the residual receptor is able to fulfill the task. It is also possible that proteins of a redundant pathway could substitute for ER function at an early age. Whether ER plays a role in early development or not, the expression of ER makes the embryo susceptible to the consequences of exposure to estrogen at unwanted times. Normally the presence of α-fetoprotein in mice and rats, which binds to estradiol and lowers the estradiol concentration in the fetus,[99] would protect the embryo from exposure to high levels of maternal estrogen during fetal development. However, other estrogenic compounds that do not bind α-fetoprotein would leave the embryos unprotected. The deleterious effect of prenatal exposure to DES provides such an example.

If ER is not important for early embryogenesis, why would the animal risk being exposed to estrogen to express ER so early? One possibility is that ER participates in the modeling of chromatin structure during development. In cells, DNA is not naked. Rather, it exists in the form of chromatin in which DNA is wrapped around histone octamers that form a regularly phased structure termed the nucleosome. Generally, the presence of nucleosomes restricts the access of transcription factors and thus represses transcription. In the promoter region of actively transcribed genes, nucleosomes are modified such that the transcription initiation complex can form on the DNA.[100,101] Because ER exerts its function as a transcription factor, the interaction of ER with the chromatin is very important. The importance of the chromatin state for ER regulation is exemplified by the following observation.[102] ER was introduced into ER-negative Rat-1 cells through stable transfection. The expression of either the endogenous prolactin gene or a transiently transfected reporter gene with the prolactin promoter was analyzed in the presence of transiently cotransfected pit-1 factor, which is a tissue-specific transcriptional factor necessary for the expression of the prolactin gene. Interestingly, only the transiently transfected gene was turned on, but not the endogenous gene. The difference between the transcriptional regulatory region of the two genes is the chromatin structure. The transiently transfected gene, having been in the cell for only a short time, would not have acquired chromatin structure. As a result, transcriptional factors such as ER and pit-1 easily could access the DNA and activate transcription. The endogenous gene, however, could be in a "closed" state such that even though the transcription factors exist, they are not able to bind to the DNA. No activation of transcription would occur. Steroid receptors have been shown to have the ability to induce changes in chromatin structure.[4,5] It was shown that ER induces DNAse hypersensitivity rapidly (within 15 min) in the presence of ligand in a yeast system.[103] Even though this could reflect the events in mammalian cells, the ligand-dependent change in chromatin structure detected might just be one of the later steps of a multistep activation process. ER might function in a ligand-independent fashion in early changes in chromatin structure. An early presence of ER may be needed to set the chromatin in a proper "open" state to ensure the access of ER at a later time. This hypothesis agrees with the finding that there appears to be a requirement for a longer presence of ER than just the moment of induction in order to regulate the nucleosome-covered endogenous gene. Transiently transfected ER was not able to turn on the endogenous PR gene in Rat-1 cells (K. Kaneko and J. Gorski, unpublished result). However, when stably transfected, the ER was able to do so. The requirement for prolonged presence was also true for PR.[104] In that case, PR was introduced into PR-negative cells either through stable transfection or transient transfection. It was shown that only stably transfected PR was able to activate the mouse mammary tumor virus (MMTV) promoter organized in nucleosome structure, although the ability to activate the transiently expressed gene was no different between transiently or stably transfected PR. It is likely that only through stable transfection would receptors have time to gain access to the chromatin of the endogenous gene and even induce changes in chromatin structure. This chromatin modulation may be crucial for the receptor to function later. A similar requirement during development could be envisioned for the regulation of certain estrogen target genes. ER may need to be present very early in development to shape the chromatin structure, which will allow the realization of regulation by estrogen later. In this regard, it will be interesting to see whether the normal response to estrogen can be fully recovered if ER is reintroduced to the ER "knock out" mice at some time later in development.

REFERENCES

1. **Walters, M. R.,** Steroid hormone receptors and the nucleus, *Endocr. Rev.,* 6, 512, 1985.

2. **Beato, M.,** Gene regulation by steroid hormones, *Cell,* 56, 335, 1989.

3. **Wahli, W. and Martinez, E.,** Superfamily of steroid nuclear receptors—positive and negative regulators of gene expression, *FASEB J.,* 5, 2243, 1991.

4. **Beato, M.,** Transcriptional control by nuclear receptors, *FASEB J.,* 5, 2044, 1991.

5. **Truss, M. and Beato, M.,** Steroid hormone receptors—interaction with deoxyribonucleic acid and transcription factors, *Endocr. Rev.,* 14, 459, 1993.

6. **Tsai, M.-J. and O'Malley, B. W.,** Molecular mechanisms of action of steroid/thyroid receptor superfamily members, *Annu. Rev. Biochem.,* 63, 451, 1994.

7. **Guyton, A. C.,** *Textbook of Medical Physiology,* W. B. Saunders, Philadelphia, 1981.

8. **Bellido, T., Girasole, G., Passeri, G., Yu, X. P., Mocharla, H., Jilka, R. L., Notides, A., and Manolagas, S. C.,** Demonstration of estrogen and vitamin D receptors in bone marrow-derived stromal cells: up-regulation of the estrogen receptor by 1,25-dihydroxyvitamin-D3, *Endocrinology,* 133, 553, 1993.

9. **Ben-Hur, H., Mor, G., Blickstein, I., Likhman, I., Kohen, F., Dgani, R., Insler, V., Yaffe, P., and Ornoy, A.,** Localization of estrogen receptors in long bones and vertebrae of human fetuses, *Calcif. Tissue Int.,* 53, 91, 1993.

10. **Masuyama, A., Ouchi, Y., Sato, F., Hosoi, T., Nakamura, T., and Orimo, H.,** Characteristics of steroid hormone receptors in cultured MC3T3-E1 osteoblastic cells and effect of steroid hormones on cell proliferation, *Calcif. Tissue Int.,* 51, 376, 1992.

11. **Mizutani, T., Nishikawa, Y., Adachi, H., Enomoto, T., Ikegami, H., Kurachi, H., Nomura, T., and Miyake, A.,** Identification of estrogen receptor in human adipose tissue and adipocytes, *J. Clin. Endocrinol. Metab.,* 78, 950, 1994.

12. **Nishikawa, Y., Ikegami, H., Sakata, M., Mizutani, T., Morishige, K., Kurachi, H., Hirota, K., Miyake, A., and Tanizawa, O.,** Ovariectomy increases the level of estrogen receptor mRNA and estrogen receptor binding sites in female rat adipose tissue, *J. Endocrinol. Invest.,* 16, 579, 1993.

13. **Pedersen, S. B., Borglum, J. D., Moller, P. T., and Richelsen, B.,** Effects of in vivo estrogen treatment on adipose tissue metabolism and nuclear estrogen receptor binding in isolated rat adipocytes, *Mol. Cell. Endocrinol.,* 85, 13, 1992.

14. **Smith, O. W.,** Diethylstilbestrol in the prevention and treatment of complications of pregnancy, *Am. J. Obstet. Gynecol.,* 56, 821, 1948.

15. **Smith, O. W. and Smith, G. van S.,** Use of diethylstilbestrol to prevent fetal loss from complications of late pregnancy, *N. Engl. J. Med.,* 241, 562, 1949.

16. **Herbst, A. L., Ulfelder, H., and Poskanzer, D. C.,** Adenocarcinoma of the vagina: association of maternal stilbestrol therapy with tumor appearance in young women, *N. Engl. J. Med.,* 241, 878, 1971.

17. **Herbst, A. L., Cole, P., Colton, T., Robboy, S. J., and Scully, R. E.,** Age-incidence and risk of diethylstilbestrol-related clear cell adenocarcinoma of the vagina and cervix, *Am. J. Obstet. Gynecol.,* 128, 43, 1977.

18. **Herbst, A. L., Kurman, R. J., and Scully, R. E.,** Vaginal and cervical abnormalities after exposure to diethylstilbestrol *in utero, Obstet. Gynecol.,* 40, 287, 1972.

19. **Bibbo, M., Al-Naqeeb, M., Baccarini, I., Gill, W., Newton, M., Sleeper, K. M., Sonex, M., and Wied, G. L.,** Follow-up study of male and female offspring of DES-treated mothers, *J. Reprod. Med.,* 15, 29, 1975.

20. **Gill, W. B., Scumacher, G. F. B., and Bibbo, M.,** Structural and functional abnormalities in the sex organs of male offspring of mothers treated with diethylstilbestrol (DES), *J. Reprod. Med.,* 16, 147, 1976.

21. **McLachlan, J. A., Newbold, R. R., and Bullock, B. C.,** Long-term effects on the female mouse genital tract associated with prenatal exposure to diethylstilbestrol, *Cancer Res.,* 40, 3988, 1980.

22. **Newbold, R. R., Bullock, B. C., and McLachlan, J. A.,** Exposure to diethylstilbestrol during pregnancy permanently alters the ovary and oviduct, *Biol. Reprod.,* 28, 735, 1983.

23. **Newbold, R. A. and McLachlan, J. A.,** Vaginal adenosis and adenocarcinoma in mice exposed prenatally or neonatally to diethylstilbestrol, *Cancer Res.,* 42, 2003, 1982.

24. **McLachlan, J. A., Newbold, R. R., and Bullock, B.,** Reproductive tract lesions in male mice exposed prenatally to diethylstilbestrol, *Science,* 190, 991, 1975.

25. **McLachlan, J. A.,** Prenatal exposure to diethylstilbestrol in mice: toxicological studies, *J. Toxicol. Environ. Health,* 2, 527, 1977.

26. **Newbold, R. R., Bullock, B. C., and McLachlan, J. A.,** Lesions of the rete testis in mice exposed prenatally to diethylstilbestrol, *Cancer Res.,* 45, 5145, 1985.

27. **Bullock, B. C., Newbold, R. R., and McLachlan, J. A.,** Lesions of testis and epididymis associated with prenatal diethylstilbestrol exposure, *Environ. Health Perspect.,* 77, 29, 1988.

28. **McLachlan, J. A., Newbold, R. R., Shah, H. C., Hogan, M. D., and Dixon, R. L.,** Reduced fertility in female mice exposed transplacentally to diethylstilbestrol (DES), *Fertil. Steril.,* 38, 364, 1982.

29. **Ostrander, P. L., Milles, K. T., and Bern, H. A.,** Long-term responses of the mouse uterus to neonatal diethylstilbestrol treatment and to later sex hormone exposure, *J. Natl. Cancer Inst.,* 74, 121, 1985.

30. **Newbold, R. R., Bullock, B. C., and McLachlan, J. A.,** Uterine adenocarcinoma in mice following developmental treatment with estrogens: a model for hormonal carcinogenesis, *Cancer Res.,* 50, 7677, 1990.

31. **Newbold, R. R., Suzuki, Y., and McLachlan, J. A.,** Müllerian duct maintenance in heterotypic organ culture after in vivo exposure to diethylstilbestrol, *Endocrinology,* 115, 1863, 1984.

32. **Hogan, B., Costantini, F., and Lacy, E.,** *Manipulating the Mouse Embryo: A Laboratory Manual,* Cold Spring Harbor Laboratory Press, Cold Spring Harbor, New York, 1986.

33. **McLaren, A.,** The embryo, in *Embryonic and Fetal Development,* 2nd ed., Austin, C. R. and Short, R. V., Eds., Cambridge University Press, Cambridge, 1982, 1.

34. **Schultz, G. A.,** Utilization of genetic information in the preimplantation mouse embryo, in *Experimental Approaches to Mammalian Embryonic Development,* Rossant, J. and Pedersen, R. A., Eds., Cambridge University Press, Cambridge, 1986, 239.

35. **Schultz, R. M.,** Regulation of zygotic gene activation in the mouse, *BioEssays,* 15, 531, 1993.

36. **Martinez-Salas, E., Linney, E., Hassell, J., and DePamphilis, M. L.,** The need for enhancers in gene expression first appears during mouse development with formation of the zygotic nucleus, *Genes Dev.,* 3, 1493, 1989.

37. **Bonnerot, C., Vernet, M., Grimber, G., Briand, P., and Nicolas, J.-F.,** Transcriptional selectivity in early mouse embryos: a qualitative study, *Nucleic Acids Res.,* 19, 7251, 1991.

38. **Bachvarova, R. and DeLeon, V.,** Polyadenylated RNA of mouse ova and loss of maternal RNA in early development, *Dev. Biol.,* 74, 1, 1980.

39. **Pedersen, R. A. and Burdsal, C. A.,** Mammalian embryogenesis, in *The Physiology of Reproduction,* 2nd ed., Knobil, E., Neill, J. D., Greenwald, G. S., Markert, C. L., and Pfaff, D. W., Eds., Raven Press, New York, 1994, 319.

40. **Braude, P. R.,** Control of protein synthesis during blastocyst formation in the mouse, *Dev. Biol.,* 68, 440, 1979.

41. **Schultz, G. A., Clough, J. R., Braude, P. R., Pelham, H. R. B., and Johnson, M. H.,** A re-examination of messenger RNA population in the preimplantation mouse embryo, in *Cellular and Molecular Aspects of Implantation,* Glasser, S. R. and Bullock, D. W., Eds., Plenum Press, New York, 1981, 137.

42. **Wu, J. T., Dickmann, Z., and Johnson, D. C.,** Effects of oestrogen and progesterone on the development, oviductal transport and uterine retention of eggs in hypophysectomized pregnant rats, *J. Endocrinol.,* 51, 569, 1971.

43. **Yoshinaga, K. and Adams, C. E.,** Delayed implantation in the spayed progesterone treated adult mouse, *J. Reprod. Fertil.,* 12, 593, 1966.

44. **Torbit, C. A. and Weitlauf, H. M.,** The effect of oestrogen and progesterone on CO_2 production by "delayed implanting" mouse embryos, *J. Reprod. Fertil.,* 39, 379, 1974.

45. **Moore, G. P. and Carter, N. B.,** Transcriptional activity of blastomeres in mouse embryos during delayed implantation and after oestradiol benzoate-induced resumption of development, *Cell Differ.,* 14, 19, 1984.

46. **Lau, N. I. F., Davis, B. K., and Chang, M. C.,** Stimulation of *in vitro* ³H-uridine uptake and RNA synthesis in mouse blastocysts by 17β-estradiol, *Proc. Soc. Exp. Biol. Med.,* 144, 333, 1973.

47. **Holmes, P. V. and Dickson, A. D.,** Estrogen-induced surface coat and enzyme changes in the implanting mouse blastocyst, *J. Embryol. Exp. Morphol.,* 29, 639, 1973.

48. **Nieder, G. L., Weitlauf, H. M., and Suda, H. M.,** Synthesis and secretion of stage-specific proteins by peri-implantation mouse embryos, *Biol. Reprod.,* 36, 687, 1987.

49. **Smith, D. M. and Smith, A. E. S.,** Uptake and incorporation of amino acids by cultured mouse embryos: estrogen stimulation, *Biol. Reprod.,* 4, 66, 1971.

50. **Harrer, J. A. and Lee, H. H.,** Differential effects of oestrogen on the uptake of nucleic acid precursors by mouse blastocysts in vitro, *J. Reprod. Fertil.,* 33, 327, 1973.

51. **Sen Gupta, J., Dey, S. K., and Dickmann, Z.,** Evidence that "embryonic estrogen" is a factor which controls the development of the mouse preimplantation embryo, *Steroids,* 29, 363, 1977.

52. **Sengupta, J., Roy, S. K., and Manchanda, S. K.,** Effect of an oestrogen synthesis inhibitor, 1,4,6-androstatriene-3,17-dione, on mouse embryo development in vitro, *J. Reprod. Fertil.,* 66, 63, 1982.

53. **Huet, Y. M. and Dey, S. K.,** A paradoxical effect of an antiestrogen, CI-628, on implantation in the mouse, *Proc. Soc. Exp. Biol. Med.,* 189, 61, 1988.

54. **Smith, D. M.,** The effect on implantation of treating cultured mouse blastocysts with oestrogen in vitro and the uptake of [3H]oestradiol by blastocysts, *J. Endocrinol.,* 41, 17, 1968.

55. **Cline, E. M., Randall, P. A., and Oliphant, G.,** Hormone-mediated oviductal influence on mouse embryo development, *Fertil. Steril.,* 28, 766, 1977.

56. **Safro, E., O'Neill, C., and Saunders, D. M.,** Elevated luteal phase estradiol:progesterone ratio in mice causes implantation failure by creating an uterine environment that suppresses embryonic metabolism, *Fertil. Steril.,* 54, 1150, 1990.

57. **Surani, M. A. H.,** Hormonal regulation of proteins in the uterine secretion of ovariectomized rats and the implications for implantation and embryonic diapause, *J. Reprod. Fertil.,* 43, 411, 1975.

58. **Surani, M. A. H.,** Uterine luminal proteins at the time of implantation in rats, *J. Reprod. Fertil.,* 48, 141, 1976.

59. **Bhatt, B. M. and Bullock, D. W.,** Binding of oestradiol to rabbit blastocysts and its possible role in implantation, *J. Reprod. Fertil.,* 39, 65, 1974.

60. **Niemann, H. and Elsaesser, F.,** Steroid hormones in early pig embryo development, in *The Mammalian Preimplantation Embryo,* Bavister, B. D., Ed., Plenum Press, New York, 1987, 117.

61. **Hou, Q. and Gorski, J.,** Estrogen receptor and progesterone receptor genes are expressed differentially in mouse embryos during preimplantation development, *Proc. Natl. Acad. Sci. U.S.A.,* 90, 9460, 1993.

62. **Wu, T. C. J., Wang, L., and Wan, Y. J. Y.,** Expression of estrogen receptor gene in mouse oocyte and during embryogenesis, *Mol. Reprod. Dev.,* 33, 407, 1992.

63. **Austin, C. R. and Short, R. V.,** *Hormonal Control of Reproduction,* Cambridge University Press, Cambridge, 1982.

64. **Furlow, J. D., Ahrens, H., Mueller, G. C., and Gorski, J.,** Antisera to a synthetic peptide recognize native and denatured rat estrogen receptors, *Endocrinology,* 127, 1028, 1990.

65. **Hou, Q. and Gorski, J.,** Immunocytochemical detection of estrogen receptor in mouse blastocysts, in *Proceedings of the 76th Annual Meeting of the Endocrine Society,* The Endocrine Society, Bethesda, MD, 1994, 636 (abstr. 1742).

66. **King, W. J. and Greene, G. L.,** Monoclonal antibodies localize oestrogen receptor in the nuclei of target cells, *Nature (London),* 307, 745, 1984.

67. **Welshons, W. V., Lieberman, M. E., and Gorski, J.,** Nuclear localization of unoccupied oestrogen receptors, *Nature (London),* 307, 747, 1984.

68. **George, F. W. and Wilson, J. D.,** Sex determination and differentiation, in *The Physiology of Reproduction,* 1st ed., Knobil, E. and Neill, J. D., Eds., Raven Press, New York, 1988, 3.

69. **Lubahn, D. B., Moyer, J. S., Golding, T. S., Couse, J. F., Korach, K. S., and Smithies, O.,** Alteration of reproductive function but not prenatal sexual development after insertional disruption of the mouse estrogen receptor gene, *Proc. Natl. Acad. Sci. U.S.A.,* 90, 11162, 1993.

70. **Donehower, L. A., Harvey, M., Slagle, B. L., McArthur, M. J., Montgomery, C. A., Jr., Butel, J. S., and Bradley, A.,** Mice deficient for p53 are developmentally normal but susceptible to spontaneous tumours, *Nature (London),* 356, 215, 1992.

71. **Johnson, R. S., Spiegelman, B. M., and Papaioannou, V.,** Pleiotropic effects of a null mutation in the c-fos proto-oncogene, *Cell,* 71, 577, 1992.

72. **Lohnes, D., Kastner, P., Dierich, A., Mark, M., LeMeur, M., and Chambon, P.,** Function of retinoic acid receptor gamma in the mouse, *Cell,* 73, 643, 1993.

73. **Dickmann, Z. and Dey, S. K.,** Steroidogenesis in the preimplantation rat embryo and its possible influence on morula-blastocyst transformation and implantation, *J. Reprod. Fertil.,* 37, 91, 1974.

74. **Dickmann, Z., Dey, S. K., and Gupta, J. S.,** A new concept: control of early pregnancy by steroid hormone originating in the preimplantation embryo, *Vitam. Horm.,* 34, 215, 1976.

75. **Wu, J. T.,** Metabolism of progesterone by hamster blastocysts and the ontogeny of progesterone metabolic capability, *Biol. Reprod.,* 33, 53, 1985.

76. **Wu, J. T.,** Metabolism of progesterone by preimplantation mouse blastocysts in culture, *Biol. Reprod.,* 36, 549, 1987.

77. **Dickmann, Z., Dey, S. K., and Gupta, J. S.,** Steroidogenesis in rabbit preimplantation embryos, *Proc. Natl. Acad. Sci. U.S.A.,* 72, 298, 1975.

78. **George, F. W. and Wilson, J. D.,** Estrogen formation in the early rabbit embryo, *Science,* 199, 200, 1977.

79. **Edgar, D. H., James, G. B., and Mills, J. A.,** Steroid secretion by human early embryos in culture, *Hum. Reprod.,* 8, 277, 1993.

80. **Dickman, Z. and Dey, S. K.,** Two theories: the preimplantation embryo is a source of steroid hormones controlling (1) morula-blastocyst transformation and (2) implantation, *J. Reprod. Fertil.,* 35, 615, 1973.

81. **Dickmann, Z., Gupta, J. S., and Dey, S. K.,** Does "blastocyst estrogen" initiate implantation? *Science,* 195, 687, 1976.

82. **Grube, K. E., Gwazdauskas, F. C., Lineweaver, J. A., and Vinson, W. E.,** Steroidogenic capabilities of the early mouse embryo, *Steroids,* 32, 345, 1978.

83. **Kaufman, M. H.,** *The Atlas of Mouse Development,* Academic Press, London, 1992.

84. **Stumpf, W. E., Narbaitz, R., and Sar, M.,** Estrogen receptors in the fetal mouse, *J. Steroid Biochem.,* 12, 55, 1980.

85. **Narbaitz, R., Stumpf, W. E., and Sar, M.,** Estrogen target cells in the larynx: autoradiographic studies with ^{3}H-diethylstilbestrol in fetal mice, *Horm. Res.,* 12, 113, 1980.

86. **Narbaitz, R., Stumpf, W. E., and Sar, M.,** Estrogen receptors in mammary gland primordia of fetal mouse, *Anat. Embryol.,* 158, 161, 1980.

87. **Sheehan, D. M. and Young, M.,** Diethylstilbestrol and estradiol binding to serum albumin and pregnancy plasma of rat and human, *Endocrinology,* 104, 1442, 1979.

88. **Keefer, D. and Holderegger, C.,** The ontogeny of estrogen receptors: brain and pituitary, *Dev. Brain Res.,* 19, 183, 1985.

89. **Holderegger, C. and Keefer, D.,** The ontogeny of the mouse estrogen receptor: the pelvic region, *Am. J. Anat.,* 177, 285, 1986.

90. **Hochner-Celnikier, D., Marandici, A., Iohan, F., and Monder, C.,** Estrogen and progesterone receptors in the organs of prenatal cynomolgus monkey and laboratory mouse, *Biol. Reprod.,* 35, 633, 1986.

91. **Friedman, W. J., McEwen, B. S., Toran-Allerand, C. D., and Gerlach, J. L.,** Perinatal development of hypothalamic and cortical estrogen receptors in mouse brain: methodological aspects, *Dev. Brain Res.,* 11, 19, 1983.

92. **Byskov, A. G.,** Primordial germ cells and regulation of meiosis, in *Germ Cells and Fertilization,* 2nd ed., Austin, C. R. and Short, R. V., Eds., Cambridge Unversity Press, Cambridge, 1982, 1.

93. **Byskov, A. G. and Hoyer, P. E.,** Embryology of mammalian gonads and ducts, in *The Physiology of Reproduction,* 2nd ed., Knobil, E., Neill, J. D., Greenwald, G. S., Markert, C. L., and Pfaff, D. W., Eds., Raven Press, New York, 1994, 487.

94. **Jost, A., Vigier, B., Prepin, J., and Perchellet, J. P.,** Studies on sex differentiation in mammals, *Recent Prog. Horm. Res.,* 29, 1, 1973.

95. **Greco, T. L.,** *A Study of the Ontogeny of Estrogen Receptors in Male and Female Fetal and Neonatal Mouse Reproductive Tracts using Immunodetection Methods,* Ph.D. thesis, University of Wisconsin-Madison, 1991.

96. **Greco, T. L., Furlow, J. D., Duello, T. M., and Gorski, J.,** Immunodetection of estrogen receptors in fetal and neonatal female mouse reproductive tracts, *Endocrinology,* 129, 1326, 1991.

97. **Greco, T. L., Furlow, J. D., Duello, T. M., and Gorski, J.,** Immunodetection of estrogen receptors in fetal and neonatal male mouse reproductive tracts, *Endocrinology,* 130, 421, 1992.

98. **Greco, T. L., Duello, T. M., and Gorski, J.,** Estrogen receptors, estradiol, and diethylstilbestrol in early development: the mouse as a model for the study of estrogen receptors and estrogen sensitivity in embryonic development of male and female reproductive tracts, *Endocr. Rev.,* 14, 59, 1993.

99. **Nunez, E. A., Benassayag, C., Savu, L., Vallette, G., and Jayle, M. F.,** Purification and comparative estrogen binding properties of different forms of rat, mouse, and human alpha-1-fetoproteins, in *Onco-Developmental Gene Expression,* Fishman, W. H. and Sell, S., Eds., Academic Press, New York, 1976, 365.

100. **Elgin, S. C. R.,** Chromatin structure and gene activity, *Curr. Opin. Cell Biol.,* 2, 437, 1990.

101. **Workman, J. L. and Buchman, A. R.,** Multiple functions of nucleosomes and regulatory factors in transcription, *TIBS,* 18, 90, 1993.

102. **Kaneko, K. J., Gelina, C., and Gorski, J.,** Activation of the silent progesterone receptor gene by ectopic expression of estrogen receptors in a rat fibroblast cell line, *Biochemistry,* 32, 8348, 1993.

103. **Pham, T. A., Hwung, Y.-P., McDonnell, D. P., and O'Malley, B. W.,** Transactivation functions facilitate the disruption of chromatin structure by estrogen receptor derivatives *in vitro*, *J. Biol. Chem.,* 266, 18178, 1991.

104. **Smith, C. L., Archer, T. K., Hamlin-Green, G., and Hager, G. L.,** Newly expressed progesterone receptor cannot activate stable, replicated mouse mammary tumor virus templates but acquires transactivation potential upon continuous expression, *Proc. Natl. Acad. Sci. U.S.A.,* 90, 11202, 1993.

Chapter 10

EFFECTS OF NUTRITION ON REPRODUCTIVE ENDOCRINE FUNCTION

Béla E. Piacsek

CONTENTS

INTRODUCTION

Reproduction in mammals is regulated by a multicomponent system that consists of the hypothalamic-pituitary-gonadal axis and the accessory structures. Endocrine control of this axis depends on the negative feedback loop between gonads and the hypothalamic-pituitary complex. Secretion of the gonadotropic hormones is inhibited by the circulating levels of gonadal steroid and/or protein hormones either directly at the level of the adenohypophysis or indirectly through changes in the secretion of hypothalamic gonadotropin-releasing hormone (GnRH). Secretion of the gonadal hormones, in turn, is dependent on stimulation by pituitary gonadotropins. In the female, this negative feedback loop is interrupted during the immediate preovulatory period when gonadal estrogen exhibits a positive stimulus on the release of pituitary gonadotropins, producing a rapid and pronounced surge in the secretion of these hormones. This event leads to ovulation and the formation of a corpus luteum from the remaining cells of the ovulated follicle.

Superimposed on this basic operative form of simple endocrine feedback loops are a number of environmental factors that can modulate the function of the axis, thereby affecting reproductive function. These modulatory influences may be exerted directly at the level of the hypothalamus or they may be received and processed through other areas of the central nervous system (CNS) before being relayed to the appropriate hypothalamic connections. Environmental variables that have been demonstrated to modify the reproductive process are photoperiod, temperature, nutrition, population density, and olfactory and acoustic stimuli. The purpose of this chapter is to present a discussion of the influence of nutritional variables on reproductive function with a focus on the endocrine changes and mechanisms through which the influence is exerted.

OUTLINE OF THE PROBLEM

A discussion of the effects of nutrition on reproductive function is complicated by a number of different variables that must be considered before any meaningful conclusions can be formulated. These variables include species, sex, and age differences of the organisms used as models to study the problem. Species that have been studied include laboratory and wild rodents, laboratory and wild lagomorphs, several domestic species, and primates, including humans. In an evaluation of the effects of nutrition on female reproductive function, one must distinguish between the pregnant and nonpregnant, as well as the prepubertal, organism. The same distinction with respect to sexual maturity also must be observed in the male. Other complications that enter into our current knowledge of this subject are the distinction between qualitatively and quantitatively modified diets. The major portion of past studies have concentrated on caloric restriction and protein deficiency. Evaluations of the effects of modified composition in terms of carbohydrate, fat, vitamins, minerals, and micronutrients are limited. Finally, even if one limits review of the available literature to single topics such as caloric restriction, experimental protocols range from short-term complete starvation to chronic moderate underfeeding. Although some generalized conclusions can be drawn on a cumulative systemic level, examination of mechanistic details yields a diversity of interpretations.

EFFECTS OF NUTRITIONAL MODIFICATION IN FEMALES

SEXUALLY IMMATURE ORGANISMS

Evaluation of the effects of prepubertal undernutrition can be ambiguous in some laboratory species. In the rat, a species that has been frequently used as a model for such studies, one must distinguish between preweaning and postweaning reduction in food intake. The preweaning period may represent 55–60% of the prepubertal life span, whereas in the human, it is only 12–15%. Studies, using variable litter size to modify preweaning food intake, have produced equivocal results regarding the timing of vaginal opening and first estrus. Early reports[1,2] indicated a delay in these parameters of sexual maturation. However, more recent observations failed to confirm such a delay,[3-5] despite the lower body weight of the underfed animals. One must also express some reservations regarding the use of litter size as a quantitative means of varying food intake. Factors other than food intake may be associated with crowding and may affect sexual maturation.

Studies on the effects of postweaning reduction in food intake on the timing of vaginal opening and first estrus have shown more consistent results than those with preweaning underfeeding as far as chronological status is concerned. There is a general agreement that a 30–50% reduction in food intake will result in a significant delay in the average age at which vaginal opening and first estrus occur in the rat.[6-10] Similar delays in sexual maturation have been shown in sheep[11] and humans.[12]

Although the chronological delay is well documented, the status of somatic development at the time of puberty in underfed females is more controversial. Some reports[1,2,6,7] indicate that in the undernourished rat vaginal opening will occur at body weights that are significantly below those of *ad libitum*-fed controls. Other investigators have not found such a difference[4,7,10] and at least one study[7] indicates that late maturing underfed rats may be heavier than controls at the time of maturation. Attempts have been made to relate the delay in sexual maturation to growth rate, which was measured in groups of rats subjected to different levels of underfeeding.[8] The timing of vaginal opening and first estrus was inversely related to growth rate.

Although caloric intake can clearly influence the timing of sexual maturation in the rat, studies with qualitatively modified diet indicate that growth rate and body size may not be the only determinants of the process. A significant increase in fat intake results in early maturation despite growth rate and body size identical to control animals.[9] On the other hand, a valine-deficient diet has been shown to delay puberty, despite a lack of difference in growth rate, thus resulting in maturation at a different body size than controls.[8] These studies suggest that attainment of critical body size or body fat percentage may not be the necessary trigger for the onset of puberty in the rat.

Delays in sexual maturation in undernourished females also have been shown in other species. In girls, reduced nutrition results in a delay of menarche.[12–14] A similar conclusion can be drawn from evidence in sheep[11] and cattle.[15] The human studies cited above do suggest a strong association between puberty and a particular lean mass-to-fat ratio in body composition. However, this relationship is correlative and a causal relation can only be speculated.

SEXUALLY MATURE ORGANISMS

Aberration and cessation of normal cycles as a result of reduced nutrition has been demonstrated in several species,[16–20,42] including humans.[21] The changes in cycles are usually the result of ovarian atrophy and lack of ovulation. These effects of reduced nutrition may not be universally observed in all mammalian species. Several feral species have been observed to breed successfully after prolonged periods of partial or even complete starvation[19] and, probably, represent special cases of adaptation to such conditions.

EFFECTS OF NUTRITIONAL MODIFICATION IN MALES

SEXUALLY IMMATURE ORGANISMS

Discussion of the influence of nutrition on reproductive function in the male according to the stage of sexual maturity is more difficult than in the female because of a lack of an easily recognizable external sign of maturation (e.g., vaginal opening and cornification in the female). The only conclusive proof of a fully mature male organism is a fertile mating. Other complications in evaluating the effects of reduced nutrition arise from the fact that in some studies the nutritional changes were initiated well before the pubertal period, but results were not evaluated until the animals were well past the normal maturation period.

A review of available studies indicates that the interstitial apparatus of the testes is more sensitive to reduction of food intake than are the seminiferous tubules. A reduction in caloric intake between 3 and 11 weeks of age did not prevent tubular development[22] in male rats, despite a limited weight gain of only 20 g per animal during the study period. On the other hand, the interstitial tissue showed marked regression. Although a reduction in caloric intake does not have a severe effect on the seminiferous tubules, results from studies with protein-deficient diets are more variable. A protein-free diet[23] has been shown to produce a reduction in tubular diameter and spermatogenic arrest at the primary spermatocyte stage after 15 days and at the spermatogonial stage following 35 days of restriction. The change in testicular morphology was accompanied by reduced accessory structure development and lower prostatic fructose levels. A more recent study,[24] using a 50% reduction in dietary protein content, showed no change in testicular histology, but did report a reduction in androgen binding protein, *in vitro* testosterone secretion, and accessory structure growth.

SEXUALLY MATURE ORGANISMS

Results of studies with modified nutrition in sexually mature males are species variable and subject to other environmental influences. Under controlled environmental conditions, in laboratory rats, chronic moderate reduction in food intake or short-term total starvation has little effect on the tubular structures of the testis or spermatogenesis,[25–27] but does result in significant impairment of Leydig cell structures. Prolonged severe reduction of food intake or extended maintenance on a protein-free diet reduces testicular weights but not the responsiveness to exogenous stimulation by gonadotropins.[28,29]

Studies in mice clearly indicate a species variability and further underscore the problem of drawing generalized conclusions about the effects of reduced food intake in reproduction.[30,31] The response of male house mice to a moderate reduction in caloric intake appears similar to that observed in laboratory rodents, showing little or no change in spermatogenic function. By contrast, deer mice show significant impairment of spermatogenesis after 5 weeks on the same daily intake as house mice in the same study.[31]

In addition to species differences, environmental variables, other than nutrition, can modify the response to a reduction of food intake. Cold temperatures notably enhance the dietary effects on litter production in house mice[32] and testicular function in deer mice.[33]

ENDOCRINE CHANGES

UNDERFED FEMALES

Information on endocrine changes and endocrine mechanisms, which may mediate nutrition-induced effects on reproduction, has expanded substantially during the past decade. However, no single primary endocrine signal has emerged that could be designated as the immediate response to a reduction in caloric intake. It is quite possible that no single endocrine change exists and that the cessation of the reproductive cycle is the cumulative result of several endocrine changes acting in parallel and at different loci. On the other hand, while the endocrine changes may be manifold, it may be a reasonable expectation that a single metabolic signal exists, such as the availability of a metabolic substrate. A significant effort on the part of several investigators has been put forth in an attempt to identify such a signal. These efforts have been extensively discussed in recent reviews.[34,35] The following discussions will concentrate on the endocrine changes and mechanisms that have been shown to participate in the nutrition-induced reproductive failure.

Endocrine Changes in Intact Organisms

Evidence available to date indicates that the defect induced by reduced caloric intake is probably contained within the hypothalamic-pituitary axis and not at the gonadal level. Early investigations indicated that the atrophied ovaries of undernourished or protein-deficient rats can be reactivated by pituitary extracts or gonadotropin preparations.[16,17,36] On the other hand, a more recent study[37] indicated that in prepubertal female rats body weight can have a significant effect on the gonadal response to pregnant mare serum gonadotropin. A small change in estradiol responsiveness by uteri of underfed female rats also has been reported.[4] However, although small differences in ovarian and uterine responsiveness to their respective tropic hormones have been shown, the cumulative evidence indicates that reduced gonadotropin, particularly luteinizing hormone (LH), secretion represents the main cause of reproductive cessation. This conclusion is supported by measurements of LH concentrations in the sera of underfed organisms. Although early studies[37–39] indicated little or no change in serum LH concentrations of underfed rats, more recent investigations evaluating the secretory dynamics of LH secretion in several species clearly point to inadequate LH secretion as a result of reduced nutrition. In young rats, where sexual maturation has been prevented by caloric restriction, no detectable pulses are present,[40,41] but only 42 h of *ad libitum* food intake restores normal pulse characteristics (Figures 1 and 2). Similar results can be demonstrated in sheep with nutritionally delayed puberty[11] and food-restricted sows.[42] The failure of earlier studies to detect significant changes in serum LH concentration of intact rats may have been due to the very low levels of this hormone, which may be near the lower limit of detection by available assay methods and, therefore, small but critical differences may not appear significant. Furthermore, early studies used single-sample measurements which do not yield information regarding secretory dynamics. Serum LH concentration in anorexic women are suppressed and the secretory pattern resembles that of the prepubertal organism.[43,44] In contrast to LH secretion, serum concentrations of follicle-stimulating hormone (FSH) in underfed females appear as high or even higher than in *ad libitum*-fed controls, and most evidence suggests that reproductive failure is not due to a deficiency in the secretion of this hormone,[37,38,45] although humans may represent an exception.[46] Interestingly, age appears to modify the FSH response to dietary restriction in humans.[47]

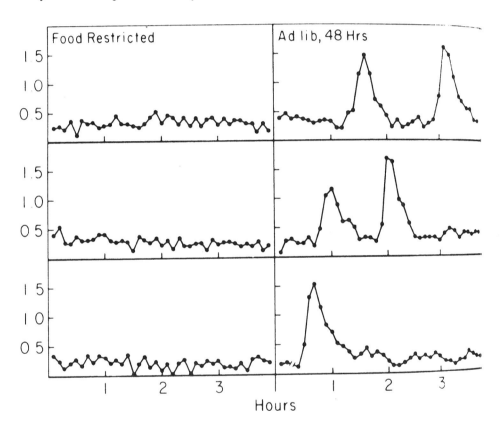

FIGURE 1. Representative pattern of change in blood levels of luteinizing hormone (LH) in 3 intact food-restricted females and 3 intact females that had been given unlimited access to food for 48 h. Each panel represents a single cannulated female whose blood was sampled every 5 min for somewhat over 3.5 h. (From Bronson, F. H., *Am. J. Physiol.*, 254, R616, 1988. With permission.)

Studies with Endocrine Manipulations

Studies with endocrine manipulations of the hypothalamic-pituitary-gonadal axis have yielded more useful information regarding the mechanistic basis of diet-induced suppression of reproductive function and strongly suggest that an increase in the negative feedback sensitivity to ovarian steroids may be, at least, partly responsible.[10,41,45,49–51] As indicated above, LH secretion in the presence of intact gonads is abnormal. On the other hand, removal of the ovaries results in a significant rise in both LH and FSH secretion in underfed female rats.[10,41,45,50,51] Although the postcastration rise of serum FSH concentration appears to be equal to that observed in controls,[10,38,52] the response in LH secretion has been reported to

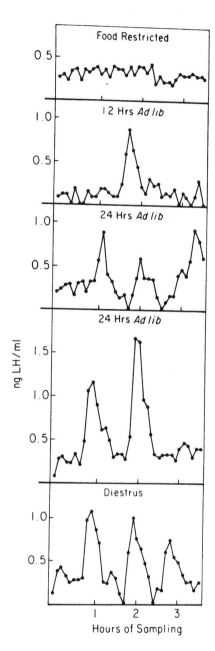

FIGURE 2. Blood levels of luteinizing hormone (LH) in sequentially collected samples obtained every 6 min from female rats. The top pattern is typical of food-restricted females. The three middle panels are typical of these females when examined 12 or 24 h after the resumption of *ad libitum* feeding. The lower panel is a typical pattern observed in normally fed adult females during the late afternoon of diestrus. (From Bronson, F. H., *Endocrinology*, 118, 2483, 1986. With permission.)

be equal[10,50–52] or slightly reduced.[38] The postcastration response for LH is also reduced in underfed hamsters.[48] The differences in the observed postcastration rise of serum LH concentration may have been due to differences in experimental protocol with respect to severity of caloric restriction, timing of ovariectomy in relation to the duration of underfeeding, and the time that blood samples were obtained after ovariectomy. The last factor may be especially important when one examines the results obtained with repeated sample collections.[10,50,53] Although the postovariectomy increase in serum LH concentration of underfed female rats will reach the same amplitude as that of *ad libitum*-fed controls, there appears to be a time lag in the response of the underfed animal.

Investigations into the LH secretory dynamics of adult ovariectomized, 48-h-fasted rats[51] showed no differences in pulse frequency and amplitude when compared to controls. On the other hand, rats with delayed puberty, as a result of chronic underfeeding, do show a decreased frequency and increased pulse amplitude (Figure 3). The difference in the response of these two animal models may have been due more to age than feeding protocol, because chronically underfed adult ovariectomized females also do not exhibit a significant change in frequency or amplitude[54] (Figure 4).

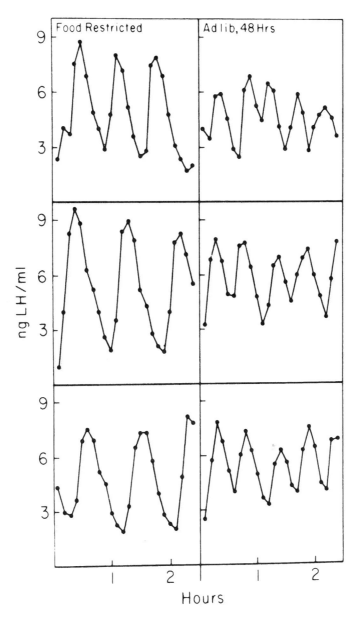

FIGURE 3. Representative temporal patterns of change in blood levels of luteinizing hormone (LH) in 3 ovariectomized, food-restricted females and 3 ovariectomized females that had been fed *ad libitum* for 48 h. Each panel represents a single cannulated female whose blood was sampled every 5 min for 2.5 h. (From Bronson, F. H., *Am. J. Physiol.*, 254, R616, 1988. With permission.)

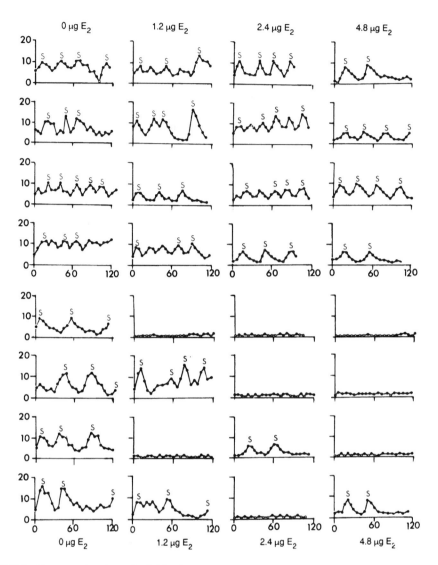

FIGURE 4. Representative plasma luteinizing hormone (LH) pulse profiles in control (top 4 rows) and underfed (bottom 4 rows) rats 12 days after ovariectomy and implantation with 0 (left-hand column), 1.2 (second column from the left), 2.4 (second column from the right), or 4.8 (far right column) μg E_2. Vertical axis represents ng LH/ml. Horizontal axis represents time in minutes. Open circles indicate LH concentrations, which were below the level of assay sensitivity. Significant pulses are indicated by the letter S. (From Spillar, P. A. and Piacsek, B. E., *Neuroendocrinology*, 53, 253, 1991. With permission.)

Perhaps the most unequivocally demonstrated effect of reduced caloric intake is the reduced LH secretion in the presence of exogenously administered estrogen (17β-estradiol or estradiol benzoate) to ovariectomized animals. Mean circulatory LH concentrations consistently have been reported to be significantly more depressed in underfed rats than in controls treated with identical doses of estradiol (Figures 5 and 6).[10,45,50,51,54]

This effect is clearly demonstrated regardless of age, feeding protocol or timing of ovariectomy and estrogen administration. Although the decrease in mean levels is unequivocally demonstrated, the reasons for this change are not as clear. In the acutely fasted ovariectomized rat, estradiol implants produced a significantly greater decrease in both frequency and amplitude of LH pulses than in comparably treated controls.[51] In chronically underfed ovariectomized rats, the decrease in LH pulses appeared to be an "all-or-none"

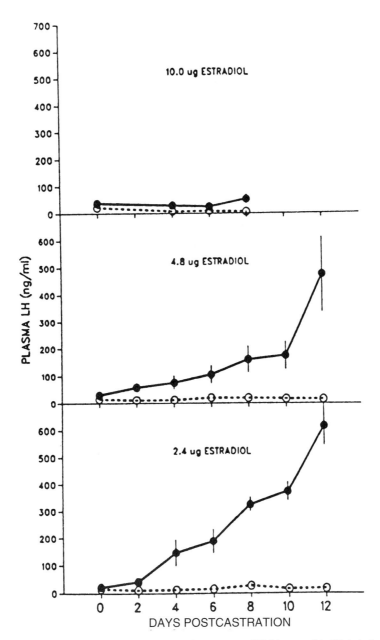

FIGURE 5. Plasma luteinizing hormone (LH) concentrations (means ± SEM) in control (solid circles) and reduced-fed (open circles) female rats following ovariectomy and implantation of capsules containing 10 μg (top panel), 4.8 μg (middle panel), or 2.4 μg (bottom panel) 17β-estradiol. (From Sprangers, S. A. and Piacsek, B. E., *Biol. Reprod.*, 39, 81, 1988. With permission.)

phenomenon.[54] Animals with detectable pulses had frequencies and amplitude similar to controls, and the decrease in mean LH concentration was the result of a complete cessation of pulsatility in proportion to the dose of estradiol administered by subcutaneous implants (Figure 4). In addition to the differences in feeding and surgical protocol, the latter study[54] utilized smaller doses of estradiol. A significant decrease in the percentage of animals showing detectable pulses (Figure 7) was obtained with doses of estradiol that produced plasma levels too low to be detected by radioimmunoassay and produced no significant increase in uterine weights. Another possible explanation may be the length of time during which samples were

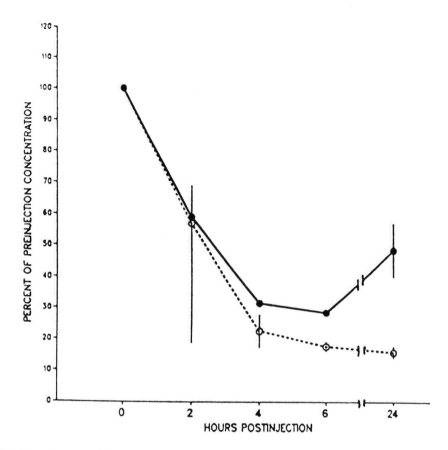

FIGURE 6. Plasma luteinizing hormone concentrations (mean ± SEM) in ovariectomized control (solid circles) and reduced-fed (open circles) rats after subcutaneous injection of 3 μg estradiol benzoate per kilogram of body weight. (From Sprangers, S. A. and Piacsek, B. E., *Biol. Reprod.*, 39, 81, 1988. With permission.)

collected, which was 3 h in the former study[51] and only 2 h in the latter.[54] Perhaps a longer collection time might have yielded a pulse. Supporting this explanation are the results obtained in underfed rats with intact ovaries where the mean frequency was only 0.4 pulses per hour, with 20% of animals showing no detectable pulses in a 3.5-h collection period.[40] Progesterone by itself or in combination with estradiol does not appear to have greater efficacy in the underfed rat.[51] The increased negative feedback efficacy of estradiol has also been confirmed in undernourished sheep.[11]

Because the above studies monitored circulating LH concentrations both for mean levels and for pulse analysis, they do shed some light on the site of the diet-induced defect. A change in mean concentration and a change in pulse amplitude may be the result of changes in GnRH secretion or a change in pituitary responsiveness to GnRH. A change in pulse frequency, on the other hand, points to a change in GnRH pulse generation.

Attempts have been made to investigate the possibility of decreased GnRH sensitivity at the level of the adenohypophysis. Results suggest a significant species variability. In the rat pituitary responsiveness to GnRH appears normal in response to a single infusion of this hormone in adult underfed, ovariectomized and estrogen/progesterone-treated rats[55] and in adult ovariectomized estrogen-treated rats.[56] In fact, when calculated as a percent increase over preinfusion levels, the rise in serum LH is greater than that observed in *ad libitum*-fed controls.[56] In intact rats with food restriction-induced delay in puberty, normal pubertal development is induced by repeated pulsing with GnRH.[40] On the other hand, in ovariectomized, estrogen/progesterone-treated immature rats, reduced food intake reduces the LH

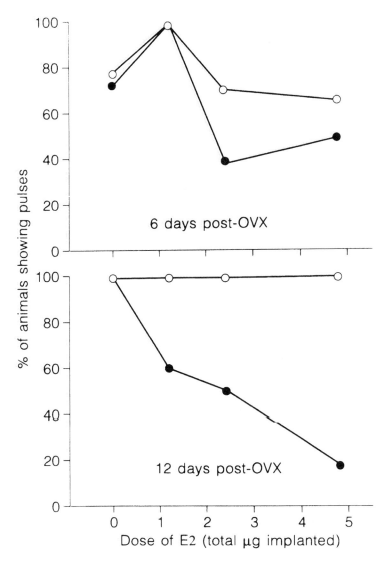

FIGURE 7. Percent of control (open circles) and underfed (solid circles) animals showing at least one luteinizing hormone (LH) pulse according to PC-Pulsar 6 days (top panel) and 12 days (bottom panel) after ovariectomy (OVX) and implantation of a pellet containing 0, 1.2, 2.4, or 4.8 μg E_2. (From Spillar, P. A. and Piacsek, B. E., *Neuroendocrinology,* 53, 253, 1991. With permission.)

response to high, but not low, doses of GnRH and the response in intact underfed, immature rats is increased when compared to controls.[57] Studies in underfed, ovariectomized sheep indicate that GnRH responsiveness is not impaired.[58] A normal response to GnRH has also been observed in underfed, ovariectomized, estrogen-maintained sheep.[59] The efficacy of GnRH to stimulate LH and FSH secretion also has been shown in sows that have been made anestrous with reduced caloric intake.[42]

The maintained pituitary responsiveness of underfed rats is also supported by indirect evidence, based on the fact that the ability to produce an LH surge, following proper steroid priming, is preserved. In adult, ovariectomized rats that have been primed with estrogen, underfeeding does not prevent the progesterone-induced LH surge.[55] Available evidence in both immature and adult underfed rats suggests that the sensitivity to the positive feedback effects of estrogen may even be increased, either at the hypothalamic level or by increased pituitary responsiveness to GnRH.[4,60] It must be noted, however, that the underfed prepubertal rats[4] were significantly older, although weight matched, than the *ad libitum*-fed controls. The above observation strongly suggests that in the rat, sheep, and pig, pituitary responsiveness is preserved in the calorically restricted female. In contrast, available evidence indicates that in humans this may not be true.[21] GnRH administration to women with severe weight loss results in no increase in either LH or FSH secretion and, during weight recovery, significant LH response was not detected until individuals were within 19% of their normal body weight.[61] Reduced pituitary responsiveness may also be present in cattle,[62] although this effect appears to be somewhat age dependent.

UNDERFED MALES

Studies on the endocrine changes in underfed males have not yielded uniform results. There is reasonably good agreement regarding serum LH and testosterone concentrations. Measurements in rats,[25,27,63,64,69] deer mice,[31] cattle,[65] and Rhesus monkeys[66–68] indicate that LH and testosterone secretion are depressed by a reduction in food intake. Estimates of serum testosterone levels in rats either by direct measurement or through measurement of accessory structure weights[25,27,68,69] indicate a strong suppressive effect of underfeeding. Similar observations have been made in deer mice.[33] In a long-term study (21–1000 days), testosterone and 5α-dihydrotestosterone did not reach the same pubertal peak in underfed rats as in controls, but the decline with age was less precipitous than in the *ad libitum*-fed controls.[69]

Serum FSH concentrations in rats show a decrease following 7 days of complete starvation,[63] but no change after 20 days of 50% food reduction.[27] Moderate underfeeding also has no effect on FSH levels in prepubertal male rats.[71]

Only limited information is available in humans.[21] With severe protein and caloric deficiency in men, there is a decline in circulating testosterone levels but a rise in both serum FSH and LH concentrations, suggesting a decrease in testicular responsiveness.

Experimental manipulation of the hypothalamic-pituitary-gonadal axis indicates that, as is the case for females, removal of the gonads results in a significant postcastration response in underfed male rats. Both FSH and LH concentrations rise in circulation. The postcastration rise in LH in protein-deficient rats appears to be normal,[24] whereas the increase in FSH levels may be equal[72] or greater[24,73] than that observed in castrate control rats. In rats with reduced caloric intake, LH levels following castration do not differ significantly from *ad libitum*-fed controls.[64,71]

In rats, the most clearly documented change in response to reduced caloric intake appears to be the increased negative feedback efficacy of testosterone on LH release.[64,71,73] By contrast, the negative feedback of testosterone on FSH secretion is not enhanced by caloric deficiency,[71,73] but it is greater in the protein-deficient animal. Caloric restriction and protein deficiency also exhibit differential effects on the *in vitro* synthesis of inhibin, which is unchanged by the former but reduced by the latter.[73]

Available evidence indicates that at least some of the effect of reduced nutrition, whether in the presence of steroid feedback or in castrate organisms, is exerted directly at the level of the hypothalamus, resulting in an apparent deficiency of GnRH release.[64] In calorically restricted male rats, GnRH content of the median eminence increases significantly compared to control animals, despite the pronounced reduction in serum LH concentration.[64] Support for this hypothesis also comes from studies in the fasted Rhesus monkey, where pituitary responsiveness to GnRH is normal in amplitude but the frequency of endogenous pulses is decreased, as indicated by decreased LH pulse frequencies.[66] On the other hand, GnRH sensitivity studies in underfed male rats also suggest that at least part of the diet-induced suppression of LH release is the result of decreased response to GnRH.[64] No decrease in testicular responsiveness to LH is present in underfed rats,[64] and with moderate reduction in food intake spermatogenesis remains normal despite reduction in the secretion of both gonadotropins.[6]

SOME RELEVANT QUESTIONS

A review of the literature published in the past 10 years indicates that significant progress has been made in exploring the endocrine mechanisms responsible for the diet-induced suppression of reproductive function. Nevertheless, there are several important areas that need further elucidation. First, the effect of reduced caloric intake on the clearance and metabolic fate of various endocrine secretions in the hypothalamic-pituitary-gonadal axis must be clarified. This is particularly germane in the case of steroid hormones because of the change in body composition (fat vs. lean mass) and because of the repeated demonstration in both females and males with exogenous steroid administration that the negative feedback efficacy of these hormones is increased with reduced nutrition.

In female rats with delayed puberty induced by restricted food intake, the disappearance rates from circulation of radiolabeled LH and estradiol do not differ from that of refed controls during the first hour following infusion.[41] Similar results were obtained for the disappearance rate of unlabeled estradiol.[74] No difference in the ratio of free to bound estradiol has been found in underfed rats.[50] Perhaps the most comprehensive study of estradiol clearance has been in the sheep.[75] This study utilized a qualitative and quantitative recovery and analysis of radioactivity from injected radiolabeled 17β-estradiol cleared through fecal and urinary routes over a 48-h period. The slower passage of ingested material in the food-restricted ewes resulted in retarded excretion of radioactivity in the feces and higher plasma concentrations of metabolites, particularly of a polar compound that remained higher in the food-restricted animal's plasma between 4 and 24 h following infusion.

A second question to be addressed is the possible role the hypothalamic-pituitary-adreno-cortical axis may play in the suppression of gonadotropin secretion. If reduced food intake, particularly a severe or complete starvation, acts as an environmental stress, there may be an increase in the activity of this axis, resulting in increased plasma levels of glucocorticoid hormones or possibly sex hormones, such as progesterone and androgens. The ability of glucocorticoids to modify gonadotropin secretion has been demonstrated both *in vivo*[76] and *in vitro*.[77] Studies in undernourished sheep suggest that, in this species, glucocorticoids do not play a significant role in mediating the effects of reduced caloric intake.[78] Basal and pulsatile cortisol release did not differ in food-restricted animals when compared to *ad libitum*-fed controls and the response to adrenocorticotropic hormone (ACTH) and stress was similar in both groups, despite suppression of pulsatile LH release. Similar conclusions can be drawn from studies in fasted male Rhesus monkeys,[79] which show no correlation between plasma cortisol levels and suppression of LH secretion and no effect of exogenous corticoid (hydrocortisone acetate) or dexamethasone on LH secretion. In the underfed female rat, no increase in adrenal progesterone secretion has been found[80] and corticosterone levels appear similar to that found in *ad libitum*-fed controls.[81]

A third question that merits some consideration concerns the possible presence of some direct neural, rather than humoral, signals from the alimentary tract that may modify hypothalamic function with respect to gonadotropin secretion. At least one report in male rats indicates that gastrointestinal filling may play a role in nutritional signaling on LH release, at least during the first 3 days of food reduction.[82] In this study, a 50% reduction in macronutrients produced a decrease in LH pulse amplitude, which was prevented by substitution of cellulose for the reduced macronutrient mass. However, by the 7th and 10th days of the study, the cellulose-substituted rats did not differ from the reduced fed.

The fourth question should address the possible role of hypothalamic neurotransmitters and neuromodulators in the diet-induced reduction of gonadotropin, particularly LH, secretion. Among these, endogenous opioid peptides and neuropeptide Y (NPY) particularly warrant attention, because both have been shown to be involved in the regulation of LH release either indirectly via GnRH or directly at the level of the adenohypophysis.

An inhibitory effect of opioid peptides on LH release has been reported in *ad libitum*-fed rats,[83,84] sheep, [85,86] rabbit,[87] hamster,[88] and primates.[89] Available evidence also indicates that this inhibitory role of endogenous opioid peptides is, at least partly, steroid dependent.[90–94] Because of this parallel between diet-induced and opioid inhibition of LH release, the opiatergic pathways would appear to be a likely candidate in mediating the effects of reduced caloric intake. However, available information offers only limited support for this hypothesis. In 72-h-fasted, ovariectomized, estrogen-treated rats, stimulation of the ventral noradrenergic tract induced a significantly lower LH release than in *ad libitum*-fed controls. Administration of naloxone elevated the response to stimulation to a level that was equal to that found in controls.[95] A more recent study in rats[51] tends to confirm the role of opioid peptides in the underfed rat. By contrast, in undernourished female lamb with delayed puberty, naloxone was found to have no effect on LH secretion.[96] Naloxone also does not reverse the anestrous condition induced in hamsters by food deprivation.[34]

Another potentially important neuropeptide, which may be involved in nutritional regulation of reproduction, is NPY. More than a decade has passed since the demonstration that NPY may play a pivotal role in the control of LH secretion in the rat.[97] The subject has been the focus of recent reviews.[98–101] It is clear from these studies that in the presence of preovulatory levels of estradiol, NPY stimulates LH release both by increasing GnRH secretion and by enhancing the stimulatory effects of GnRH at the pituitary level. By contrast, in the gonadectomized rat, NPY is an inhibitor of LH release.[97,102] Equally important is the knowledge that NPY is a potent appetite stimulator[97,103] and the fact that its hypothalamic content changes following manipulation of food intake.[104,105] Despite this apparent relevance, only a few studies have attempted to relate NPY to both food intake and reproduction. Measurement of serum LH concentrations and NPY concentrations in four selected hypothalamic loci in growth-retarded ewes showed a significant reduction in both mean LH levels and LH pulse frequency but a rise of NPY levels in all four hypothalamic sites. The greatest increase was in the median eminence area.[106] Another study with underfed sheep also showed the expected decrease in mean serum LH levels and LH pulse frequency, but also demonstrated an increase in hypothalamic NPY mRNA, with no change in GnRH mRNA.[107]

The role of two other peptides, one of neural origin, the other of intestinal origin, has been explored. In fasted female rats, evidence from the use of corticotropic hormone-releasing hormone (CRH) antagonists suggests that this peptide may be involved in the diet-induced suppression of pulsatile LH secretion.[108] The hypothesis that gastrointestinal cholecystokinin (CCK) may serve as a signal following food intake also has been tested in male Rhesus monkeys.[109] Although CCK can stimulate LH release, it does not appear to be involved in the resumption of LH release during refeeding of fasted animals.

The final question that obviously must be addressed is the nature of the metabolic signal responsible for the induction of endocrine changes resulting in decreased reproductive function. This subject has been extensively reviewed recently.[34,35]

SUMMARY

Dietary restriction (caloric or protein) in most mammalian species results in reduction or complete cessation of reproductive function. Some exceptions to this generalization may be found among feral species. Furthermore, the effects of such dietary restrictions on the hypothalamic-pituitary-gonadal axis can vary significantly with species, age, sex, and environmental factors, such as temperature and photoperiod. It is also apparent that some of the equivocal conclusions drawn from different studies are the result of variations in the feeding protocol, ranging from moderate chronic reductions in caloric intake to total starvation which may be acute (24–72 h) or extended (1 week).

Despite these differences and the diversity of experimental protocols employed, some consensus has emerged regarding the effects of reduced food intake and the mechanisms that may mediate these effects in the hypothalamic-pituitary-gonadal axis. Although both sexes are sensitive to reduced caloric intake based on gonadal morphology and function, females appear to have a more pronounced response to the same degree of food reduction than males. This is not surprising if one considers the energy cost of an ensuing pregnancy and lactation to the female. Nevertheless, adequate behavioral studies should be conducted to compare the impact of underfeeding on reproductive success between the sexes. In females, underfeeding results in cessation of reproductive cycles, reduced ovarian follicular development, and lack of ovulation, and, in the young, a delay in puberty. In males, the impact of caloric restriction on interstitial cell function is greater than on the seminiferous tubules and spermatogenesis.

It now is reasonably certain that with moderate underfeeding the responsiveness of the gonads to pituitary gonadotropins is not compromised. Therefore, inadequate gonadotropin secretion is the most likely explanation of reproductive failure. The effect of reduced nutrition on LH release has been unequivocally established. The effect on FSH secretion does not appear to be as pronounced as on LH secretion.

Most evidence points to a lack of adequate GnRH release from the hypothalamus, rather than a reduced pituitary responsiveness to GnRH, as the reason for reduced circulating LH levels, but some exceptions can be cited. The hypothalamic defect is also supported by a decrease in LH pulse frequency or a complete cessation of pulsatile LH release in the calorically challenged organism.

The reduced GnRH release, as monitored by serum LH pulsatility, appears to have a steroid-dependent and steroid-independent component, although the former has been more unequivocally documented than the latter. Although the increased negative feedback efficacy of estradiol and testosterone have been clearly established, progesterone by itself or in the presence of estradiol does not appear to be more potent in the underfed animal than in *ad libitum*-fed controls.

The reasons for the increased negative feedback efficacy of gonadal steroid hormones is not known. The synthesis of GnRH appears not to be affected and the lack of release into portal circulation appears to be the principal defect in the underfed organism.

Among hypothalamic neurotransmitters and neuromodulators, the endogenous opioid peptides, NPY and CRH have been implicated in the mediation of diet-induced reproductive failure. The effect of CRH appears to be direct because involvement of glucocorticoid hormones has not been demonstrated.

REFERENCES

1. **Kennedy, G. C. and Mitra, J.,** Body weight and food intake as initiating factors for puberty in the rat, *J. Physiol. (London)*, 166, 408, 1963.
2. **Widdowson, E. M. and McCance, R. A.,** Some effects of accelerating growth. I. General somatic development, *Proc. R. Soc. London Ser. B*, 152, 188, 1960.
3. **Bakke, J. L., Lawrence, N. L., Bennett, J., and Robinson, S.,** Late effects of neonatal undernutrition and overnutrition on pituitary-thyroidal and gonadal function, *Biol. Neonate*, 27, 259, 1975.
4. **Ronnekliev, O. K., Ojeda, S. R., and McCann, S. M.,** Undernutrition, puberty, and development of estrogen positive feedback in the female rat, *Biol. Reprod.*, 19, 414, 1978.
5. **Piacsek, B. E.,** unpublished data, 1983.
6. **Glass, A. R. and Swerdloff, R. S.,** Nutritional influences on sexual maturation in the rat, *Fed. Proc.*, 39, 2360, 1980.
7. **Wilen, R. and Naftolin, F.,** Pubertal food intake and body length, weight and composition in the feed-restricted female rat: comparison with well-fed animals, *Pediatr. Res.*, 12, 263, 1978.
8. **Glass, A. R., Harrison, R., and Swerdloff, R. S.,** Effect of undernutrition and amino acid deficiency on the timing of puberty in rats, *Pediatr. Res.*, 10, 951, 1976.
9. **Glass, A. R., Dahms, W. T., and Swerdloff, R. S.,** Body fat at puberty in rats: alterations by changes in diet, *Pediatr. Res.*, 13, 7, 1979.

10. **Piacsek, B. E.,** Altered negative feedback response to ovariectomy and estrogen in prepubertal restricted-diet rats, *Biol. Reprod.,* 32, 1062, 1985.

11. **Foster, D. L. and Olster, D. H.,** Effect of restricted nutrition on puberty in the lamb: patterns of tonic luteinizing hormone (LH) secretion and competency of the LH surge system, *Endocrinology,* 116, 375, 1985.

12. **Frisch, R. E.,** Pubertal adipose tissue: is it necessary for normal sexual maturation? Evidence from the rat and human female, *Fed. Proc.,* 39, 1295, 1980.

13. **Frisch, R. E. and Revelle, R.,** Height and weight at menarche and a hypothesis of menarche, *Arch. Dis. Child.,* 46, 695, 1971.

14. **Frisch, R. E.,** Weight at menarche: similarity for well-nourished and undernourished girls at differing ages, and evidence for historial constancy, *Pediatrics,* 50, 445, 1972.

15. **Petitclerc, D., Chapin, L. T., Emery, R. S., and Tucker, H. A.,** Body growth, growth hormone, prolactin and puberty response to photoperiod and plane of nutrition in Holstein heifers, *J. Anim. Sci.,* 57, 892, 1983.

16. **Marrian, G. F. and Parkes, A. S.,** The effect of anterior pituitary preparations administered during dietary anoestrus, *Proc. R. Soc. London Ser. B,* 105, 248, 1929.

17. **Mulinos, M. G. and Pomerantz, L.,** Pseudohypophysectomy, a condition resembling hypophysectomy, produced by malnutrition, *J. Nutr.,* 19, 493, 1940.

18. **Piacsek, B. E. and Meites, J.,** Reinitiation of gonadotropin release in underfed rats by constant light or epinephrine, *Endocrinology,* 81, 535, 1967.

19. **Widdowson, E. M.,** The role of nutrition in mammalian reproduction, in *Environmental Factors in Mammal Reproduction,* Gilmore, D. and Cook, B., Eds., Macmillan, London, 1981, 145.

20. **Doney, J. M. and Gunn, R. G.,** Nutritional and other factors in breeding performance of ewes, in *Environmental Factors in Mammal Reproduction,* Gilmore, D. and Cook, B., Eds., Macmillan, London, 1981, p.1969.

21. **Warren, M. P.,** Effect of undernutrition on reproductive function in the human, *Endocr. Rev.,* 4, 363, 1983.

22. **Widdowson, E. M., Mavor, W. O., and McCance, R. A.,** The effect of undernutrition and rehabilitation on the development of the reproductive organs: rats, *J. Endocrinol.,* 29, 119, 1964.

23. **Tripathi, S. S., Roy, S. K., and Kar, A. B.,** Effect of protein deficiency on genital organs and fertility of male rats, *Indian J. Exp. Biol.,* 6, 195, 1968.

24. **Glass, A. R., Mellitt, R., Vigersky, R. A., and Swerdloff, R. S.,** Hypoandrogenism and abnormal regulation of gonadotropin secretion in rats fed a low protein diet, *Endocrinology,* 104, 438, 1979.

25. **Grewal, T., Mickelsen, O., and Hafs, H. D.,** Androgen secretion and spermatogenesis in rats following semi-starvation, *Proc. Soc. Exp. Biol. Med.,* 138, 723, 1971.

26. **Negro-Vilar, A., Dickerman, E., and Meites, J.,** Effects of starvation on hypothalamic FSH-RF and pituitary FSH in male rats, *Endocrinology,* 188, 1246, 1971.

27. **Howland, B. E.,** The influence of feed restriction and subsequent re-feeding on gonadotrophin secretion and serum testosterone levels in male rats, *J. Reprod. Fertil.,* 44, 429, 1975.

28. **Berliner, D. L. and Ellis, L. C.,** The effect of irradiation on endocrine cells. V. A comparison between the effects of inanition and irradiation on androgen production by murine testicular tissue, *Radiat. Res.,* 24, 572, 1965.

29. **Leathem, J. H., II,** Hormones in growth and development. Hormones and protein nutrition, *Recent Prog. Horm. Res.,* 14, 141, 1958.

30. **Blank, J. L. and Desjardins, C.,** Spermatogenesis is modified by food intake in mice, *Biol. Reprod.,* 30, 410, 1984.

31. **Blank, J. L. and Desjardins, C.,** Differential effects of food restriction on pituitary-testicular function in mice, *Am. J. Physiol.,* 248, R181, 1985.

32. **Pryor, S. and Bronson, F. H.,** Relative and combined effects of low temperature, poor diet, and short daylength on the productivity of wild house mice, *Biol. Reprod.,* 25, 734, 1981.

33. **Desjardins, C. and Lopez, M. J.,** Environmental cues evoke differential responses in pituitary-testicular function in deer mice, *Endocrinology,* 112, 1398, 1983.

34. **Wade, G. N. and Schneider, J. E.,** Metabolic fuels and reproduction in female mammals, *Neurosci. Biobehav. Rev.,* 16, 235, 1992.

35. **Friedman, M. I.,** Making sense out of calories, in *Handbook of Behavioral Neurobiology,* Stricker, E. M., Ed., Plenum Press, New York, 1990, 513.

36. **Srebnik, H. H., Nelson, M. M., and Simpson, M. E.,** Response to exogenous gonadotropins in the absence of dietary protein, *Proc. Soc. Exp. Biol. Med.,* 99, 57, 1958.

37. **Howland, B. E.,** Gonadotropin levels in female rats subjected to restricted feed intake, *J. Reprod. Fertil.,* 27, 467, 1971.

38. **Ibrahim, E. A. and Howland, B. E.,** Effect of starvation on pituitary and serum follicle-stimulating hormone and luteinizing hormone following ovariectomy in the rat, *Can. J. Physiol. Pharmacol.,* 50, 768, 1972.

39. **Srebnik, H. H., Nelson, M. M., and Simpson, M. E.,** Follicle stimulating hormone (FSH) and interstitial-cell stimulating hormone (ICSH) in pituitary and plasma of intact and ovariectomized protein deficient rats, *Endocrinology,* 68, 317, 1961.

40. **Bronson, F. H.,** Food-restricted, prepubertal female rats: rapid recovery of luteinizing hormone pulsing with excess food, and recovery of pubertal development with gonadotropin releasing hormone, *Endocrinology,* 118, 2483, 1986.

41. **Bronson, F. H.,** Effect of food manipulation on the GnRH-LH-estradiol axis of young female rats, *Am. J. Physiol.,* 254, R616, 1988.

42. **Armstrong, J. D. and Britt, J. H.,** Nutritionally-induced anestrus in gilts: metabolic and endocrine changes associated with cessation and resumption of estrous cycles, *J. Anim. Sci.,* 65, 508, 1987.

43. **Boyar, R. M., Katz, J., Finkelstein, J. W., Kapen, S., Weiner, H., Weitzman, E., and Hellman, L.,** Anorexia nervosa: immaturity of the 24 hour luteinizing hormone secretory pattern, *N. Engl. J. Med.,* 291, 861, 1974.

44. **Vigersky, R. A., Andersen, A. E., Thompson, R. H., and Loriaux, D. L.,** Hypothalamic dysfunction in secondary amenorrhea associated with simple weight loss, *N. Engl. J. Med.,* 297, 1141, 1977.

45. **Howland, B. E. and Ibrahim, E. A.,** Increased LH suppressing effect of oestrogen in ovariectomized rats as a result of underfeeding, *J. Reprod. Fertil.,* 35, 545, 1973.

46. **Warren, M. P.,** Effects of undernutrition on reproductive function in the human, *Endocr. Rev.,* 363, 1983.

47. **Schweiger, U., Laessle, R., Pfister, H., Hoehl, C., Schwingenschloegel, M., Schweiger, M., and Pirke, K. M.,** Diet-induced menstrual irregularities: effects of age and weight loss, *Fertil. Steril.,* 48, 746, 1987.

48. **Howland, B. E. and Skinner, K. R.,** Effect of starvation on LH levels in male and female hamsters, *J. Reprod. Fertil.,* 32, 505, 1973.

49. **Walker, R. F. and Frawley, L. S.,** Gonadal function in underfed rats. II. Effect of estrogen on plasma gonadotropins after pinealectomy or constant light exposure, *Biol. Reprod.,* 17, 630, 1977.

50. **Sprangers, S. A. and Piacsek, B. E.,** Increased suppression of luteinizing hormone secretion by chronic and acute estradiol administration in underfed adult female rats, *Biol. Reprod.,* 39, 81, 1988.

51. **Cagampang, F. R., Maeda, K. I., Tsukamura, H., Ohkura, S., and Ota, K.,** Involvement of ovarian steroids and endogenous opioids in the fasting-induced suppression of pulsatile LH release in ovariectomized rats, *J. Endocrinol.,* 129, 321, 1991.

52. **Stewart, S. F., Kopia, S., and Gawlak, D. L.,** Effect of underfeeding, hemigonadectomy, sex and cyproterone acetate on serum FSH levels in immature rats, *J. Reprod. Fertil.,* 45, 173, 1975.

53. **Knuth, U. A. and Friesen, H. G.,** Starvation induced anoestrus: effect of chronic food restriction on body weight, its influence on estrous cycle and gonadotropin secretion in rats, *Acta Endocrinol.,* 104, 402, 1983.

54. **Spillar, P. A. and Piacsek, B. E.,** Underfeeding alters the effect of low levels of estradiol on luteinizing hormone pulsatility in ovariectomized female rats, *Neuroendocrinology,* 53, 253, 1991.

55. **Howland, B. E.,** Gonadotropin release induced by GnRH or progesterone in female rats maintained on high or low levels of feed intake, *J. Reprod. Fertil,.* 47, 137, 1976.

56. **Spillar, P. A., Lively, K. M., and Piacsek, B. E.,** Increased luteinizing hormone (LH) secretion in response to gonadotropin releasing hormone (GnRH) in two different models of restricted-fed female rats, *Biol. Reprod.,* 38 (Suppl.), 161, 1988.

57. **Lively, K. M. and Piacsek, B. E.,** Gonadotropin-releasing hormone sensitivity in underfed prepubertal female rats, *Am. J. Physiol.,* 255, E482, 1988.

58. **Foster, D. L., Ebling, F. J. P., Micka, A. F., Vannerson, L. H., Bucholtz, D. C., Wood, R. I., Suttie, J. M., and Fenner, D. E.,** Metabolic interface between growth and reproduction. I. Nutritional modulation of gonadotropin, prolactin, and growth hormone secretion in the growth-limited female lamb, *Endocrinology,* 125, 342, 1989.

59. **Kile, J. P., Alexander, B. M., Moss, G. E., Hallford, D. M., and Nett, T. M.,** Gonadotropin-releasing hormone overrides the negative effect of reduced dietary energy on gonadotropin synthesis and secretion in ewes, *Endocrinology,* 128, 843, 1991.

60. **Sprangers, S. A. and Piacsek, B. E.,** Estradiol feedback in gonadotropin secretion in the underfed female rat, *Biol. Reprod.,* 36 (Suppl.), 151, 1987.

61. **Warren, M. P., Jewelewicz, R., Dyrenfurtle, I., Aus, R., Khalaf, S., and Vande Wiele, R. L.,** The significance of weight loss in the evaluation of pituitary response to LH-RH in women with secondary amenorrhea, *J. Clin. Endocrinol. Metab.,* 40, 601, 1975.

62. **Day, M. L., Inakawa, K., Zalesky, D. D., Kitlok, R. J., and Kinder, J. E.,** Effects of restriction of dietary energy intake during the prepubertal period on secretion of luteinizing hormone and responsiveness of the pituitary to luteinizing hormone releasing hormone in heifers, *J. Anim. Sci.,* 62, 1641, 1986.

63. **Howland, B. E. and Skinner, K. R.,** Effect of starvation on gonadotropin secretion in intact and castrated male rats, *Can. J. Physiol. Pharmacol.,* 51, 759, 1973.

64. **Pirke, K. M. and Spyra, B.,** Influence of starvation on testosterone-luteinizing hormone feedback in the rat, *Acta Endocrinol.,* 96, 413, 1981.

65. **Gauthier, D. and Berbigier, P.,** The influence of nutritional levels and shade structure on testicular growth and hourly variations of plasma LH and testosterone levels in young Creole bulls in a tropical environment, *Reprod. Nutr. Dev.,* 22, 793, 1982.

66. **Cameron, J. L. and Nosbisch, C.,** Suppression of pulsatile luteinizing hormone and testosterone secretion during short term food restriction in the adult male Rhesus monkey (*Macaca mulatta*), *Endocrinology*, 128, 1532, 1991.

67. **Schreihofer, D. A., Parfitt, D. B., and Cameron, J. L.,** Suppression of luteinizing hormone secretion during short-term fasting in male Rhesus monkeys: the role of metabolic versus stress signals, *Endocrinology*, 132, 1881, 1993.

68. **Schreihofer, D. A., Amico, J. A., and Cameron, J. L.,** Reversal of fasting-induced suppression of luteinizing hormone (LH) secretion in male Rhesus monkeys by intragastric nutrient infusion: evidence for rapid stimulation of LH by nutritional signals, *Endocrinology*, 132, 1890, 1993.

69. **Merry, B. J. and Holehan, A. M.,** Serum profiles of LH, FSH, testosterone and 5 alpha-DHT from 21 to 1000 days of age in *ad libitum* and dietary restricted rats, *Exp. Gerontol.*, 16, 431, 1981.

70. **Smith, S. R., Chhetri, M. K., Johansen, A. J., Radfar, N., and Migeon, C. J.,** The pituitary-gonadal axis in men with protein-caloric malnutrition, *J. Clin. Endocrinol. Metab.*, 41, 60, 1975.

71. **Piacsek, B. E., Bonifer, T. M., and Tan, R. C.,** Altered testosterone feedback in pubertal male rats raised in reduced caloric intake, *J. Androl.*, 7, 292, 1986.

72. **Root, A. W. and Russ, R. D.,** Short-term effects of castration and starvation upon pituitary and serum levels of luteinizing hormone and follicle stimulating hormone in male rats, *Acta Endocrinol. (Copenhagen)*, 70, 665, 1972.

73. **Glass, A. R., Steinberger, A., Swerdloff, R., and Vigersky, R. A.,** Pituitary testicular function in protein-deficient rats. Follicle-stimulating hormone hyperresponse to castration and supersensitivity of gonadotropin secretion to androgen negative feedback, *Endocrinology*, 110, 1542, 1982.

74. **Sprangers, S. A. and Piacsek, B. E.,** Estrogen and luteinizing hormone (LH) interactions in adult female rats on restricted food intake, *Biol. Reprod.*, 34 (Suppl.), 184, 1986.

75. **Adams, N. R., Abordi, J. A., Briegel, J. R., and Sanders, M. R.,** Effect of diet on the clearance of estradiol-17β in the ewe, *Biol. Reprod.*, 51, 668, 1994.

76. **Ringstrom, S. J., Suter, D. E., Hostetter, J. P., and Schwartz, N. B.,** Cortisol regulates secretion and pituitary content of the two gonadotropins differentially in female rats: effects of gonadotropin-releasing hormone antagonist, *Endocrinology*, 130, 3122, 1992.

77. **D'Agostine, J., Valadka, R. J., and Schwartz, N. B.,** Differential effects of *in vitro* glucocorticoids on luteinizing hormone and follicle-stimulating hormone secretion: dependence on sex of pituitary donor, *Endocrinology*, 127, 891, 1990.

78. **I'Anson, H., Quiet, E. H., Wood, R. I., England, B. G., and Foster, D. L.,** Adrenal axis and hypogonadotropism in the growth-restricted female lamb, *Biol. Reprod.*, 50, 137, 1994.

79. **Helmreich, D. L., Mattem, L. G., and Cameron, J. L.,** Lack of a role of the hypothalamic-pituitary-adrenal axis in the fasting-induced suppression of luteinizing hormone secretion in adult male Rhesus monkeys (*Macaca mulatta*), *Endocrinology*, 132, 2427, 1993.

80. **Becker, G. M. and Piacsek, B. E.,** Role of progesterone in diet-induced suppression of LH secretion in adult female rats, *Biol. Reprod.*, 48 (Suppl.), 154, 1993.

81. **Becker, G. M. and Piacsek, B. E.,** unpublished data, 1993.

82. **Dong, Q., Rintala, H., and Handelsman, D. J.,** Effect of gastrointestinal filling during undernutrition on pulsatile LH secretion in mature male rats, *Proc. 9th Int. Congr. Endocrinol.*, 411 (Abstr. #12.03.003), 1992.

83. **Ieiri, T., Ureu, H. T., and Meites, J.,** Effects of morphine and naloxone on serum levels of luteinizing hormone and prolactin in prepubertal male and female rats, *Neuroendocrinology*, 29, 288, 1979.

84. **Babu, G. N., Mario, J., Bona-Gallo, A., and Gallo, R. V.,** Steroid-independent endogenous opioid peptide suppression of pulsatile luteinizing hormone release between estrus and diestrus in the rat estrous cycle, *Brain Res.*, 416, 235, 1987.

85. **Brooks, A. N., Lamming, G. E., Lees, P. D., and Haynes, N. B.,** Opioid modulation of LH secretion in the ewe, *J. Reprod. Fertil.*, 76, 693, 1986.

86. **Ebling, F. J. P., Schwartz, M. L., and Foster, D. L.,** Endogenous opioid regulation of pulsatile luteinizing hormone secretion during sexual maturation in the female sheep, *Endocrinology*, 125, 369, 1989.

87. **Orstead, K. M. and Spies, H. G.,** Inhibition of hypothalamic gonadotropin-releasing hormone release by endogenous opioid peptides in the female rabbit, *Neuroendocrinology*, 46, 14, 1987.

88. **Donham, R. S., Sarafidin, E. H., and Stetson, M. H.,** Naloxone administration to female hamsters advances puberty by enhancing luteinizing hormone release, *Proc. Soc. Exp. Biol. Med.*, 182, 291, 1986.

89. **Orstead, K. M., Hess, D. L., and Spies, H. G.,** Opiatergic inhibition of pulsatile luteinizing hormone release during the menstrual cycle of Rhesus macaques, *Proc. Soc. Exp. Biol. Med.*, 184, 312, 1987.

90. **Gabriel, S. M., Simpkins, J. W., and Kalra, S. P.,** Modulation of endogenous opioid influence on LH secretion by progesterone and estrogen, *Endocrinology*, 113, 1806, 1983.

91. **Yang, K., Haynes, N. B., Lamming, G. E., and Brooks, A. N.,** Ovarian steroid hormone involvement in endogenous opioid modulation of LH secretion in mature ewes during the breeding and non-breeding seasons, *J. Reprod. Fertil.*, 83, 129, 1988.

92. **Whisnant, C. S. and Goodman, R. L.,** Effect of an opioid antagonist on pulsatile luteinizing hormone secretion in the ewe vary with changes in steroid negative feedback, *Biol. Reprod.*, 39, 1032, 1988.

93. **Bhanot, R. and Wilkinson, M.,** Opiatergic control of LH secretion is eliminated by gonadectomy, *Endocrinology*, 112, 3993, 1983.

94. **Bhanot, R. and Wilkinson, M.,** The inhibitory effect of opiates on gonadotropin secretion is dependent upon gonadal steroids, *J. Endocrinol.*, 102, 133, 1984.

95. **Dyer, R. G., Mansfield, S., Corbet, L. H., and Dean, A. D. P.,** Fasting impairs LH secretion in female rats by activating an inhibitory opioid pathway, *J. Endocrinol.*, 105, 91, 1984.

96. **Ebling, F. J. P., Wood, R. I., Karsch, F. J., Vannerson, L. A., Suttie, J. M., Bucholtz, D. C., Schall, R. E., and Foster, D. L.,** Metabolic interfaces between growth and reproduction. III. Control mechanisms controlling pulsatile luteinizing hormone secretion in the nutritionally growth-limited female lamb, *Endocrinology*, 126, 2719, 1990.

97. **Kalra, S. P. and Crowley, W. R.,** Norepinephrine-like effects of neuropeptide-Y on LH release in the rat, *Life Sci.*, 35, 1173, 1984.

98. **Kalra, S. P. and Crowley, W. R.,** Neuropeptide-Y: a novel neuroendocrine peptide in the control of pituitary hormone secretion, and its relation to luteinizing hormone, *Front. Neuroendocrinol.*, 13, 1, 1992.

99. **Levine, J. E., Bauer-Dautoin, A. C., Besecke, L. M., Conaghan, L. A., Legan, S. J., Meredith, J. M., Strobl, F. J., Urban, J. H., Vogelsong, K. M., and Wolfe, A.W.,** Neuroendocrine regulation of the luteinizing hormone releasing hormone pulse generation in the rat, *Recent Prog. Horm. Res.*, 47, 97, 1992.

100. **Freeman, M. E.,** Editorial: neuropeptide-Y: a unique member of the constellation of gonadotropin-releasing hormones, *Endocrinology*, 133, 2411, 1993.

101. **Kalra, S. P., Sahn, A., Kalra, P. S., and Crowley, W. R.,** Hypothalamic neuropeptide-Y: a circuit in the regulation of gonadotropin secretion and feeding behavior, *Ann. N.Y. Acad. Sci.*, 611, 273, 1990.

102. **Kerkerian, L., Guy, J., Lefevre, G., and Pelletier, G.,** Effects of neuropeptide-Y (NPY) on the release of anterior pituitary hormones in the rat, *Peptides*, 6, 1201, 1985.

103. **Leibowitz, S. F.,** Hypothalamic neuropeptide-Y in relation to energy balance, *Ann. N.Y . Acad. Sci.*, 611, 284, 1990.

104. **Sahu, A., Swinsky, C. A., Kalra, P. S., and Kalra, S. P.,** Neuropeptide concentration in microdissected hypothalamic regions and *in vitro* release from the medial basal hypothalamus-preoptic area of streptozotocin-diabetic rats with and without insulin therapy, *Endocrinology*, 126, 192, 1990.

105. **Beck, B., Jhanwar-Uniyal, M., Burlet, A., Chapleur-Chateau, M., Leibowitz, S. T., and Burlet, C.,** Rapid and localized alterations of neuropeptide-Y in discrete hypothalamic nuclei with feeding status, *Brain Res.*, 528, 245, 1990.

106. **Ober, J. H. and Malven, P. V.,** Effect of growth retardation on pituitary luteinizing hormone and hypothalalmic neuropeptide-Y in ovariectomized sheep, *Neuroendocrinology*, 56, 331, 1992.

107. **McShane, T. M., Petersen, S. L., McCrane, S., and Keisler, D. H.,** Influence of food restriction on neuropeptide-Y, proopiomelanocortin, and luteinizing hormone-releasing hormone gene expression in sheep hypothalami, *Biol. Reprod.*, 49, 831, 1993.

108. **Maeda, K., Cagampang, F. R., Coen, C. W., and Tsukamura, H.,** Involvement of the catecholaminergic input to the paraventricular nucleus and of corticotropin-releasing hormone in the fasting-induced suppression of luteinizing hormone release in female rats, *Endocrinology*, 134, 1718, 1994.

109. **Schreihofer, D. A., Golden, G. A., and Cameron, J. L.,** Cholecystokinin (CCK)-induced stimulation of luteinizing hormone (LH) secretion in adult male Rhesus monkeys: examination of the role of CCK in nutritional regulation of LH secretion, *Endocrinology*, 132, 1553, 1993.

Chapter 11

THE TESTIS

Joachim Braun and Rudolf Stolla

CONTENTS

MORPHOLOGY AND FUNCTIONS

DEVELOPMENTAL ASPECTS
Sexual Differentiation

The undifferentiated gonad originates from the mesenchyme on the medioventral surface of the mesonephric ridges. In humans, the developing gonad experiences a sexually indifferent period of approximately 7–10 days that occurs at 6 weeks of gestation. During this period, primordial germ cells (PGCs) arrive at the gonad after migration from their initial location close to the yolk sac endoderm. In addition, the indifferent gonad consisting of loose mesenchymal tissue is invaded by cells from the mesonephros and is covered by coelomic epithelium.[1]

At this stage, sex differentiation is initiated under the influence of the testis determining factor (TDF) located on the Y chromosome. During the 1970s and early 1980s a gene for the H-Y antigen (histocompatibility-Y antigen) was postulated to be the factor determining testicular differentiation.[2] However, the hypothesis was abandoned when it was discovered that a certain strain of mice which had testes lacked the H-Y antigen.[3] Page et al.[4] identified a gene that encodes a zinc-finger-containing protein (ZFY). This gene was claimed to be a second candidate for TDF until it was reported that ZFY is absent in many 46XX males.[5] In 1990 a single-copy gene was isolated on the short arm of the Y chromosome that proved to be necessary for male sex determination.[6,7] It was named SRY in humans and Sry in mice, for the gene in the sex determination region of the Y chromosome. Direct evidence that SRY is the primary testis determinant was obtained when the mouse Sry was introduced into XX mouse embryos and was demonstrated to give rise to normal testes development in chromosomally female transgenic mice.[8] However, it cannot be ruled out that other genes are involved in the process of sex determination in mammals, and that SRY is only the beginning of a gene regulatory cascade.[9,10]

In an XY embryo TDF commits the primitive gonad to testicular development, resulting first in Sertoli and later in Leydig cell differentiation. The origin of Sertoli cells is still uncertain. They may develop from mesenchymal cells or mesonephrogenic blastema. During early gonadal development the Sertoli cells surround the germ cells to form the testicular cords, the precursors of the seminiferous tubules.[1] Sertoli cells are responsible for the secretion of the anti-müllerian hormone (AMH), also termed müllerian-inhibiting hormone (for review see Cate and Wilson[11]). Leydig cells develop shortly after gonadal sex differentiation has taken place, correlating with the onset of testosterone production. The origin of the fetal Leydig cell precursor cells has not yet been clarified. They may arise from mesenchymal cells or from mesonephric cells. The differentiating Leydig cells rapidly gain the typical morphological appearance of steroid-producing cells. The rise in testosterone secretion by the testis is closely correlated with cytodifferentiation and increase in size and number of Leydig cells. Similarly, testosterone secretion declines when Leydig cells dedifferentiate during late fetal life.[12]

Testosterone and AMH produced by the fetal testes are required for all subsequent male sex differentiation. It was established by the pioneer work of Jost[13] that the development of the female urogenital tract occurs in the absence of gonadal hormones, whereas hormonal secretion of the fetal testes is necessary to induce the male phenotype in eutherian mammals. AMH causes regression of the paired müllerian ducts (the female internal genital tract precursor structure), whereas testosterone causes differentiation of the wolffian ducts into the male internal genital tract (for review see Byskov and Hoyer,[12] George and Wilson[14]).

AMH has been shown to be a glycoprotein with structural similarities to inhibin and transforming growth factor-β (TGF-β). The müllerian duct is sensitive to AMH for only a short period after gonadal sex differentiation. In some species, however, AMH is produced in abundant amounts for an extended period. It has been suggested that AMH secretion after gonadal sex differentiation may be important for other purposes, e.g., inhibition of meiosis and initiation of testicular descent.[1,12,14]

AMH acts independently of testosterone as demonstrated in castrated fetuses, in which the müllerian duct persists and the wolffian duct does not develop. Development of the wolffian duct can be induced by injections of testosterone, but this treatment leaves the müllerian duct unaffected and the two systems develop side by side. In intact fetuses treated with cyproteron-acetate, a potent antiandrogen, the wolffian duct does not develop due to the lack of androgen effects, but the müllerian duct regresses normally. These individuals have testes but no other sexual organs.[15]

It seems that testosterone itself rather than its derivative dihydrotestosterone (DHT) is responsible for differentiation of the wolffian duct, although DHT may be important for the development of the epididymis.[12] The actions of testosterone and DHT are mediated by a specific intracellular androgen receptor.[16] Whether testosterone production is regulated by fetal and/or maternal gonadotropins is not clear. Receptors for luteinizing hormone (LH) have been shown to be present in the fetal rabbit testis at the time of initial testosterone synthesis. However, onset of testosterone synthesis and the resulting differentiation of the genital tract in rabbits occurs in the absence of gonadotropic stimulation. Later in embryogenesis testosterone synthesis is regulated by gonadotropin. Whether gonadotropin is critical for the initiation of testosterone synthesis in the human fetal testis is uncertain.[14]

In the male fetus, the first step of differentiation of the urogenital tract is the regression of the müllerian ducts. As this regression begins, the wolffian ducts undergo differentiation. The cranial part of the wolffian duct develops into the epididymis, the central portion becomes the vas deferens, and the caudal part gives rise to the seminal vesicle and the ejaculatory duct.[12] Development of the urethra, the accessory organs, and the external genitalia begins after the onset of virilization of the wolffian ducts. Studies in rat, rabbit, guinea pig, and human embryos indicate that DHT is responsible for the differentiation of the male urethra, prostate, and external genitalia, whereas testosterone mediates the virilization of the wolffian ducts.[14]

Descent of the Testis

In most mammals, including man, the descent of testis is completed by the time of birth or shortly afterwards. The mechanisms of testicular descent and the possible hormonal control of the process are not yet fully understood. It was proposed that the whole process of testicular descent from the posterior abdominal wall to the scrotum occurs in three phases:[1] first, the cranial movement of the metanephros causing the testis to acquire a more caudal position, then the transabdominal movement of the testis to the inguinal ring, and third, the descent through the inguinal canal to the scrotum. Increasing intraabdominal pressure during the second phase is believed to cause a herniation in the abdominal wall (the processus vaginalis) along the course of the inguinal portion of the gubernaculum. Descent of the testis into the scrotum in the final stage probably involves a progressive degeneration of the proximal part of the gubernaculum.[14,17]

Much controversy still exists about the hormonal control of the testicular descent. Two theories based on animal experimental work have been proposed.[18] The first suggests that androgens mediate descent possibly via stimulation by fetal gonadotropins and epididymal growth.[19,20] The other main theory is more complex and proposes a biphasic mechanism.[21] During the first phase, a nonandrogenic testicular factor, possibly AMH, induces gubernacular enlargement and descent of the testis as far as the internal ring, as this step still occurs in mice and humans with androgen resistance. This view is supported by observations that antiandrogens given during this phase do not significantly block testicular descent, and oestrogens given during this phase block descent and cause retained müllerian ducts and gubernacular atrophy, possibly via inhibition of AMH. The second phase of gubernacular regression is dependent on androgens, as exogenous testosterone restores gubernacular regression in orchidectomized animals, and as oestrogen inhibits this phase of descent, possibly because of its antiandrogenic action. This inhibition may be reversed by DHT (for review see Kiely[18]). However, the role of androgens in the second phase of descent has been questioned by the finding that flutamide, a nonsteroidal antiandrogen, blocked testicular descent in rats only when given prenatally, which is coincident with the first phase of descent.[22]

ANATOMY OF THE TESTIS
Location
In most mammals, the testes are located outside of the abdomen in the scrotum, either periodically (during the time of reproductive activity), e.g., in some seasonal breeders, or permanently, e.g., in domestic mammals and man. The position of the scrotum in relation to the abdomen shows considerable variation between the species. Also, the size of the testes varies depending on the species. Their weight increases manifold at puberty and in some seasonal breeders at the beginning of the breeding season. In humans, it slightly decreases with age.[17]

Scrotum
The scrotum is part of a temperature regulating system, keeping the temperature of the gonads several degrees lower than the temperature inside the body cavity. This is of particular importance because in species with a scrotum spermatogenesis is particularly sensitive to temperature.[23] However, in many eutherian mammals without a scrotum spermatogenesis occurs without any change in temperature.[24] Several physiological mechanisms enable the scrotum to actively control its own temperature: smooth muscle fibers in the skin of the scrotum, the tunica dartos muscles, the cremaster muscle, sweat glands, and pigmentation of the skin. Thermal receptors within the scrotal skin respond to rising temperatures. As a result, the tunica dartos relaxes and scrotal sweating increases (for details see Setchell et al.[17]). An additional component of this temperature controlling system is the pampiniform plexus (see below).

Blood and Nerve Supply
The testis is supplied with blood by the internal spermatic artery, which arises from the abdominal aorta. The artery runs directly to the testis where it branches in animals with abdominal testes. In animals with scrotal testes, the artery runs along the body wall, passes through the inguinal canal, and coils extensively before it reaches the testicular surface. The veins leaving the testis divide near the dorsal pole to form a venous complex, called the pampiniform plexus. These venous branches surround the coiled artery in mammals. The pampiniform plexus acts as a very efficient countercurrent heat exchanger so that the arterial blood is cooled by the venous blood; at the same time, the venous blood is warmed to body temperature by the arterial blood. In addition, by this arrangement the pulse is almost eliminated from the arterial blood as it flows through the cord. Arteriovenous anastomoses have been demonstrated to exist in the spermatic cord of several mammals. Studies of hormone secretion from the testis show a considerable reduction of testosterone concentrations when levels in venous blood sampled from below the pampiniform plexus are compared with the

levels higher up the spermatic cord.[25] These anastomoses are believed to provide a transfer of arterial blood to the venous drainage of the pampiniform plexus, thereby diluting the venous concentrations above the pampiniform plexus (for review see Setchell et al.[17]).

The nerve supply is derived from the superior spermatic nerve of lumbosacral origin and consists mainly of sympathetic fibers. The nerves follow the spermatic arteries to the surface of the testis, where they branch into the testicular parenchyma. In the testis, adrenergic nerves can be found in the interstitial tissue in association with blood vessels. Vascular tone in the testis is under nervous control. Leydig cells appear to have β-adrenergic binding sites.[26] Stimulation of cultured Leydig cells with catecholamines has been shown to increase their production of testosterone,[27] whereas blockade of sympathetic activity reduced testosterone levels and the response to human chorionic gonadotropin (hCG).[28] No nerves penetrate the seminiferous tubules, but axons bearing synaptic vesicles were found on the basal lamina in humans.[29]

There were some suggestions in the early literature that denervation causes dilatation of testicular blood vessels and degeneration of germ cells in the seminiferous tubules;[30] however, these effects may have been secondary to vascular effects or to interference with transport of sperm and fluid through the epididymis.[17] Transection of the main vascular and nervous supply of the testes of young piglets had no effect on their subsequent development, and section of the testicular nerves of adult rams caused no deterioration in seminal quality during the next 6 weeks.[31,32] It has been suggested that the short-term effects of vasoligation or unilateral castration on plasma concentrations of follicle-stimulating hormone (FSH), LH, and prolactin provide evidence for a direct neural connection between the testes and the central nervous system.[33,34]

Structure of the Testis

The testis has an ovoid shape and is encased by a tough capsule, the tunica albuginea. There are relatively few blood vessels and smooth muscle fibers in the tunica albuginea. The muscle cells are capable of rhythmic contractions which seem to be important for the transport of spermatozoa out of the testis in the epididymis as well as for maintaining the interstitial pressure inside the testis.[35-37] The testicular parenchyma consists of seminiferous tubules and interstitial tissue. Most of the testis is made up by the seminiferous tubules, which are cylindrical, highly convoluted, and densely packed, having only small interstitial spaces. The amount of interstitial tissue in relation to the testicular volume varies from about 10% in the rat to about 60% in the boar.[38,39] In the human testis about one third of the parenchyma is taken up by the loose connective tissue surrounding the seminiferous tubules.[40] The spermatozoa are produced inside the seminiferous tubules. Usually both ends of the tubules open into the rete testis via the short tubuli recti (Figure 1).

Interstitial Tissue

The interstitial tissue includes blood vessels, lymphatic vessels, nerves, connective tissue, and Leydig cells (Figure 2). In most mammals, including man, the Leydig cells are arranged in clusters. Also found there are mast cells and macrophages. The close association of these macrophages with Leydig cells suggests some functional association; however, their role(s) in the testis is yet to be established.[17]

Seminiferous Tubules

The seminiferous epithelium is a complex stratified epithelium containing tall columnar Sertoli cells and various populations of germ cells (Figure 3). The seminiferous tubule is limited by a lamina propria consisting of fibroblasts, myoid cells, collagen fibers, and a layer of endothelial cells. Rhythmic contractions of the myoid cells presumably help to move spermatozoa and fluids from the seminiferous tubules.[41] Testosterone receptors seem to be present in the myoid cells.[42] The Sertoli cells lie immediately inside the tubule wall, their cytoplasm extending from the tubule wall to the lumen. The remaining space between the

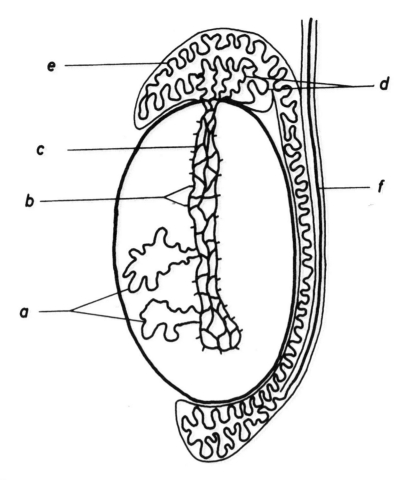

FIGURE 1. The efferent duct system of the testis and the epididymis (schematic). a, seminiferous tubules; b, tubuli recti; c, rete testis; d, ductuli efferentes; e, ductus epididymis; f, ductus deferens.

tubule wall and the lumen is occupied by the germinal cells, the spermatogonia along the tubule wall, and the more mature germ cells toward the lumen. Germ cells are either completely or partly surrounded by the Sertoli cells. In most mammalian species, the tubules are two-ended, with both ends opening into the rete testis.[17]

Rete Testis and Efferent Ducts

At each end of the seminiferous tubules, where they open into the rete testis, there is a short transitional zone lined with cells resembling Sertoli cells. The transitional zone is joined to the rete testis by a tubulus rectus (Figure 1). These straight tubules are the first component of the passageway through which spermatozoa pass from the seminiferous epithelium to the epididymis. Straight tubules converge in the cranial two thirds of the testis in an area termed the rete testis, which is a complicated network of intercommunicating channels. Tubules of the intratesticular rete testis penetrate the tunica albuginea and continue as an extratesticular rete. Eventually, each rete tubule fuses with the efferent ducts (ductuli efferentes testis) that lead to the epididymal duct (ductus epididymis).[17]

Epididymis

The epididymal duct is a single highly convoluted duct, closely applied to the surface of the testis extending from the anterior to the posterior pole of the organ.[17] The epididymis is divided anatomically into three parts: caput, corpus, and cauda. From a functional point of

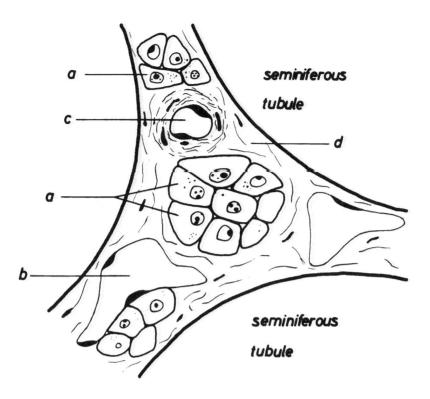

FIGURE 2.   The interstitial tissue (schematic). a, Leydig cells; b, lymphatic sinusoid; c, artery; d, connective tissue.

view, the epididymis has three segments.[43,44] Epithelia of the efferent ducts plus the initial segment of the caput are involved in resorption of most of the fluid and solutes entering from the testis.[45] The middle segment includes major portions of the caput and corpus epididymis and is involved in spermatozoal maturation. The terminal segment is composed of the cauda epididymis and proximal deferent duct and is involved in storage of fertile spermatozoa.

The ductus deferens (Figure 1) arises from the epididymal duct and extends from the cauda epididymis through the spermatic cord to the pelvic urethra.

CYTOLOGY OF THE TESTIS
Leydig Cells

The Leydig cells are the site of androgen production. They are rich in smooth endoplasmic reticulum. Together with mitochondria containing tubular cristae and cytoplasmic lipid inclusions, these three components are concerned with steroidogenic functions. Although the small quantity of rough endoplasmic reticulum probably contributes the necessary enzymes that catalyze these steroidogenic pathways, the role of Golgi complex, liposomes, and large crystals of Reinke remain largely unknown. It is suggested that these crystalline inclusions represent a form of storage material when the biosynthetic activity of the Leydig cells is reduced. It is assumed that testosterone diffuses out of the Leydig cell into the surrounding extracellular tissue because there are no secretory vesicles visible in the cytoplasm.[46] Leydig cell morphology changes with the seminiferous cycle being most dramatic at stages VII and VIII.[47] In addition to studies with normal testes, examination of damaged or abnormal testes has revealed that damage of seminiferous tubule function causes abnormal cytological features and functions in adjacent Leydig cells.[48,49] These morphological studies of both normal and abnormal testes implied that a regulatory interaction may exist between Sertoli cells and Leydig cells. Leydig cells have been shown to have junctional interactions between themselves, but there is no physical contact between Sertoli cells and Leydig cells.[50,51]

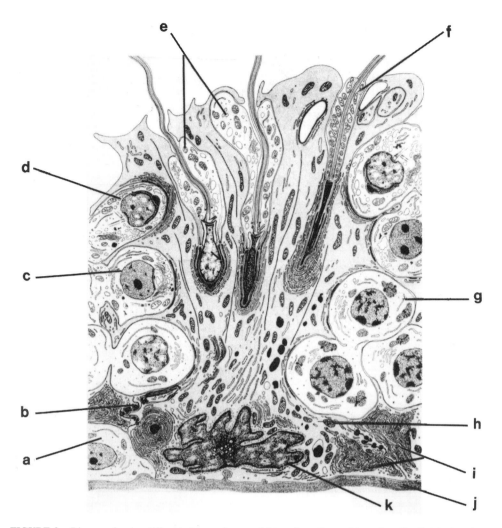

FIGURE 3. Diagram showing different phases of spermatid transformation and inter-Sertoli cell tight junctions. a, spermatogonium; b, tight junctions between Sertoli cells forming a boundary between the basal and the adluminal compartment; c, spermatid (Golgi phase); d, spermatid (cap phase); e, spermatid (acrosome phase); f, spermatid (maturation phase); g, primary spermatocyte with cytoplasmic bridge; h, cytoplasm of the Sertoli cell; i, endoplasmic reticulum; j, basal lamina; k, nucleus. (From Liebich, H.-G., *Funktionelle Histologie,* 2nd ed., Schattauer, Stuttgart, New York, 1993. With permission.)

Recent quantitative analysis of Leydig cells suggests that a gradual decline in androgen levels with advancing age is associated with a progressive disappearance of the Leydig cells.[46] Young men have approximately twice as many Leydig cells when compared with men of 60 or more years of age. At present it is not known how Leydig cells are removed from the testis, although phagocytosis of degenerating cells by the macrophages is a possible mechanism.[52]

Sertoli Cells

In humans, the Sertoli cell occupies about 38% of the seminiferous epithelium.[40] Sertoli cells contain large and irregular nuclei, usually situated in the basal position of the cell (Figure 3). The voluminous cytoplasm usually displays a polar distribution, with the organelles and inclusions more abundant in the basal trunk than in the apical portion, and the reverse distribution for glycogen, mitochondria, and the smooth endoplasmic reticulum. There is a relatively low proportion of rough endoplasmic reticulum in the cell cytoplasm, which also lacks vesicles or large granules usually associated with the transport and secretion of proteins. Sertoli cells contain much smooth endoplasmic reticulum, small quantities of mitochondria, liposomes, and Golgi membranes, and a variable number of lipid inclusions.[46,53] In the basal region of the seminiferous epithelium the plasma membranes of adjacent Sertoli cells form specialized junctional complexes which constitute the structural basis of the blood-testis barrier. These tight junctions provide a barrier to the passage of large molecular weight substances into the seminiferous tubules and thereby create a basal and an adluminal compartment within the epithelium. Spermatogonia reside in the basal compartment and the spermatocytes and spermatids develop in the adluminal compartment. This arrangement is thought to provide separate physiological environments in support of the process of meiotic maturation and spermiogenesis.[46]

Various specific anatomical interrelationships exist between Sertoli cells and all germ cell classes. They include ectoplasmic specializations, desmose-like contacts, gap junctions, and tubular bulbo complexes.[53,54] An individual Sertoli cell can be in contact with 5 adjacent Sertoli cells at the basal surface of the cell and 47 adjacent germinal cells at various stages of development.[51] This extremely elaborate network between Sertoli cells and germinal cells is involved in attachment, displacement, cell shaping, and cell-cell transfer of molecules and cellular materials. The unique strategic position of the Sertoli cell allows this cell type to receive, integrate, and limit all the signals required for the spermatogonic process to or from the extratubular compartment.[53]

The presence of the basal lamina of the seminiferous tubule, which separates peritubular cells and Sertoli cells, prevents junctional contacts between the cells. Therefore, the metabolic cooperation observed *in vitro* between the cells is likely not present *in vivo*.[51]

Although it is conventionally accepted that Sertoli cells do not divide after puberty, there are some indications that in seasonal breeders like the stallion Sertoli cells may proliferate as the breeding season approaches.[55] Because each Sertoli cell accommodates about the same number of germ cells throughout life, the decline in daily sperm production observed in men between the age of 20 and 80 years is probably a result of a loss of Sertoli cells.[56]

Germ Cells and Spermatogenesis

The spermatogenic process is a series of complex cellular changes, which results in the formation of the male haploid gamete, the spermatozoon.[57,58] In many mammals sperm cells are produced continuously from puberty to senescence. In some species, e.g., in seasonal breeders, it is interrupted into a series of distinct phases based on environmental cues that are transduced into hormonal signals stimulating or inhibiting spermatogenesis.[59]

The development of spermatozoa in the seminiferous epithelium includes three main phases: spermatogonial multiplication, meiosis, and spermiogenesis. Four basic cell types can be recognized during these phases: the spermatogonia, the spermatocytes (primary and secondary), the spermatids, and the spermatozoa (Figure 3). Spermatogonia multiply by mitotic division. The last generation produces the primary spermatocytes. DNA is synthesized for the last time during spermatogenesis by these primary spermatocytes. The diploid primary spermatocytes undergo the first meiotic division, producing the haploid secondary spermatocytes which divide at the second meiotic division. After the second meiotic division, one primary spermatocyte gives rise to four haploid spermatids. During spermiogenesis the young spermatids are transformed into mature sperm cells with their characteristic form.

Spermatogenesis follows basically the same rules in all mammals, including man. Because the divisions and the transformation of cells during spermatogenesis are well coordinated, the germ cells are always found in special associations. The associations are usually classified into stages, according to the morphological characteristics of the acrosome or the developing cells. In different animal species the number of stages may vary depending on the arbitrary criteria used for their identification. In the human, six stages were identified.[60] At any one part of a tubule, spermatogenesis passes through all stages until the initial association reappears. A complete set of cell associations forms the germinal epithelial cycle. The cycle is repeated, forming consecutive waves of spermatogenesis along the long axis of the tubules.

The duration of the germinal epithelial cycle varies from 8.3 to 16 days in the investigated mammalian species: man has the longest cycle (16 days) and the boar the shortest (8.3 days). The duration of spermatogenesis, that is, the development of a sperm cell starting from the origin of the stem spermatogonium, is 74 days in man.[61]

In most mammals, the entire tubule cross-section is in the same stage of the seminiferous cycle, whereas in the human testis the position of the stages seen in a single cross-section of a tubule gives the impression of a random pattern of germ cell development.[62] Therefore, it was assumed that human spermatogenesis is irregular or at least is subjected to a lesser extent to principles of synchronism and coordination than in most nonhuman mammals.[63] However, Schulze and Rehder[64] proposed that the stages of the human seminiferous cycle formed an orderly sequence orientated in a helical pattern.

The mechanism by which the remarkable organization of the seminiferous cycle is achieved is not fully understood. In the early literature, it was speculated that synchronization was dependent on external factors.[65] It was assumed that the Sertoli cell exerts a coordinating influence via its specialized contacts with the germ cells.[66] However, the observation that in hypophysectomized rats the Sertoli cells are regressed yet the germ cell stages maintain their characteristic associations and other observations discounted the Sertoli cell as a coordinating factor.[67] Clermont[67] concluded that the synchronized development of germ cells depends on the precise rate of each stage of development because of inherent timing devices. The nature of this timing devices has not been resolved, but more recent studies indicate that the extensive links between germ cells are the likely mechanism to allow their coordinated development.[68] This coordination is likely the result of cytoplasmic transport of coordinating molecules like actin.[69,70]

HORMONES OF THE TESTIS

ANDROGENS

One of the first experiments in endocrinology was performed by Berthold in 1849.[71] He demonstrated that castration of the cock was followed by regression of the comb, and that the size of the comb was maintained after transplantation of the testes to a new site. Test-osterone was first isolated and synthesized in 1935.[72]

Considerable progress has been made in elucidating the mechanism of action of androgens as sensitive and reliable assays for measuring androgens became available. More recently, genes encoding enzymes involved in the steroidogenic pathway have been cloned and their structures identified. These findings have revealed a much more complicated mechanism than previously anticipated by which steroidogenesis is controlled at the molecular level.

Biochemistry of Androgens

All steroid hormones, including androgens, have a common cyclopentanoperhydro-phenanthrene nucleus (Figure 4). This is a completely reduced structure with 17 carbon atoms arranged in three six-membered rings (A, B, and C) and a five-membered ring (D). Androgens are named systematically by reference to a parent structure, androstane, a steroid with methyl groups (CH_3) on carbon atoms 10 and 13. Naturally occurring androgens possess additional substitutions on carbon atoms 3 and 17 in the form of a hydroxy (OH) or oxy (=O) group.

The formula of a steroid hormone cannot adequately represent its structure, because the carbon atoms are orientated in space in the so-called chair form and the substituents may be above the ring (β form) or below the ring (α form). The conformation determines the degree of androgenic activity on target organs.

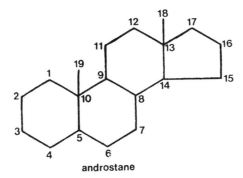

FIGURE 4. Basic structure of androgens.

Substrate for Androgen Production

Cholesterol is the starting substrate for steroidogenesis, thus providing the basic steroid ring structure. Depots of cholesterol (lipid droplets) can be found in the cytoplasm of Leydig cells; when androgens are synthesized at an increased rate, the number of lipid droplets in Leydig cells is significantly reduced.[73]

The most important source of cholesterol for testicular androgen production is *de novo* synthesis.[74] Cholesterol is synthesized from acetyl-CoA, either derived from blood or formed during metabolism of glucose. Synthesis is thought to occur primarily in the smooth endoplasmic reticulum, as is the case in other tissues.[75] In the rat, experimental evidence has been presented that cholesterol biosynthesis takes place within the mitochondria.[76]

The first step during biosynthesis of cholesterol is the formation of a C_6 compound, mevalonic acid, from three molecules of acetyl-CoA. Coupling of six molecules of mevalonic acid produces the C_{30} hydrocarbon squalene, which is transformed by cyclization to lanosterol, the first cyclic cholesterol precursor. Cholesterol is formed after removal of three methyl groups.[77]

In addition to *de novo* synthesis of cholesterol, Leydig cells can take up plasma lipoprotein cholesterol by endocytosis, which may be used directly for steroid synthesis or stored in lipid droplets in the cytoplasm. The contribution of each source differs from species to species. By feeding ^{14}C-cholesterol, the contribution of plasma cholesterol to the production of testicular androgens was found to be 13% in the guinea pig and approximately 40% in the rat.[74,78] *In vitro* incorporation of ^{14}C-acetate into testosterone occurred in rabbit but not in rat testes.[79,80]

Site of Androgen Production

Almost all testicular androgens are synthesized and secreted by the Leydig cells. Excised seminiferous tubules could not produce androgens from cholesterol *in vitro*.[81] A physiologically relevant secretion of androgens from seminiferous tubules *in vivo* has not been demonstrated so far.

Cholesterol may be stored in lipid droplets within the cytoplasm of Leydig cells in an unesterified form or is present as cholesterol esters. A cholesterol ester hydrolase that can be stimulated by hCG has been detected in murine testes.[82] Because hCG has a LH-like activity, cholesterol ester hydrolase stimulation may be LH dependent. Transport of free cholesterol to the outer membrane of the mitochondria is achieved by a sterol carrier protein (SCP-2).[83] The enzymes for the first step in androgen synthesis (the conversion of cholesterol to pregnenolone, commonly referred to as side chain cleavage) are located at the inner mitochondrial membrane. A small peptide (30 amino acids) has been described that is thought to act as a promotor for the transport within the mitochondrial membranes.[84] Further conversion of pregnenolone occurs mainly in the microsomes of the endoplasmic reticulum.

Conversion of Cholesterol to Pregnenolone

The conversion of cholesterol to pregnenolone is referred to as the side chain cleavage of cholesterol (Figure 5). It is thought that cholesterol is hydroxylated first at C-20 or C-22. In either case the resulting compound is hydroxylated further to form 20α,22-dihydroxycholesterol. The side chain is then cleaved between C-20 and C-22, producing the side chain fragment isocaproic aldehyde and the C-21 steroid pregnenolone. This process requires reducing equivalents from NADPH, molecular oxygen, and an enzyme system containing cytochrome P450scc. Mitochondrial cytochrome P450 uses an adrenodoxin reductase (flavoprotein) and a nonheme iron-sulfur-containing protein (adrenodoxin). In man, a single gene has been detected on chromosome 15 that is encoding for cytochrome P450ssc. This enzyme has only a single binding site and catalyzes all three reactions during the conversion from cholesterol to pregnenolone. The intermediate compounds are tightly bound to the enzyme and therefore almost no free intermediates exist.[85]

Conversion of Pregnenolone to Testosterone

The conversion of pregnenolone to testosterone takes place in microsomes of the smooth endoplasmic reticulum. Two pathways have been discovered: the so-called Δ^5 pathway involves intermediates with a double bond in ring B (17α-hydroxypregnenolone, dehydroepiandrosterone, and androstenediol) and the Δ^4 pathway (double bond in ring A) via progesterone and 17α-hydroxyprogesterone to 4-androstenedione and testosterone (Figure 6). In the adult human testis the Δ^5 pathway appears to be the most important, whereas a prevalence for the Δ^4 pathway has been observed in the human fetal testis.[86] The preferred pathway may also vary between species; e.g., the Δ^4 pathway via progesterone is preferred in the adult rat testis.[87]

The conversion of C-21 steroids to C-19 steroids involves 17α-hydroxylation to 17α-hydroxyprogesterone or 17α-hydroxypregnenolone and a C-17–20 lyase reaction, leading to dehydroepiandrosterone or androstenedione. There is good evidence that both reactions are catalyzed by a single microsomal enzyme, P450c17, which is virtually identical to that found in the mitochondria of Leydig cells promoting C-27 side chain cleavage.[88] Obviously, the association with certain cell organelles determines the actual enzymatic activity of this enzyme. This is demonstrated also by the apparent differences between adrenal and testicular steroid hormone production. It has been demonstrated that a single gene encodes for both adrenal and testis P450c17.[89] However, pregnenolone is converted in the adrenal mainly to the C-21 steroid cortisol by 17α-hydroxylation whereas C-17–20 lyase activity is low. Factors influencing this key branching point of steroidogenesis may be the lipid composition of the microsomal membranes or activity of P450 reductase in the adrenal and testis, respectively.

A special feature of the last step of the Δ^5 and Δ^4 pathways, conversion of dehydroepiandrosterone or androstenedione to androstenediol or testosterone, respectively, is its reversibility. The microsomal enzyme involved is a 17β-hydroxysteroid dehydrogenase and NAD$^+$ is required. The activity of this enzyme is not a rate-limiting factor for the production of testosterone, but may be modulated by product activation.[90]

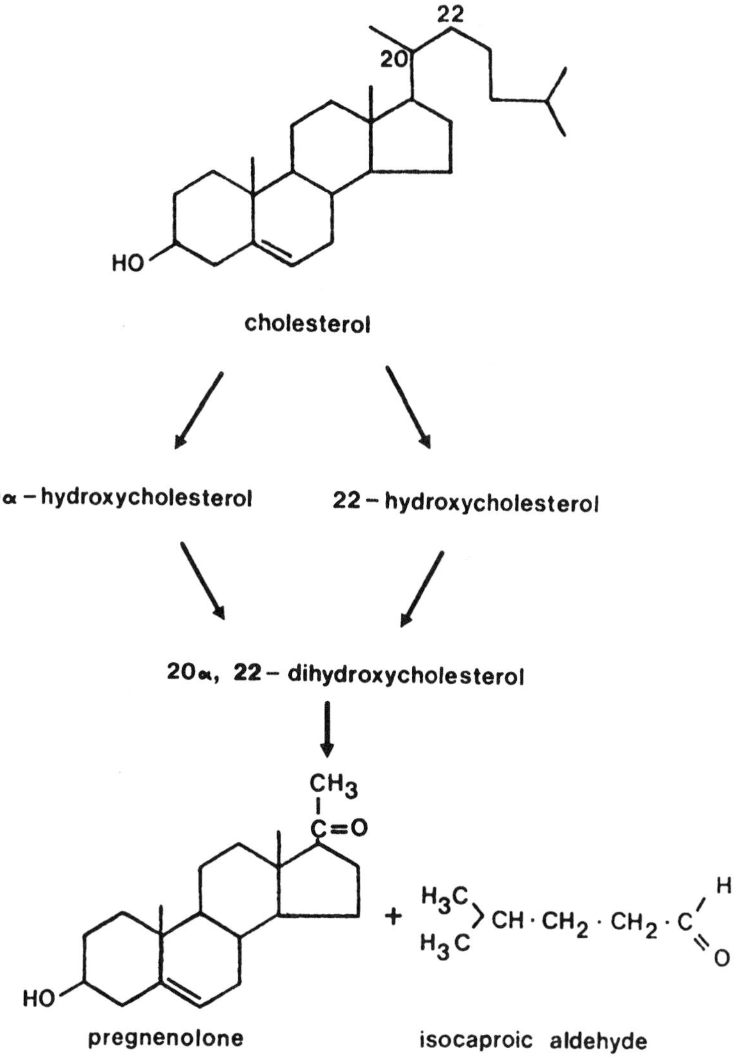

FIGURE 5. Conversion of cholesterol to pregnenolone. (Modified from Gower, D. B., in *Biochemistry of Steroid Hormones,* Makin, H. L. J., Ed., Blackwell Scientific, Oxford, 1975, 47.)

The conversion from the Δ^4 pathway to the Δ^5 pathway can take place at any stage of the pregnenolone side-chain cleavage. This is achieved by oxidation of the 3β-hydroxyl group to a Δ^4-3-keto structure (dehydrogenation) and rearrangement of the double bond (isomerization). These reactions are catalyzed by 3β-hydroxysteroid dehydrogenase, an enzyme which has yet to be completely purified. Although a single protein derived from cDNA for human placental 3β-hydroxysteroid dehydrogenase was able to convert C-21 and C-19 steroids, experiments with bovine adrenal cortex suggest that there are two enzyme systems for C-21 and C-19 substrates, respectively.[91,92]

Secretion, Transport, and Catabolism of Androgens

Androgens are released from Leydig cells into the seminiferous tubules, into the testicular lymph and via bloodstream to the rest of the body. The concentration of androgens in the lymph and in the rete testis fluid is higher than in the spermatic venous blood, but the flow rate of blood exceeds that of the other fluids by approximately 100-fold. Therefore, the major

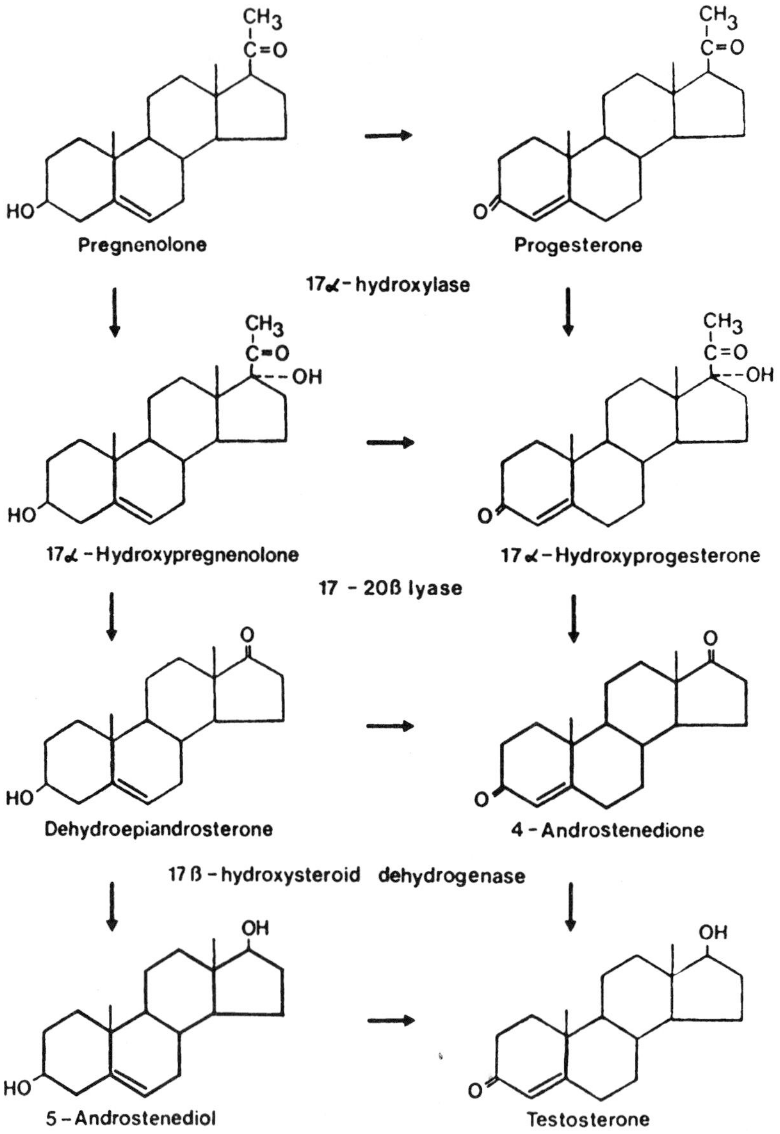

FIGURE 6. "5-en-3-hydroxy" (left-hand column) and "4-en-3-oxo" (right-hand column) pathway from pregnenolone to testosterone. (Modified from Eik-Nes, K. B., *Handbook Physiology Section 7, Endocrinology,* Vol. 5, Hamilton, D. W. and Greep, R. O., Eds., American Physiological Society, Washington, D.C., 1975, 95.)

portion of androgens leaves the testis via the spermatic venous blood. However, sulfated steroids leave the testis via the lymph.[93]

The single, very long, and tightly coiled testicular artery is intimately associated with the testicular veins (pampiniform plexus) in the spermatic cord. Transfer of substances from the pampiniform plexus to the testicular artery by a passive diffusion has been postulated; an obvious candidate is testosterone, but the increase in the concentration in the arterial blood is insignificant.[94] The large and consistent reduction of testosterone levels as blood passes from the testis up the spermatic cord can be explained by arteriovenous anastomoses between the testicular artery and the pampiniform plexus. These anastomoses have been demonstrated in domestic animals and may be present also in primates and humans.[95,96] Flow in these anastomoses appears to be from the artery to the vein, with up to 60% of arterial blood passing directly to the veins. The dilution of the venous blood probably accounts for most of the reduction of testicular-derived factors present therein.

The concentration of testosterone in peripheral blood in different species such as humans, monkey, dog, rat, ram, bull, and boar is in the range of 2 to 5 ng/ml.[97] Testosterone concentrations in peripheral blood show a circadian rhythm with the lowest concentrations around midnight and the highest values in the morning. This can be demonstrated in humans, rhesus monkey, pig, and horse. In ruminants, irregular fluctuations of testosterone concentration but no consistent diurnal rhythm could be demonstrated.

Testosterone is transported in peripheral blood attached to carrier proteins by a weak and reversible binding. In man, about 60% is bound to the so-called testosterone-binding globulin (TeBG), 38% to albumin or cortisol-binding globulin, and a mere 2% is free. TeBG also binds 5α-dihydrotestosterone (5α-DHT) and 17β-estradiol to some extent. The TeBG or sex hormone-binding globulin (SHBG) is formed in the liver and is chemically and immunologically indistinguishable from the androgen-binding protein produced by Sertoli cells. Because only unbound testosterone can enter sex accessory tissue, androgenic activity is regulated in part by the extent of binding to proteins in the plasma and by the amount of binding protein available. In humans, a close relationship between plasma TeBG and circulating steroids has been demonstrated.[98] These studies suggest that TeBG has two binding sites: one for the steroid hormone and a second binding site for the plasma membrane of sex hormone target cells. "Free" TeBG can attach to membrane receptors and then bind sex hormones which activate a second messenger. Thus it is possible that steroid hormones exert their effects on target cells without actually activating the steroid hormone receptor.

The liver and to some extent the intestine catabolize free testosterone to androstenedione in the presence of 17β-hydroxysteroid dehydrogenase by the oxidation of the 17β-hydroxy group (Figure 7). Further reduction of this compound leads to the A-saturated steroids, 5α- and 5β-androstane-3,17-diones. The two androstanediones are converted to four isomeric 17-oxosteroids. These are conjugated as sulfates or glucuronides and excreted in the urine or feces. In a similar way, testosterone can be reduced to isomeric androstenediols, which are conjugated to glucuronides prior to excretion.[99]

The clearance of testosterone by the liver is not as complete as that of many other steroids. The binding of circulating testosterone to the TeBG prevents it from being inactivated completely during one passage through the liver. Androstenedione, which is only nonspecifically bound to albumin, is cleared more effectively.[100]

OTHER TESTICULAR HORMONES

Although testosterone is the major androgen leaving the testis, other androgens are also known to be released from the testis. Production of androgens such as androstenedione and androsterone may greatly vary between immature and mature individuals, as has been demonstrated in the rat and the bull.[101,102] The concentration of androstenedione was high in bulls before puberty whereas testosterone was the principal androgen in the adult bull. In the bull, production of androstenedione in the testis seems to be closely related to testosterone production because GnRH application increased peripheral concentration of both compounds.[103]

The testes of the boar produce 16-unsaturated C-19 steroids, which are concentrated in the body fat and the salivary glands (Figure 8). They act as pheromones. Pheromones are agents used for communication among individuals of the same species. The most active compounds in the boar are, 5α-androst-16-en-3-on, 5α-androst-16-en-3α-ol, and 5-androst-16-3β-ol. These steroids are derived from pregnenolone or progesterone. They do not possess any detectable androgenic potency.[104]

Estrogens

An interesting phenomenon of testicular steroidogenesis is aromatization of androstenedione, testosterone, or 19-hydroxy-androstenedione to estradiol-17β or estrone, the two resulting

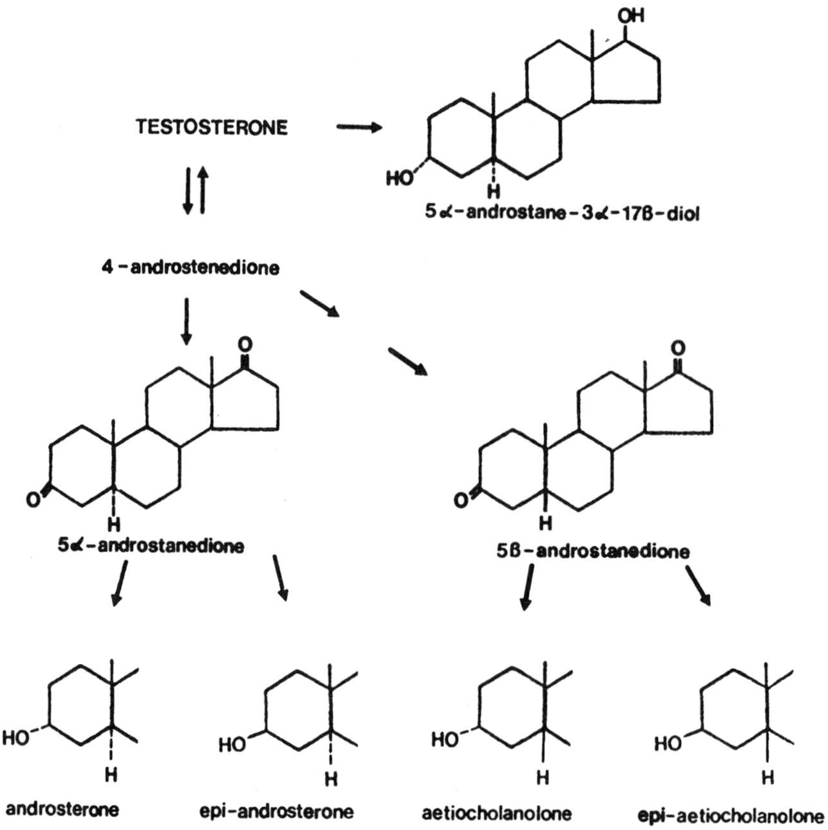

FIGURE 7. Catabolic pathway of testosterone. (Modified from Gower, D. B., in *Steroid Hormones,* Croom Helm, London, 1979, 50.)

products being interconvertible (Figure 9). Production of estrogens by the testis has been demonstrated in several species, e.g., humans, dog, rat, pig, cattle, and horse.[104-108] The C-19 steroids are transformed to C-19 steroids by removing the 19-methyl group. This reaction is catalyzed by P450 together with NADPH reductase. The exact site where estrogen production occurs inside the testes is not known. Cultured Sertoli cells produced small amounts of estradiol in response to FSH; other experiments indicated that 17β-estradiol synthesis occurs in cultured Leydig cells but not in Sertoli cells.[109,110]

In humans, approximately 20% of total estrogens in the peripheral plasma are contributed from testicular production, the major portion being derived from the peripheral conversion which may take place in adipose tissue.[105] The boar and the stallion are unique among domestic animal species in excreting large quantities of estrogens from the testes. Purified Leydig cells of mature boars produced estrogens *in vitro* and application of hCG to intact stallions led to a prolonged increase of testosterone and estrone sulfate in the peripheral blood, suggesting that Leydig cells are a significant source of testicular estrogens in these species.[111,112] Concentrations of estrogens in peripheral blood plasma of boars may even exceed those of testosterone and are much higher compared to sows in oestrus. Considerable amounts of estrogens have been detected in semen samples from the boar with about half of the estrogens bound to spermatozoa.[113] It has been shown that seminal plasma estrogens stimulate the myometrial contraction frequency of sows in estrus via release of prostaglandin $F_{2\alpha}$ ($PGF_{2\alpha}$) from the endometrium.[114] In the stallion, high concentrations of estradiol-17β (73.4 pg/ml), estrone (257.1 pg/ml), and estrone sulfate (4116.1 pg/ml) were found in seminal plasma, yet the physiological role of these steroids in equine species has yet to be elucidated.[115]

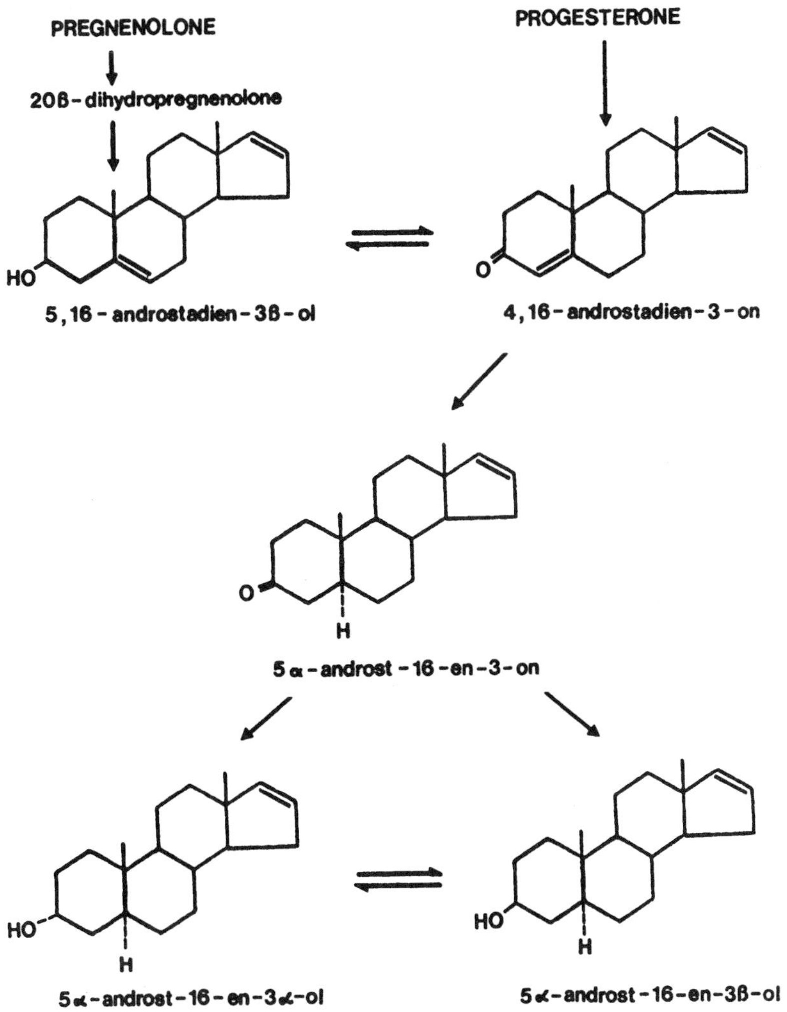

FIGURE 8. Biosynthesis of 16-unsaturated C-19 steroids. (Modified from Claus, R., *Mammalian Pheromones with Special Reference to the Boar Taint Steroid and Its Relationship to Other Testicular Steroids,* Paul Parey, Hamburg, 1979.)

Inhibin and Related Peptides

The concept of a nonsteroidal factor, formed by the testes and regulating pituitary FSH secretion, emerged more than 60 years ago.[116,117] Since then, a FSH antagonist has been hypothesized, but unequivocal evidence for the existence of inhibin was obtained just recently, when the exact nature of this hormone had been reported in 1985.[118] The term "inhibin" was originally defined by McCullagh.[117] Inhibin is a glycoprotein, a disulfide-linked heterodimer consisting of dissimilar subunits, α and either β_A (inhibin A) or β_B (inhibin B). It has been isolated as a 58 or 30–32 kDa form in follicular fluid or rete testis fluid in cattle, pig, sheep, and rat.[119] The different forms of inhibin can be explained by the existence of potential cleavage sites in the α subunit (e.g., at residue 167), leading to a variety of fragments of the precursor molecule. In general, posttranslational processing of inhibin subunits may be responsible for the generation of multiple monomeric or dimeric forms.

Amino acid sequences for the α and β chains show significant homology within and between species. An interspecies homology of about 85% was found for the primary structure of the α subunit, nearly 100% for the β_A subunit, and more than 95% for the β_B subunit. The

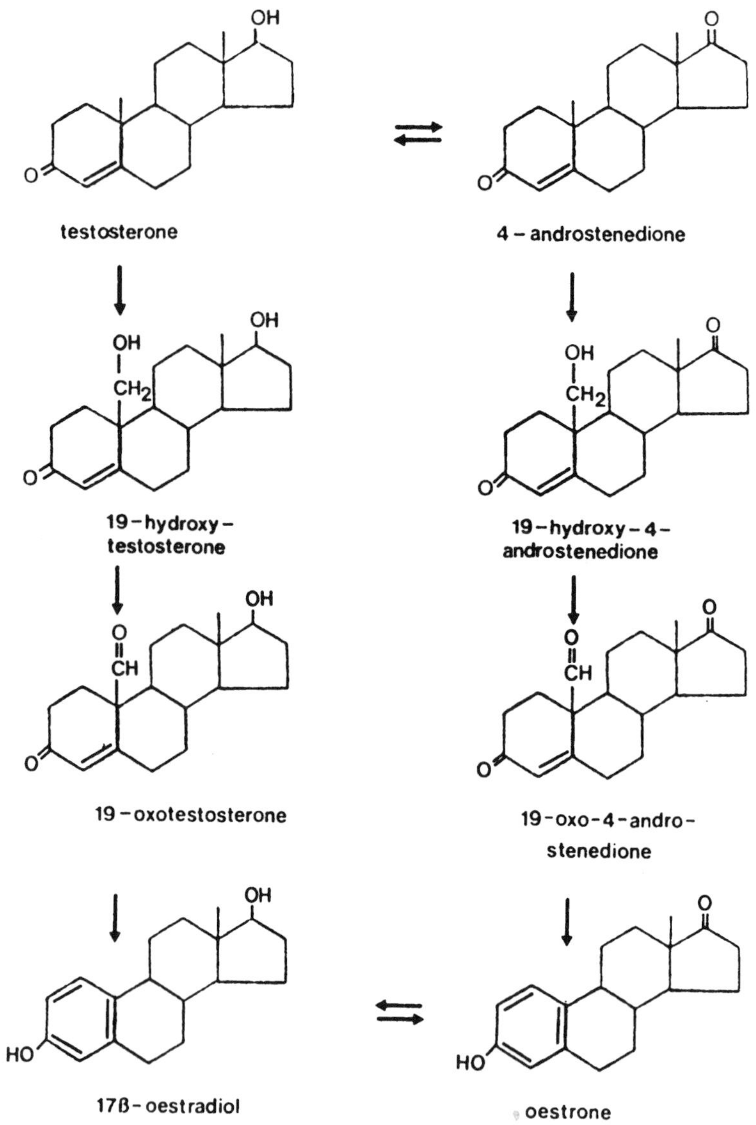

FIGURE 9. Possible pathways of testosterone to estrogens. (Modified from Gower, D. B., in *Steroid Hormones,* Croom Helm, London, 1979, 31.)

β subunit shares considerable homology with a range of cell differentiation proteins including TGF-β, müllerian-inhibiting substance, and activin, which is able to stimulate FSH secretion *in vivo.*[120]

Inhibin produced by male and female gonads is probably identical as demonstrated in the sheep: inhibins from rete testis fluid and follicular fluid were shown to be structurally similar.[121] Most studies about inhibin have concentrated on the role of inhibin in female reproduction, partly due to the fact that follicular fluid is the richest and easily accessible source for gonadal inhibin. The extent to which inhibin plays a role in male reproduction is far from clear. It is generally accepted that the Sertoli cells are the major cellular compartment that produces inhibin. Evidence for this assumption has been obtained by immunohistochemical studies and by localization of mRNA to α, β$_A$, and β$_B$ subunit in Sertoli cell nuclei.[122] Inhibin is released from Sertoli cells in a bidirectional manner via the apex of the cell into the lumen of the seminiferous tubules and through the base of the Sertoli cell into the interstitial spaces and the vascular system. In the adult ram, concentration of immunoreactive inhibin α subunit in the rete testis fluid was 25 times the level in testicular lymph which drains the interstitium and more than 500 times the concentration in testicular blood.[123]

The nature of inhibin as a FSH antagonist in the male has been proven by *in vitro* and *in vivo* studies. Isolated seminiferous tubule segments from adult male rats responded to FSH stimulation with secretion of immunoactive inhibin in a stage-specific manner.[124] Human recombinant inhibin was effective in lowering elevated FSH levels of castrated rams to a level commonly observed in intact rams; LH plasma concentrations were not affected by this treatment.[125] However, several lines of evidence suggest that control of FSH by inhibin is not achieved by a simple dual feedback mechanism. Inhibin has been shown to be secreted not only by Sertoli cells, but also by rat Leydig cells *in vitro*, and a significant amount of mRNA for inhibin has been detected in nongonadal tissues.[126] *In vivo* studies suggest that testosterone may be involved in control of inhibin production. Administration of a Leydig cell cytotoxin (ethane dimethane sulfonate) to either intact or cryptorchid animals caused a significant decrease of circulating testosterone followed by a rise of FSH.[127,128]

Recently, inhibin β subunit dimers (either β_A–β_A or β_A–β_B) have been isolated from follicular fluid.[129] Due to the stimulating effect on the FSH secretion of pituitary cells *in vitro*, the term "activin" has been chosen for these inhibin related proteins. A further striking homology was observed between inhibin subunit sequences. TGF-β is produced and secreted by peritubular cells as well as Sertoli cells and may play a role in peritubular cell differentiation and contractility.[130] The role of these and other inhibin related proteins in testicular function is far from clear. They may act as local regulators in an autocrine and/or paracrine fashion.

EFFECTS OF ANDROGENS
Molecular Aspects of Androgen Action

Binding of steroids to receptors in target tissues or cells is an essential intermediate step in the molecular expression of steroid-induced responses. Testosterone, the principal androgen secreted by the testes, enters target cells by passive diffusion. In the cell, testosterone can either bind immediately to the androgen receptor or be converted to dihydrotestosterone by a 5α-reductase enzyme. Earlier evidence suggested that the different effects of testosterone and dihydrotestosterone might be mediated by two different androgen receptor molecules present in the cytoplasm and the nucleus, respectively.[131] This hypothesis has been supported by the fact that these hormones serve different biological functions. Testosterone is necessary for gonadotropin regulation, spermatogenesis, and the wolffian phase of male sexual differentiation, whereas virilization of the urogenital sinus and external genitalia as well as sexual maturation at puberty is dihydrotestosterone dependent.[132] However, the hypothesis of a second androgen receptor has not been substantiated, and the two hormones clearly bind to the same receptor. The androgen receptor was among the last major receptors of the thyroid/steroid class to be cloned. Its structure is similar to other steroid binding receptors: a hormone-binding region, a hinge region, a DNA binding domain, and an N-terminal domain.[133] The encoding gene is linked to the X chromosome and codes for 917 amino acid proteins.

DHT binds to this receptor with a greater affinity than testosterone and forms a more stable complex with the androgen receptor.[134] The resulting hormone-receptor complex interacts with acceptor sites of nuclear genes, resulting in a changed chromatin activity. Ultimately new mRNA reaches the cytoplasm of the cell and new proteins are synthesized. Inactivation of testosterone or DHT probably takes place in the cytoplasm by further reduction to 5α-androstane-3α,17β-diol and 5α-androstane-3,17β-diol. Both compounds possess considerably less androgenic potency than DHT.[135]

Effect on Spermatogenesis

LH stimulates the Leydig cells to produce the androgens required for spermatogenesis. The significance of testosterone for spermatogenesis is highlighted by very high levels of testosterone within the testis when compared to levels in peripheral blood and the failure of 5α-reductase antagonists to impair spermatogenesis.[136] Values for testosterone up to 400 ng/ml in the interstitial fluid from intact rats have been reported, in contrast to a range of 1 to 3 ng/ml in peripheral blood. However, recent experiments indicate that DHT may play a role in maintenance of spermatogenesis as well; spermatogenesis was maintained quantitatively in rats receiving DHT implants.[137] The minimal average intratesticular concentration of DHT associated with the quantitative maintenance of spermatogenesis was approximately 50% of the testosterone concentration shown previously to be required.

Although it was generally accepted that testosterone is important for spermatogenesis, the mechanism of action on spermatogenesis remained controversial. Recent studies suggest that the most important androgen-dependent phase is the transformation of round spermatids to spermatozoa.[138] Lower doses of testosterone were necessary for the survival of round spermatids whereas higher doses were required for the development to spermatozoa. Because functional androgen receptors have not been found so far on germ cells, actions of androgens on spermatogenesis are probably mediated by Sertoli cells; e.g., binding of spermatids to Sertoli cells was reported to be testosterone dependent *in vivo*.[139] In addition, peritubular myoid cells are prime candidates for modulating actions of androgens on tubular function (see "Local Control Mechanisms"). More recently, there is growing evidence for a role of androgen binding protein (ABP) as a modulator of androgen action on spermatogenesis, thus providing an androgen-receptor-independent mechanism.[98] Transport of testosterone to the germ cells bound to ABP or the interaction of testosterone with ABP could play a role in germ cell development.

Epididymis

The most important functional change the spermatozoa undergo in the epididymis is the acquisition of the ability to fertilize ova. This functional maturation and the ability of the epididymis to store spermatozoa in a mature state are androgen dependent. A large number of studies has tested the effects of castration and replacement with testosterone on a wide array of epididymal functions. Androgens stimulate the secretory activity of the epididymis. The products interact with spermatozoa to bring about changes required for their maturation and survival. The source of androgens necessary for epididymal function is most likely the testes. It has been shown that in species such as rabbit and sheep or cattle, the epididymis can synthesize testosterone either *de novo* or from precursor steroids.[140,141] However, the steroidogenic capacity of the epididymis must be minimal because atrophy of the epididymis occurs after removal of the testis.[142] Testosterone can enter the epididymis in two ways, directly by a luminal pathway bound to ABP and from the circulating blood.

When radioactive testosterone is administered peripherally, the radioactive steroid found in the epididymis is DHT.[143] This corresponds well with the fact that mediation of androgen action in many target tissues requires the formation of DHT. In the rat, the concentration of testosterone declined from 18 to 5 ng/ml between the rete testis and the caput epididymis while that of DHT increased from 2.5 to 59 ng/ml.[144] These experiments imply that DHT is formed from testosterone inside the epididymis. Activity of the 5α-reductase enzyme, responsible for converting testosterone to DHT, is higher in the caput than in the cauda epididymis in most species examined thus far.

Although it is generally accepted that androgens are necessary for epididymal function, the mechanism of androgen action is far less clear. In the epididymis, androgens can bind to androgen receptors as well as ABP. ABP is synthesized by Sertoli cells and enters the epididymis via the efferent ducts. A possible role for ABP may be the regulation of

5α-reductase activity. Unilateral orchidectomy led to a fall of 5α-reductase activity selectively on the side where the testis had been removed.[145]

Accessory Sex Glands

The actions of androgens on male accessory sex glands are detected by changes following castration in adults, or by the failure to develop particular characteristics after prepubertal castration. Normal development of the accessory organs of the male reproductive tract is closely correlated with physical and testicular growth. In the adult, secretions from the accessory sex glands are under control of androgens, e.g., fructose and citric acid.[146] Most of our knowledge concerning endocrine control of sex accessory tissue comes from studies in the rat prostate.

Although testosterone is the primary plasma androgen, it appears to function as a pro-hormone in male accessory sex glands where metabolism to DHT occurs. Both testosterone and DHT can be found in the peripheral blood, but testosterone levels are approximately 11-fold higher than those of DHT. In addition to its low plasma concentration, tight binding to plasma proteins further diminishes its direct effect. The formation of DHT in the cell is under control of the enzyme 5α-reductase (Figure 10). This enzyme is tightly bound to the membranes of the nuclear envelope and the endoplasmic reticulum, and the enzyme has never been solubilized or purified in an active form. The cDNA-encoding human 5α-reductase has been cloned and expressed in the form of a hydrophobic protein containing 259 amino acids with an estimated molecular weight of 29 kDa.[147] Cloning of this enzyme with a pH optimum around 8 was followed by the discovery of a pH 5.5 enzyme; in the prostate, the principal 5α-reductase activity is due to the pH 5.5 enzyme.

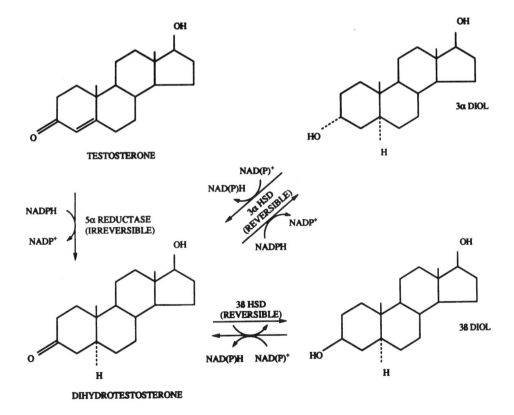

FIGURE 10. Formation of dihydrotestosterone and further metabolites from testosterone in peripheral tissues.

The prostate is unique among the sex accessory glands in as much as it is prone to abnormal growth. It is also remarkable that benign prostatic hypertrophy and prostatic cancer are common only to humans and dogs. Androgens seem to play a role in promoting prostate growth by preventing cell death rather than by stimulating cell proliferation. A variety of endocrine approaches to treat prostate cancer have been developed. Hormonal therapy is directed at lowering circulating testosterone levels or blocking androgen action.[148]

Sexual Behavior

Individuals castrated before puberty fail to develop adult patterns of sexual behavior unless given androgens. After castration of adults, sexual activity may persist for a variable time. The duration depends on the involvement of psychic elements in libido. Castration also produces more general changes in behavior such as reduced aggression, and this effect was probably the main reason for introducing castration in male domestic animals. Rising androgen levels during puberty can be associated with increased aggressiveness in boys, but androgen levels beyond the physiological range do not induce aggressive behavior in adults.[149,150]

General Effects

Testosterone is the most important testicular secretory product in the induction and maintenance of male secondary sex characteristics. This has been well known since ancient times through the effects observed after castration. Besides castration, a vast number of pathological conditions can cause hypogonadism followed by androgen deficiency. Tumors of the hypothalamus, pituitary, or the testis itself can result in a suppressed androgen production. Disorders of target tissues may also lead to defects in virilization. During the past years, several syndromes of androgen resistance, caused by deficiency in 5α-reductase or defects in the androgen receptor, have been described.[151] The age of onset of androgen deficiency critically influences the clinical features in androgen-deficient individuals. Prepubertal androgen deficiency results in continued growth of the long bones and an unbroken and high-pitched voice, a phenomenon well known in humans and animal husbandry.[152] In postpubertal individuals, a lack of androgens will lead to atrophy of muscles, a feminine body fat distribution, and in some cases gynecomastia, although the voice remains deep.

Androgens exert anabolic effects, such as increase of muscle protein. This is reflected in a higher level of urinary creatinine and a decrease in urinary nitrogen excretion. The anabolic activity of androgens is not related to their androgenic potency. These effects have led to a widespread abuse of androgens among top-level athletes as well as amateurs. Combinations of two or more steroids, oral and injectable, are used in excess doses in order to achieve the desired effects. A total steroid dose of 3 g has been suggested as a minimal effective dose for a significant effect on lean body mass.[153] It is doubtful that excess doses of anabolic steroids act via muscle androgen receptors because these receptors become saturated at physiological levels of testosterone.[154]

Clinical Use of Androgens

In accordance with the observed effects of androgens on a variety of physiological functions in the male, androgens can be used to prevent the long-term consequences of androgen deficiency. Currently, replacement of androgens is a standard therapy in cases of male hypogonadism and delayed puberty; potential indications such as osteoporosis and senescence are under investigation.[155] Because free testosterone is metabolized rapidly, the parent molecule has to be modified in order to achieve a short-, medium-, or long-acting compound. Testosterone esters such as testosterone enanthate or undecanoate are slowly released from oily vehicles thus providing the basis for injectable depots of testosterone. Absorbed esters are hydrolyzed to testosterone so that these drugs act in the same way as the endogenous hormone, including conversion to DHT. Orally active compounds result from alkylation of testosterone at the C_{17} or C_1 position.[156] Constant levels in the circulation can be obtained by implants of crystalline testosterone, transdermal application, or testosterone encapsulated in biodegradable microspheres.

CONTROL OF TESTICULAR FUNCTION

THE HYPOTHALAMO-PITUITARY-GONADAL AXIS

The nervous system is involved to a varying degree in almost every aspect of the physiology of reproduction. A major part of neural involvement is the regulation of gonadal function by the brain through hypothalamic control of anterior pituitary gonadotropin secretion. Current ideas regarding hypothalamic control of reproduction are based on the discovery of neurosecretion and of the functional significance of the hypophyseal portal vasculature. The hypothalamus releases GnRH, a decapeptide composed of 10 amino acids, which is transported to the anterior pituitary. GnRH is synthesized in the hypophysiotropic area, transported by axonal processes to the median eminence, and released into the hypophyseal portal system to reach the pars distalis of the adenohyophysis where it stimulates the output of LH and FSH.

The target tissues for FSH and LH are different components of the testes. FSH exerts an effect primarily on the Sertoli cells and the seminiferous tubules, whereas LH influences the Leydig cells. The steroids secreted by the gonads act as feedback signals. The signals are mediated by specific steroid binding proteins or by steroid receptors present in hypothalamic neurons and in pituitary cells. These feedback signals influence FSH and LH secretion and thereby maintain a state of dynamic equilibrium between the secretion of hypothalamic gonadotropin-releasing hormone (GnRH), pituitary gonadotropins (LH, FSH), and gonadal steroids. This system of interdependent endocrine organs is referred to as the hypothalamo-pituitary-gonadal axis (Figure 11).

Hypothalamic Gonadotropin-Releasing Hormone (GnRH)

In 1977, two scientists, Schally and Guillemin, shared the Nobel prize for their independent research on the chemical structures of hypothalamic hormones controlling pituitary functions. Using porcine hypothalamus or ovine hypothalamus, they isolated a decapeptide with combined LH-RH and FSH-RH activity and having the sequence p-Glu-His-Trp-Ser-Tyr-Gly-Leu-Arg-Pro-Gly-NH2.[157,158] Neither was able to separate a substance with only LH-RH or FSH-RH activity, and so have failed all attempts so far to characterize two distinct releasing hormones for the gonadotropins LH and FSH. This decapeptide, called GnRH, can be synthesized, and was found to release gonadotropic hormones as effectively as the natural product. GnRH is secreted into the hypothalamic-hypophyseal portal vessels in a pulsatile pattern. Pulsatile release of GnRH, mediated by neural elements within the mediobasal hypothalamus, is essential for optimal pubertal maturation and normal reproductive function.[159] The GnRH neurones are in turn regulated by feedback of gonadal steroid hormones as well as by local control mechanisms. The hypothalamic neurons are capable of certain autonomous functions. This has been shown by experiments in which the hypothalamo-pituitary complex has been isolated from the rest of the brain.[160] The pulsatile rhythm of basal FSH and LH remained unaffected.

Although some function of the hypothalamus can occur in isolation, stimulatory and inhibitory inputs from higher nerve centers are necessary for the full functioning. The limbic system is probably the most important among the nerve centers that influence the hypothalamic control of the gonadotropin secretion. Structures of the mesencephalon, especially the formatio reticularis, are also involved. Stimulatory and inhibitory effects such as light or darkness, temperature, stress, peripheral nerve reflexes, and various other internal or external factors, are factors influencing GnRH secretion. Neurotransmitters play an important role in modulating release of GnRH. It is generally accepted that GnRH pulses are generated primarily by noradrenaline.[161]

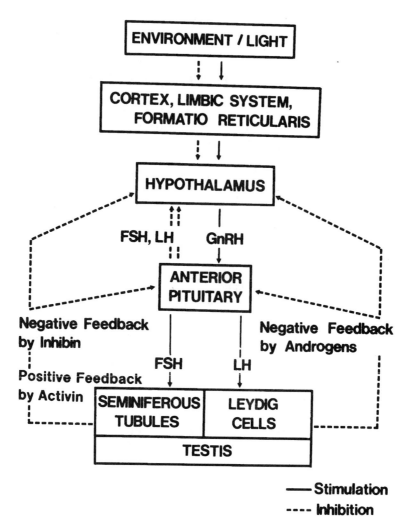

FIGURE 11.   Neuroendocrine regulation of testicular function.

Gonadotropins

The pituitary gland consists of the neurohypophysis and the adenohypophysis. The neurohypophysis can be subdivided into the median eminence, the infundibular stem, and the infundibular process, the two latter parts commonly referred to as posterior lobe. The adenohypophysis or glandular lobe consists of the pars intermedia, pars tuberalis, and pars distalis. The term anterior pituitary (or anterior lobe) describes the pars tuberalis and the pars distalis. The gonadotropic hormones FSH and LH, also known as ICSH (interstitial cell-stimulating hormone), are synthesized in and released from the anterior pituitary under the influence of GnRH. They are produced in the basophil cells of the pars distalis. Both hormones are glycoproteins with a molecular weight of approximately 29,000 and consist of two dissimilar peptide chains, referred to as α and β subunit. Individual subunits have little if any biological activity. The α subunit is common to both hormones and it is the β subunit that determines the specific mode of action.

Luteinizing Hormone

The importance of the anterior pituitary for the maintenance of testicular function has long been known. Much knowledge about the effects of the gonadotropins has been aquired with experiments on hypophysectomized animals. Extensive testicular atrophy occurs following hypophysectomy, and the synthesis of androgens proceeds at a greatly reduced rate. LH provides the most important stimulus for the production of androgens by the testes.[162]

The control of steroid production in Leydig cells is achieved by interaction with the cell surface LH receptor. The structure of the LH receptor has been recently determined: a large extracellular domain, with seven transmembrane segments and a cytoplasmic tail.[163] The receptor for LH also recognizes hCG. The rat LH receptor gene has been cloned and consists of 11 exons; the first 10 encode the extracellular domain, and the 11th encodes the transmembrane domain.[164] There is a considerable homology between LH receptors in different species. The human LH receptor is 85% identical to the rat LH receptor and 87% identical to the porcine LH receptor. The most homologous region is the transmembrane domain, and the least similar region is the intracellular domain. Each Leydig cell in the rat contains approximately 20,000 receptors.[165] Receptor binding activates a stimulatory GTP-binding protein, which, in turn, stimulates the adjoining adenylate cyclase (Figure 12). Two major messengers have been discovered to convert blood-borne stimuli into cellular responses, namely cyclic AMP and Ca^{2+}. The role of cAMP as an obligatory second messenger for LH-stimulated steroidogenesis is generally accepted, whereas the role of Ca^{2+} is not yet fully understood. Cyclic AMP stimulates a cAMP-dependent protein kinase, which eventually activates proteins by phosphorylation.[166] One protein affected by this form of posttranslational modification is cholesterol ester hydrolase, an enzyme responsible for releasing free cholesterol from lipid droplets. As a result of the actions of one or more proteins, cholesterol is transported from the outer to the inner mitochondrial membrane where C_{27} side chain cleavage occurs. The two processes of transport to and within the mitochondria appear to be the site of LH action on the process of steroidogenesis.

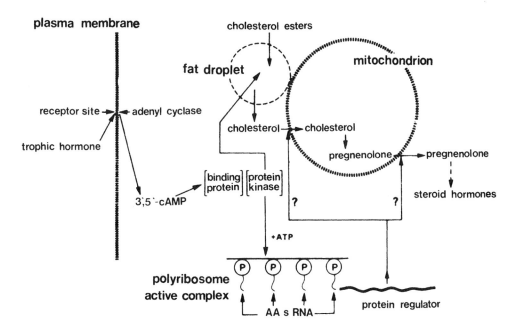

FIGURE 12. Control of steroidogenesis. (From Rommerts, F. F. G., Cooke, B. A., and van der Molen, H. J., *J. Steroid. Biochem.*, 5, 279, 1974. With permission.)

When a single injection of LH is administered, an acute response is detectable within seconds, and a slower response, namely increased production of testosterone, can be observed over a period of hours. If LH stimulation is maintained for longer periods, the ability to respond with increased androgen production is limited by the development of refractory changes.[156] A well-known model for this adaptive response is to administer LH twice. In many cases, a second injection produces a smaller response than the first—a phenomenon commonly referred to as down-regulation. The term down-regulation describes a decrease in the number of LH receptors following an injection of LH (or hCG). Occupied receptors are presumably internalized, followed by dissociation of LH, which may be degraded. Eventually, free receptors return to the cell surface, but for a given period of time the cell cannot give an adequate response to LH.[167] Under physiological conditions, down-regulation of the LH receptor appears to be part of the normal cellular processing of receptors. Down-regulation may be necessary to prevent depletion of LH receptors by LH pulses.

Follicle-Stimulating Hormone

FSH is important in the initiation of the spermatogenic process and may be important in the mature individual for the maintenance of optimal testicular function. The major target for FSH within the testis is the Sertoli cell. This view is substantiated by the fact that FSH receptors could be demonstrated on Sertoli cells only. It could be demonstrated that the number of FSH receptors varied at different stages of the seminiferous cycle, being greatest at stages XII–II.[168] The FSH receptor is very similar to the LH receptor. It possesses the same large extracellular domain, seven transmembrane helices, and a cytoplasmic tail. Following binding to the membrane receptor, FSH stimulates adenylate cyclase and G protein. This results in an increased intracellular accumulation of cAMP and stimulates the catalytic activity of a cAMP-dependent protein kinase.

Secretion of FSH from the anterior pituitary is modulated by inhibins and activins produced in Sertoli cells. Whereas activin was shown to increase FSH secretion, inhibin suppresses serum FSH concentrations. The availability of recombinant inhibin made it possible to further explore the influence of inhibin on FSH secretion. When inhibin was administered to adult castrated rats, a dose-dependent suppression of FSH secretion occurred.[169] The full FSH suppressing effect of inhibin could be detected about 8 h post-treatment. These results obtained *in vivo* are concomitant with *in vitro* experiments: addition of bovine inhibin to cultured rat pituitary cells led to a dose-dependent suppression of various parameters of FSH production and secretion.[170] Although the target of circulating inhibin is the anterior pituitary, LH secretion is not affected by the level of inhibin. The inverse relationship of serum FSH and testicular inhibin concentrations is consistent with the concept that inhibin exerts negative feedback control on FSH secretion. However, several lines of evidence suggest a more complex mechanism by which FSH secretion is regulated. Although Sertoli cells are the principal source of inhibin, Leydig cells can synthesize inhibin as well. A number of studies have demonstrated interactions between testosterone and inhibin in the regulation of FSH secretion. Finally, the recent evidence of local production of activin within the pituitary will require reevaluation of the mechanisms responsible for control of FSH secretion.

Sertoli cells synthesize a number of secretory products (proteins, peptides, energy substrates, etc.) that are thought to be under control of FSH. The first Sertoli cell protein to be discovered was ABP in the rat; this protein is immunologically related to the TeBG.[171] Because rats do not possess TeBG, ABP can be identified easily in this species. Rat ABP is a dimeric glycoprotein with a native molecular weight of 85,000. ABP is thought to be a carrier of testosterone within the Sertoli cell as well as a carrier to maintain high concentrations of androgens in seminiferous tubules and the epididymis. ABP levels are increased *in vivo* by chronic FSH treatment; likewise, accumulation of ABP *in vitro* occurs only several hours after stimulation with FSH.[172] These and other observations imply that the effects of FSH on Sertoli cell secretory functions are mediated by paracrine or autocrine mechanisms. In the case of ABP, testosterone from Leydig cells is thought to play a role.

The amount of ABP synthesized by Sertoli cells in culture is minimal when compared to that of transferrin, a metal binding protein; production of transferrin is positively regulated by FSH.[173] It has been postulated that Sertoli cells secrete this protein into the seminiferous tubules in order to transport Fe^{3+} to developing germ cells. FSH also influences Sertoli cell energy metabolism. Binding of FSH to the cell surface receptor results in stimulation of glucose uptake and lactate production.[174] Because germ cells depend on lactate as an energy source, the resulting increase in lactate and pyruvate secretion may play a role in their nourishment.[175]

LOCAL CONTROL MECHANISMS

The existence of regulatory feedback mechanisms between the hypothalamus, the pituitary, and the testis is generally accepted. During the past years, increasing evidence has been accumulated that these extratesticular mechanisms are complemented by local control systems within the testis. The action of testosterone, produced in the Leydig cells and transported to the seminiferous tubules is a well-known example of such a paracrine mechanism. However, androgens are not the only locally produced factors involved in regulation of testis function. This chapter will focus on regulatory actions between the interstitial compartment and the seminiferous tubules and vice versa (Figure 13).

Control of Tubular Function

Androgens play a significant role in initiating and maintaining spermatogenesis. Earlier studies in hypophysectomized rats had shown that high doses of testosterone given at the time of surgery maintain spermatogenesis.[176] More recently, Huang et al. were able to demonstrate that spermatogenesis can be reinitiated by testosterone alone after long-term regression in hypophysectomized rats.[177] However, quantitative studies revealed that spermatogenesis can be maintained at only 80% of normal by this treatment, and daily sperm production progressively falls with time in such animals.[178,179] The subnormal maintenance of spermatogenesis in hypophysectomized rats lends further support to the hypothesis that spermatogenesis is maintained by testosterone and a pituitary factor, most likely FSH. It has now been established that androgens are necessary for a specific stage of spermiogenesis, namely the transformation of round spermatids to spermatozoa.[138] Both FSH and testosterone may support the cellular contact between Sertoli cells and developing spermatids.[180] In order to exert its biological effect, testosterone must bind to the androgen receptor. Such receptors have been demonstrated in Sertoli and peritubular cells, but not in germ cells.[181]

The action of androgens on tubular function is complemented by other regulatory peptides, produced by the Leydig cells. Secretion of opioid peptides from Leydig cells has been demonstrated recently and the target of these peptides may be the Sertoli cells.[182] Receptors for opioids have been found on Sertoli cells; moreover, secretion of ABP from isolated Sertoli cells could be inhibited by opioids.[183] The source and function of oxytocin in control of tubular contractility is not yet fully understood.

The interactions between the interstitial and the tubular compartment are mediated in part by peritubular cells. In particular, two proteins, referred to as PModS proteins with a molecular weight of 56,000 and 59,000, respectively, have been isolated in a peritubular cell conditioned medium; PModS has been found to have a more pronounced *in vitro* effect on Sertoli cell functions than any other currently known agent.[184] These proteins are involved in the stimulatory effect of androgens on the capability of Sertoli cells to secrete ABP, inhibin, and other secretory products. Transforming growth factors, TGF-α and TGF-β, may also serve as important mediators for peritubular cell-Sertoli cell interactions.[130,185]

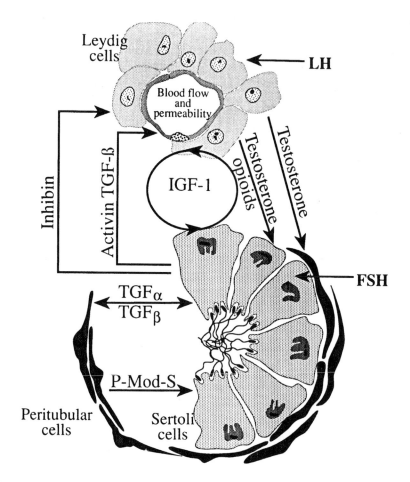

FIGURE 13.   Local control mechanism in the testis. (Modified from Verhoeven, G., in *Baillière's Clinical Endocrinology and Metabolism, The Testes,* de Kretser, D. M., Ed., Baillière Tindall, London, 1992, 313.)

Control of Leydig Cells by Paracrine Mechanisms

It has been demonstrated in several experiments that the endogenous FSH levels influence the production and secretion of testosterone. Because Sertoli cells but not Leydig cells possess FSH receptors, a paracrine action of Sertoli cells can be assumed. The ability of Sertoli cells to affect Leydig cell function was initially postulated from observations that Leydig cell morphology was altered by tubules with abnormal function.[186] Examination of normal testis has revealed morphological changes of Leydig cells synchronous to the seminiferous cycle.[187]

A number of secretory products from Sertoli cells has been isolated that can potentially influence Leydig cells. Inhibin and its related protein activin both can influence androgen production in Leydig cells.[188] However, Leydig cells have also been shown to produce these hormones. The role of inhibin and activin in regulation of steroidogenesis remains to be elucidated. Because Sertoli cells can aromatize androgens to estrogens, Sertoli cell-derived estrogen may mediate inhibitory actions on testosterone production. Other substances potentially involved in regulatory interactions between Sertoli and Leydig cells are interleukin-1 and TGF-α and -β. A better defined regulatory role could be demonstrated for insulin-like growth factor I (IGF-I). Although secretion of IGF-I into the basal compartment has not been demonstrated so far, indirect evidence suggests that IGF-I acts as an autocrine as well as a paracrine agonist. During coculture of Leydig and Sertoli cells, a more than additive increase of IGF-I production was found, and immunoneutralization of IGF-I prevented the stimulatory effect of Sertoli cells on steroidogenesis.[189,190]

In conclusion, a number of paracrine and autocrine factors has been demonstrated to mediate interactions between testicular compartments as well as cell-cell interactions. The response of Leydig cells to LH initiates a cascade of events that involves peritubular cells and Sertoli cells. Likewise, Sertoli cells appear to produce FSH-dependent factors necessary for the regulation of Leydig cell function. Although the significance of androgens for paracrine mechanisms has been demonstrated, the mode of androgen actions is far from clear. The physiological relevance and importance of most of the above-mentioned factors remain to be elucidated.

PHOTOPERIODISM

Photoperiodism is a major factor regulating reproduction especially in moderate and high latitudes with the distinct differences in seasons. The seasonal, photoperiodically dependent variation of gonadal activity is responsible for the parturition of many species at a certain time of year offering the optimal chance of survival for offspring. Species sensitive to photoperiodism can be divided in two groups. Those responding to increasing day length are referred to as "long-day species" because the onset of the breeding season is controlled by increasing light periods. Those responding to short day length are "short-day species."[191] Many mammals are long-day species (e.g., horse, mink, cat, and ferret), others are short-day species (e.g., sheep, goat, and deer), and for some species photoperiodism is of little or no importance (e.g., humans, cattle, and dog).

Photoperiodic control of reproduction depends on the presence of photoreceptors. In mammals, the obvious photoreceptor is the eye. A direct connection between the retina and the hypothalamus, separate from the optic nerve, is provided by the retinohypothalamic tract. Within the hypothalamus, the suprachiasmatic nucleus (SCN) is the driving oscillator acting as pacemaker for circadian rhythms in mammals. SCN neurons project to the superior cervical ganglia via presympathetic preganglionic neurons. Axons from the superior cervical ganglia terminate in the pineal gland and transmit signals via norepinephrine.[192] The pineal gland plays an essential role in reproductive responses to both stimulatory and inhibitory photoperiods. Photoperiodic information is transduced by the pineal gland by means of a diurnal rhythm of melatonin secretion. The role of the pineal gland in circadian regulation was further underlined by the discovery of pineal light sensitivity in the enzymes that synthesize melatonin, namely *N*-acetyltransferase and hydroxyindole-*O*-methyltransferase.[193] Pineal and plasma melatonin concentrations are at their daily nadir during the light phase and peak during portions of the dark phase. The duration of the nocturnal elevation of melatonin synthesis and secretion is related proportionally to the length of the dark phase. The duration of melatonin secretion varies therefore between long and short days, and this constitutes a neuroendocrine signal to the hypothalamo-pituitary axis. The demonstration that melatonin can account for the pineal mediation of both inductive and inhibitory day lengths raises an important question: How can one hormone have opposite effects on the same reproductive endpoint? Although no definite answers can be given, the differences in response to photoperiods may be due to differences in the processing and/or interpretation of the melatonin signal.

Melatonin not only triggers changes in the secretory pattern of gonadotropic hormones, it also modulates secretion of prolactin. The majority of seasonally breeding mammals show a seasonal pattern of prolactin secretion with peak concentrations in summer and a nadir in winter. Whether the seasonal change in prolactin secretion is an endocrine mediator of a biological rhythm of reproduction remains in contention. A clear reproductive role has been demonstrated in a number of species that show embryonic diapause. In the western spotted skunk, increasing prolactin concentrations in spring are luteotrophic and terminate embryonic diapause.[194] However, there is considerably less evidence for a role of prolactin in the control of seasonally testicular activity. In domesticated breeds of sheep, a role for the seasonal change in prolactin secretion is yet to be defined or may not exist.

The secretory pattern of the gonadotropic hormones LH and FSH has been extensively studied in the Soay sheep, in which a change in the frequency of pulsatile release of GnRH from the hypothalamus has been observed.[195] GnRH pulses are most frequent (>1 pulse every 2 h) during the breeding season (autumn), which is reflected by a high frequency and magnitude of LH pulses. The levels of FSH do not show such a distinct pulsatile pattern; however, a steady increase parallels the redevelopment of the testes and full enlargement of gonads is preceded by maximum levels some weeks earlier.[196] The levels of testosterone increase and decrease according to the LH secretion. The seasonal increase of testosterone levels can be attributed to an increased responsiveness to LH, a higher number of LH receptors, and increased activity of cell organelles associated with steroidogenesis.[197,198]

The structural and functional changes of the testis related to season have been investigated in a vast number of species. The extent of seasonal effects ranges from very subtle changes concerning only aspects of cell morphology to cases where males are infertile for part of the year. The decrease of tubular function is closely reflected by changes of the daily sperm production; because seminiferous tubules constitute the bulk of testicular tissue, testis size and weight are decreasing as well. The extent to which the testosterone secretion by the testis changes with season determines the effect on accessory sex glands, secondary sex characteristics, and sexual behavior.[59]

REFERENCES

1. **Müller, J. and Skakkebaek, N. E.,** The prenatal and postnatal development of the testis, in *Baillière's Clinical Endocrinology and Metabolism, The Testes,* Vol. 6/2, de Kretser, D. M., Ed., Baillière Tindall, London, 1992, 251.
2. **Wachtel, S. S.,** *H-Y Antigen and the Biology of Sex Determination,* Grune & Stratton, New York, 1983.
3. **McLaren, A., Simpson, E., Tomonari, K., Chandler, K., and Hogg, H.,** Male sex differentiation in mice lacking H-Y antigen, *Nature,* 312, 552, 1984.
4. **Page, D. C., Mosher, R., Simpson, E. M., Fisher, E. M. C., Mardon, G., Pollack, J., McGillivray, B., De la Chapelle, A., and Brown, L. G.,** The sex-determining region of the human Y chromosome encodes a finger protein, *Cell,* 51, 1091, 1987.
5. **Palmer, M. S., Sinclair, A. H., Berta, P., Goodfellow, P. N., Ellis, N. A., Abbas, N. E., and Fellous, M.,** Genetic evidence that ZFY is not the testis determining factor, *Nature,* 342, 937, 1989.
6. **Gubbay, J., Collignon, J., Koopman, P., Capel, B., Economou, A., Münsterberg, A., Vivian, N., Goodfellow, P., and Lovell-Badge, R.,** A gene mapping to the sex-determining region of the mouse Y chromosome is a member of a novel family of embryonically expressed genes, *Nature,* 346, 245, 1990.
7. **Sinclair, A. H., Berta, P., Palmer, M. S., Hawkins, J. R., Griffiths, B. L., Smith, M. J., Foster, J. W., Frischauf, A.-M., Lovell-Badge, R., and Goodfellow, P. N.,** A gene from the human sex-determining region encodes a protein with homology to a conserved DNA-binding motif, *Nature,* 346, 240, 1990.
8. **Koopman, P., Gubbay, J., Vivian, N., Goodfellow, P., and Lovell-Badge, R.,** Male development of chromosomally female mice transgenic for Sry, *Nature,* 351, 117, 1991.
9. **Müller, J., Schwartz, M., and Skakkebaek, N. E.,** Analysis of the sex-determining region of the Y chromosome (SRY) in sex reversed patients: point-mutation in SRY causing sex-reversion in a 46,XY female, *J. Clin. Endocrinol. Metab.,* 75, 331, 1992.
10. **Pao, C. C., Kao, S.-M., Hor, J. J., and Chang, S. Y.,** Lack of mutational alteration in the conserved regions of ZFY and SRY genes of 46,XY females with gonadal dysgenesis, *Hum. Reprod.,* 8, 224, 1993.
11. **Cate, R. L. and Wilson, C. A.,** Müllerian-inhibiting substance, in *Genes in Mammalian Reproduction,* Gwatkin, R. B. L., Ed., Wiley-Liss, New York, 1993, 185.
12. **Byskov, A. G. and Hoyer, P. E.,** Embryology of mammalian gonads and ducts, in *The Physiology of Reproduction,* Knobil, E. and Neill, J. D., Eds., Raven Press, New York, 1994, 487.
13. **Jost, A.,** A new look at the mechanism controlling sexual differentiation in mammals, *Johns Hopkins Med. J.,* 130, 38, 1972.
14. **George, F. W. and Wilson, J. D.,** Sex determination and differentiation, in *The Physiology of Reproduction,* Knobil, E. and Neill, J. D., Eds., Raven Press, New York, 1994, 3.

15. **Neumann, F., Elger, W., and Steinbeck, H.,** Drug induced intersexuality in mammals, *J. Reprod. Fertil.,* 7 (Suppl.), 9, 1969.

16. **Batch, J. A., Williams, D. M., Davies, H. R., Brown, B. D., Evans, B. A. J., Hughes, I. A., and Patterson, M. N.,** Role of the androgen receptor in male sexual differentiation, *Horm. Res.,* 38, 226, 1992.

17. **Setchell, B. P., Maddocks, S., and Brooks, D. E.,** Anatomy, vasculature, innervation, and fluids of the male reproductive tract, in *The Physiology of Reproduction,* Knobil, E. and Neill, J. D., Eds., Raven Press, New York, 1994, 1063.

18. **Kiely, E. A.,** Scientific basis of testicular descent and management implications for cryptorchidism, *Br. J. Clin. Pract.,* 48, 37, 1994.

19. **Hadziselimovic, F. and Kruslin, E.,** The role of the epididymis in descensus testis and the topographical relationship between the testis and epididymis from the sixth month of pregnancy until immediately after birth, *Anat. Embryol.,* 155, 191, 1979.

20. **Rajfer, J.,** Hormonal regulation of testicular descent, *Eur. J. Pediatr.,* 146, S6, 1987.

21. **Hutson, J. M.,** A biphasic model for the hormonal control of testicular descent, *Lancet,* 2, 419, 1985.

22. **Husman, D. A. and McPhaul, M. J.,** Time-specific androgen blockade with flutamide inhibits testicular descent in the rat, *Endocrinology,* 129, 1409, 1991.

23. **Steinberger, E. and Dixon, W. G.,** Some observations on the effect of heat on the testicular germinal epithelium, *Fertil. Steril.,* 10, 578, 1959.

24. **Waites, G. M. H.,** Temperature regulation and the testis, in *The Testis,* Vol. 1, Johnson, A. D., Gomes, W. R., and Vandemark, N. L., Eds., Academic Press, New York, 1970, 241.

25. **Maddocks, S. and Sharpe, R. M.,** Dynamics of testosterone secretion by the rat testis: implications for measurement of the intratesticular levels of testosterone, *J. Endocrinol.,* 122, 323, 1989.

26. **Anakwe, O. O., Murphy, P. R., and Moger, W. H.,** Characterization of β-adrenergic binding sites on rodent Leydig cells, *Biol. Reprod.,* 33, 815, 1985.

27. **Cooke, B. A., Golding, M., Dix, C. J., and Hunter, M. G.,** Catecholamine stimulation of testosterone production via cyclic AMP in mouse Leydig cells in monolayer culture, *Mol. Cell. Endocrinol.,* 27, 221, 1982.

28. **Damber, J. E.,** The effect of guanethidine treatment of testicular blood flow and testosterone production in rats, *Experientia,* 46, 486, 1990.

29. **Nistal, M., Paniagua, R., and Abaurrea, M. A.,** Varicose axons bearing "synaptic" vesicles on the basal lamina of the human seminiferous tubules, *Cell Tissue Res.,* 226, 75, 1982.

30. **Hodson, N.,** Sympathetic nerves and reproductive organs in the male rabbit, *J. Reprod. Fertil.,* 10, 209, 1965.

31. **Noordhuizen-Stassen, E. N. and Wensing, C. J. G.,** The effect of transection of the main vascular and nervous supply of the testis on the development of spermatogenic epithelium in the pig, *J. Pediatr. Surg.,* 18, 601, 1983.

32. **Martin, I. C. A., Lapwood, K. R., and Kitchell, R. L.,** The effects of specific neurectomies and cremaster muscle sectioning on semen characteristics and scrotal thermoregulatory responses of rams, in *Reproduction in Sheep,* Lindsey, D. R. and Pearce, D. T., Eds., Australian Academy of Science, Cambridge University Press, Cambridge, 1984, 73.

33. **Mizunuma, H., DePalatis, L. R., and McCann, S. M.,** Effect of unilateral orchidectomy on plasma FSH concentration: evidence for a direct neural connection between testes and CNS, *Neuroendocrinology,* 37, 291, 1983.

34. **Preslock, J. P. and McCann, S. M.,** Short-term effects of vasoligation upon plasma follicle-stimulating hormone, luteinizing hormone and prolactin in the adult rat: further evidence for a direct neural connection between the testes and the central nervous system, *Biol. Reprod.,* 33, 1120, 1985.

35. **Davis, J. R. and Langford, G. A.,** Comparative responses of the isolated testicular capsule and parenchyma to autonomic drugs, *J. Reprod. Fertil.,* 26, 241, 1971.

36. **Ellis, L. C., Buhrley, L. E., and Hargrove, J. L.,** Species differences in contractility of seminiferous tubules and tunica albuginea as related to sperm transport through the testis, *Arch. Androl.,* 1, 139, 1978.

37. **Rikimaru, A., Maruyama, T., Shirai, M., and Dendo, I.,** Pressure recording of contraction of the dog testis, *Tohoku J. Exp. Med.,* 108, 305, 1972.

38. **Stolla, R. and Leidl, W.,** Quantitative histological studies of testicular growth of bulls after puberty, *Zbl. Vet. Med. A,* 18, 563, 1971.

39. **Fawcett, D. W., Neaves, W. B., and Flores, M. D.,** Comparative observations on intertubular lymphatics and the organization of interstitial tissue of the mammalian testis, *Biol. Reprod.,* 9, 500, 1973.

40. **Russel, L. D., Ren, H. P., Sinha Hikim, I., Schulze, W., and Sinha Hikim, A. P.,** A comparative study in twelve mammalian species of volume densities, volumes, and numerical densities of selected testis components, emphasizing those related to the Sertoli cell, *Am. J. Anat.,* 188, 21, 1990.

41. **Clermont, Y.,** Contractile elements in the limiting membrane of the seminiferous tubules of the rat, *Exp. Cell Res.,* 15, 438, 1958.

42. **Sar, M., Stumpf, W. E., McLean, W. S., Smith, A. A., Hansson, V., Nayfeh, S. N., and French, F. S.,** Localization of androgen target cells in the rat testis: autoradiographic studies, *Curr. Top. Mol. Endocrinol.,* 2, 311, 1975.

43. **Glover, T. D. and Nicander, L.,** Some aspects and functions in the mammalian epididymis, *J. Reprod. Fertil.,* 13 (Suppl.), 39, 1971.

44. **Amann, R. P.,** Function of the epididymis in bulls and rams, *J. Reprod. Fertil.,* 34 (Suppl.), 115, 1987.

45. **Schefels, W. and Stolla, R.,** Resorption of sperm from the epididymis of the boar, *Zbl. Vet. Med. A,* 22, 302, 1975.

46. **Kerr, J. B.,** Functional cytology of the human testis, in *Baillière's Clinical Endocrinology and Metabolism, The Testes,* Vol. 6/2, de Kretser, D. M., Ed., Baillière Tindall, London, 1992, 235.

47. **Bergh, A.,** Local differences in Leydig cell morphology in the adult rat testis: evidence for a local control of Leydig cells by adjacent seminiferous tubules, *Int. J. Androl.,* 5, 325, 1982.

48. **Rich, K. A., Kerr, J. B., and de Kretser, D. M.,** Evidence for Leydig cell dysfunction in rats with seminiferous tubule damage, *Mol. Cell. Endocrinol.,* 13, 123, 1979.

49. **Kerr, J. B., Rich, K. A., and de Kretser, D. M.,** Alterations of the fine structure and androgen secretion of the interstitial cells in the experimentally cryptorchid rat testis, *Biol. Reprod.,* 20, 409, 1979.

50. **Nagano, T. and Suzuki, F.,** Freeze fracture observations on the intercellular junctions of Sertoli-cells and of Leydig cells in the human testis, *Cell Tissue Res.,* 166, 37, 1976.

51. **Skinner, M. K.,** Cell-cell interactions in the testis, *Endocr. Rev.,* 12, 45, 1991.

52. **Neaves, W. B., Johnson, L., and Petty, C. S.,** Age-related change in numbers of other interstitial cells in testes of adult men: evidence bearing on the fate of Leydig cells lost with increasing age, *Biol. Reprod.,* 33, 259, 1985.

53. **Jégou, B.,** The Sertoli-germ cell communication network in mammals, *Int. Rev. Cytol.,* 147, 25, 1993.

54. **Russel, L. D.,** Sertoli-germ cell interrelations: a review, *Gamete Res.,* 3, 179, 1980.

55. **Amann, R. P.,** Functional anatomy of the adult male, in *Equine Reproduction,* McKinnon, A. O. and Voss, J. L., Eds., Lea & Febiger, Philadelphia, 1993, 645.

56. **Johnson, L., Zane, R. S., Petty, C. S., and Neaves, W. B.,** Quantification of the human Sertoli cell population: its distribution, relation to germ cell numbers and age-related decline, *Biol. Reprod.,* 31, 785, 1984.

57. **Ortavant, R., Courot, M., and Hocherau-de Reviers, M. T.,** Spermatogenesis in domestic mammals, in *Reproduction in Domestic Animals,* Cole, H. H. and Cupps, P. T., Eds., Academic Press, New York, 1977, 203.

58. **de Kretser, D. M. and Kerr, J. B.,** The cytology of the testis, in *The Physiology of Reproduction,* Knobil, E. and Neill, J. D., Eds., Raven Press, New York, 1994, 1177.

59. **Lincoln, G. A.,** Seasonal aspects of testicular function, in *The Testis,* Burger, H. G. and de Kretser, D. M., Eds., Raven Press, New York, 1989, 329.

60. **Clermont, Y.,** The cycle of the seminiferous epithelium in man, *Am. J. Anat.,* 112, 35, 1963.

61. **Courot, M., Hocherau-de Reviers, M. T., and Ortavant, R.,** Spermatogenesis, in *The Testis, Development, Anatomy, and Physiology,* Vol. 1, Johnson, A. D., Gomes, W. R., and Vandemark, N. L., Eds., Academic Press, New York, 1970, 339.

62. **Leidl, W. and Waschke, B.,** Comparative aspects of the kinetics of the spermiogenesis, in *Morphological Aspects of Andrology,* Holstein, A. F. and Horstmann, E., Eds., Grosse, Berlin, 1970, 21.

63. **Chowdhury, A. K. and Marshall, C. T.,** Irregular pattern of spermatogenesis in the baboon (Papio anubis) and its possible mechanism, in *Testicular Development, Structure and Function,* Steinberger, A. and Steinberger, E., Eds., Raven Press, New York, 1980, 129.

64. **Schulze, W. and Rehder, U.,** Organization and morphogenesis of the human seminiferous epithelium, *Cell Tissue Res.,* 237, 395, 1984.

65. **Roosen-Runge, E. C. and Giesel, L. O.,** Quantitative studies on spermatogenesis in the albino rat, *Am. J. Anat.,* 87, 1, 1950.

66. **Cleland, K. W.,** The spermatogenic cycle of the guinea pig, *Aust. J. Biol. Sci.,* 4, 344, 1951.

67. **Clermont, Y.,** Kinetics of spermatogenesis in mammals: seminiferous epithelium cycle and spermatogonial renewal, *Physiol. Rev.,* 52, 198, 1972.

68. **Dym, M. and Fawcett, D. W.,** Further observations on the numbers of spermatogonia, spermatocytes and spermatids connected by intercellular bridges in the mammalian testis, *Biol. Reprod.,* 4, 195, 1971.

69. **Russel, L. D., Vogl, A. W., and Weber, J. E.,** Actin localization in male germ cells intercellular bridges in the rat and ground squirrel and disruption of bridges by cytochalasin D, *Am. J. Anat.,* 180, 25, 1987.

70. **Weber, J. E. and Russel, L. D.,** A study of intercellular bridges during spermatogenesis in the rat, *Am. J. Anat.,* 180, 1, 1987.

71. **Berthold, A. A.,** Transplantation der Hoden, *Arch. Anat. Physiol. Wissensch. Med.,* 16, 42, 1849.

72. **Butenandt, A. and Harrisch, G.,** Ein Weg zur Testosteron-Umwandlung des Dehydroandrostendions in Androstendiol und Testosteron, *Z. Physiol. Chem.,* 237, 89, 1935.

73. **Christensen, A. K.,** Leydig cells, in *Handbook of Physiology,* Sect. 7, Vol. 5, Greep, R. O. and Astwood, E. B., Eds., American Physiological Society, Washington, D.C., 1975, 21.

74. **Morris, M. D. and Chaikoff, I. L.,** The origin of cholesterol in liver, small intestine, adrenal gland and testis of the rat: dietary versus endogenous contribution, *J. Biol. Chem.,* 234, 1095, 1959.

75. **Tsai, S. C., Ying, B. P., and Gaylor, J.,** Testicular sterols. I. Incorporation of mevalonate and acetate into sterols by testicular tissue from rats, *Arch. Biochem. Biophys.,* 105, 329, 1964.

76. **Pignataro, O. P., Radicella, J. P., Calvo, J. C., and Charreau, E. H.,** Mitochondrial biosynthesis of cholesterol in Leydig cells from rat testis, *Mol. Cell. Endocrinol.,* 33, 53, 1983.

77. **Goad, L. J.,** Cholesterol biosynthesis and metabolism, in *Biochemistry of Steroid Hormones,* Makin, H. L. J., Ed., Blackwell Scientific, Oxford, 1975, 17.

78. **Werbin, H. and Chaikoff, I. L.,** Utilization of adrenal gland cholesterol for synthesis of cortisol by the intact normal and the ACTH-treated guinea pig, *Arch. Biochem. Biophys.,* 93, 476, 1961.

79. **Hall, P. F. and Eik-Nes, K. B.,** The action of gonadotropic hormones upon rabbit testis in vitro, *Biochim. Biophys. Acta,* 63, 411, 1962.

80. **Sandler, R. and Hall, P. F.,** The response of rat testis to interstitial cell-stimulating hormone in vitro, *Comp. Biochem. Physiol.,* 19, 833, 1966.

81. **Hall, P. F., Irby, D. C., and de Kretser, D. M.,** Conversion of cholesterol to androgens by rat testes: comparison of interstitial cells and seminiferous tubules, *Endocrinology,* 84, 488, 1969.

82. **Albert, D. H., Ascoli, M., Puett, D., and Coniglio, J. G.,** Lipid composition and gonadotropin-mediated lipid metabolism of the M5480 murine Leydig cell tumor, *J. Lipid Res.,* 21, 862, 1980.

83. **Van Noort, M., Rommerts, F. F. G., van Amerongen, A., and Wirtz, K. W. A.,** Intracellular redistribution of SPC2 in Leydig cells after hormonal stimulation may contribute to increased pregnenolone, *Biochem. Biophys. Res. Commun.,* 154, 60, 1988.

84. **Mertz, L. M. and Pedersen, R. C.,** The kinetics of steroidogenesis activator polypeptide in the rat adrenal cortex, *J. Biol. Chem.,* 264, 15274, 1989.

85. **Hall, P. F.,** Testicular steroid synthesis: organization and regulation, in *The Physiology of Reproduction,* Vol. 1, Knobil, E. and Neill, J. D., Eds., Raven Press, New York, 1993, 1335.

86. **Yanaihara, T. and Troen, P.,** Studies of the human testis. I. Biosynthetic pathways for androgen formation in human testicular tissue in vitro, *J. Clin. Endocrinol. Metab.,* 34, 783, 1972.

87. **Samuels, L. T., Bussman, L., Matsumoto, K., and Huseby, R.A.,** Organization of androgen biosynthesis in the testis, *J. Steroid Biochem.,* 6, 291, 1975.

88. **Nakajin, S., Shively J. E., Yuan, P. M., and Hall, P. F.,** Microsomal cytochrome P-450 from neonatal pig testis: two enzymatic activities (17α-hydroxylase and c17,20 lyase) associated with one protein, *Biochemistry,* 20, 4037, 1981.

89. **Matteson, K. J., Picardo-Leonard, J., Chung, B., Mohandas, T. K., and Miller, W. L.,** Assignment of the gene for adrenal P450c17 (steroid 17α-hydroxylase/17,20-lyase) to human chromosome 10, *J. Clin. Endocrinol. Metab.,* 63, 789, 1986.

90. **Oshima, H. and Ochi, A. I.,** On testicular 17β-hydroxy-steroid oxidoreductase: product activation, *Biochim. Biophys. Acta,* 306, 227, 1973.

91. **Lorence, M. C., Murray, B. A., Trant, J. M., and Mason, J. I.,** Human 3β-hydroxysteroid dehydrogenase/Δ5-4-isomerase from placenta: expression in non-steroidogenic cells of a protein that catalyzes the dehydrogenation/isomerization of C21 and C19 steroids, *Endocrinology,* 126, 2493, 1990.

92. **Penning, T. M. and Covey, D. F.,** Inactivation of Δ5-3-ketosteroid isomerase(s) from beef adrenal cortex by acetylenic ketosteroids, *J. Steroid Biochem.,* 16, 691, 1982.

93. **Setchell, B. P., Laurie, A. P. F., Flint, A. P. F., and Heap, R. B.,** Transport of free and conjugated steroids from the boar testis in lymph, venous blood and rete testis fluid, *J. Endocrinol.,* 96, 127, 1983.

94. **Free, M. J.,** Blood supply to the testis and its role in local exchange and transport of hormones, in *The Testis,* Vol. 4, Johnson, A. D. and Gomes, W. R., Eds., Academic Press, New York, 1977, 39.

95. **Noordhuizen-Stassen, E. N., Charbon, G. A., deJong, F. H., and Wensing, C. J. G.,** Functional arterio-venous anastomoses between the testicular artery and the pampiniform plexus in the spermatic cord of rams, *J. Reprod. Fertil.,* 75, 193, 1985.

96. **Maddocks, S., Hargreave, T. B., Reddie, K., Fraser, H. M., Kerr, J. B., and Sharpe, R. M.,** Intratesticular hormone levels and the route of secretion of hormones from the testis of the rat, guinea pig, monkey and human, *Int. J. Androl.,* 16, 272, 1993.

97. **Setchell, B. B.,** *The Mammalian Testis,* Paul Elek, London, 1978.

98. **Rosner, W.,** The function of corticosteroid-binding globulin and sex hormone-binding globulin: recent advances, *Endocr. Rev.,* 11, 80, 1990.

99. **Gower, D. B.,** Catabolism and conjugation, in *Steroid Hormones,* Croom Helm, London, 1979, 50.

100. **Corvol, P. and Bardin, C. W.,** Species distribution of testosterone-binding globulin, *Biol. Reprod.,* 8, 277, 1973.

101. **Tapanainen, T., Kuopio, T., Pelliniemi, L. J., and Huhtaniemi, I.,** Rat testicular endogenous steroids and number of Leydig cells between the fetal period and sexual maturity, *Biol. Reprod.,* 31, 1027, 1984.

102. **Lindner, H. R.,** Androgens and related compounds in the spermatic vein blood of domestic animals. I. Neutral steroids secreted by the bull testis, *J. Endocrinol.,* 23, 139, 1961.

103. **Möstl, E., Choi, H. S., Kruip, Th. A. M., and Bamberg, E.,** Androstendion, Epitestosteron, Testosteron und Luteinisierungshormon im Blutplasma von Stieren vor und nach Verabreichung von Gn-RH (Lutal®), *Zbl. Vet. Med. A,* 30, 429, 1983.

104. **Claus, R.,** *Mammalian Pheromones with Special Reference to the Boar Taint Steroid and its Relationship to Other Testicular Steroids,* Paul Parey, Hamburg, 1979.

105. **Kelch, R. P., Jenner, M. R., Weinstein, R., Kaplan, S. L., and Gumbach, M. M.,** Estradiol and testosterone secretion by human, simian and canine testes, in males with hypogonadism and in male pseudohermaphrodites with feminizing testes syndrome, *J. Clin. Invest.,* 51, 824, 1972.

106. **DeJong, F. H., Hey, A. H., and van der Molen, H. J.,** Effects of gonadotropins on the secretion of oestradiol-17β and testosterone by the rat testis, *J. Endocrinol.,* 57, 277, 1973.

107. **Amann, R. P. and Ganjam, V. K.,** Steroid production by the bovine testis and steroid transfer across the pampiniform plexus, *Biol. Reprod.,* 15, 695, 1976.

108. **Savard, K. and Goldzieher, J. W.,** Biosynthesis of steroids in stallion testes tissue, *Endocrinology,* 66, 617, 1960.

109. **Dorrington, J. H. and Armstrong, D. T.,** Follicle stimulating hormone stimulates estradiol-17β synthesis in cultured Sertoli cells, *Proc. Natl. Acad. Sci. U.S.A.,* 72, 2677, 1975.

110. **Tcholakian, R. K. and Steinberger, A.,** In vitro metabolism of testosterone by Sertoli cells and interstitial cells and the effect of FSH, in *Testicular Development, Structure and Function,* Steinberger, A. and Steinberger, E., Eds. Raven Press, New York, 1980, 177.

111. **Raeside, J. I. and Renaud, R. L.,** Estrogen and androgen production by purified Leydig cells of mature boars, *Biol. Reprod.,* 28, 727, 1983.

112. **Cox, J. E. and Redhead, P. H.,** Prolonged effect of a single injection of human chorionic gonadotrophin on plasma testosterone and oestrone sulphate concentrations in mature stallions, *Equine Vet. J.,* 22, 36, 1990.

113. **Claus, R., Schopper, D., and Hoang-Vu, C.,** Contribution of individual compartments of the genital tract to oestrogen and testosterone concentrations in ejaculates of the boar, *Acta Endocrinol.,* 109, 281, 1985.

114. **Claus, R., Meyer, H.-D., Gimenez, T., Hoang-Vu, C., and Münster, E.,** Effect of seminal oestrogens of the boar on prostaglandin F2α release from the uterus of the sow, *Anim. Reprod. Sci.,* 23, 143, 1990.

115. **Claus, R., Dimmick, M. A., Gimenez, T., and Hudson, L. W.,** Estrogens and prostaglandin F2α in the semen and blood plasma of stallions, *Theriogenology,* 38, 687, 1992.

116. **Mottram, J. C. and Cramer, W.,** Report on the general effects of exposure to radium on metabolism and tumor growth in the rat and the special effects on testis and pituitary, *J. Exp. Physiol.,* 13, 209, 1923.

117. **McCullagh, D. R.,** Dual endocrine activity of the testis, *Science,* 79, 19, 1932.

118. **Knight, P. G.,** Identification and purification of inhibin and inhibin-related proteins, *J. Reprod. Fertil.,* 43 (Suppl.), 11, 1991.

119. **de Kretser, D. M., Au, C. L., and Roberston, D. M.,** The physiology of inhibin in the male, in *Inhibin: Non-Steroidal Regulation of Follicle Stimulating Hormone Secretion,* Vol. 42, Burger, H. G., de Kretser, D. M., Findlay, J. K., and Igarashi, M., Eds., Serono Symp., Raven Press, New York, 1987, 149.

120. **McLachlan, R. I., Dahl, K. D., Bremner, W. J., Schwall, R., Schmelzer, C. H., Mason, A. J., and Steiner, R. A.,** Recombinant activin-A stimulates basal FSH and GnRH-stimulated FSH and LH release in the adult male macaque, Macaca fascicularis, *Endocrinology,* 125, 2787, 1989.

121. **Bardin, C. W., Morris, P. L., Chen, C. L., Shaha, C., Voglmayr, J., Rivier, J., Spiess, J., and Vale, W. W.,** Testicular inhibin: structure and regulation by FSH, androgens and EGF, in *Inhibin: Non-Steroidal Regulation of Follicle Stimulating Hormone Secretion,* Vol. 42, Burger, H. G., de Kretser, D. M., Findlay, J. K., and Igarashi, M., Eds., Serono Symp., Raven Press, New York, 1987, 179.

122. **Roberts, V., Meunier, H., Sawchenko, P. E., and Vale, W.,** Differential production and regulation of inhibin subunits in rat testicular cell types, *Endocrinology,* 125, 2350, 1989.

123. **Voglmayr, J. K., Jolley, D., Vale, W., Willoughby, D., Moser, A., So, C.-K., Chen, C.-L., and Bardin, C. W.,** Effects of follicle-stimulating hormone on inhibin release by different testicular compartments in the adult ram, *Biol. Reprod.,* 47, 573, 1992.

124. **Gonzales, G. F., Risbridger, G. P., and Ishida, H.,** Stage-specific inhibin secretion by rat seminiferous tubules, *Reprod. Fertil. Dev.,* 1, 275, 1989.

125. **Tillbrook, A. J., de Kretser, D. M., and Clarke, I. J.,** Human recombinant A suppresses plasma follicle-stimulating hormone to intact levels but has no effect on luteinizing hormone in castrated rams, *Biol. Reprod.,* 49, 779, 1993.

126. **Meunier, H., Rivier, C., Evans, R. M., and Vale, W.,** Gonadal and extragonadal expression of inhibin α, βA and βB subunits in various tissues predicts diverse function, *Proc. Natl. Acad. Sci. U.S.A.,* 85, 247, 1988.

127. **Jackson, C. M. and Morris, I. D.,** Gonadotrophin levels in male rats following impairment of Leydig cell function by ethylene dimethane sulphonate, *Andrologia,* 9, 29, 1977.

128. **Gonzales, G. F., Risbridger, G. P., and de Kretser, D. M.,** In vivo and in vitro production of inhibin by cryptorchid testis from adult rats, *Endocrinology,* 59, 179, 1989.

129. **Vale, W., Rivier, J., Vaughan, J., McClintock, R., Corrigan, A., Woo, W., Karr, D., and Spiess, J.,** Purification and characterization of an FSH releasing protein from porcine ovarian follicular fluid, *Nature,* 321, 776, 1986.

130. **Ailenberg, M., Tung, P. S., and Fritz, I. B.,** Transforming growth factor-β elicits shape changes and increases contractility of testicular peritubular cells, *Biol. Reprod.,* 42, 499, 1990.

131. **Wagner, R. K. and Hughes, A.,** Current view on androgen receptors and mechanism of androgen actions, in *Androgen II and Antiandrogens,* Eichler, O., Farah, A., Herken, H., and Welch, W. D., Eds., Springer-Verlag, Berlin, 1974, 1.

132. **George, F. W. and Peterson, K. G.,** 5α-Dihydrotestosterone formation is necessary for embryogenesis of the rat prostate, *Endocrinology,* 122, 1159, 1988.

133. **Chang, C., Katoris, J., and Liao, S.,** Molecular cloning of human and rat complementary DNA encoding androgen receptors, *Science,* 240, 327, 1988.

134. **Grino, P. B., Griffin, J. E., and Wilson, J. D.,** Testosterone at high concentrations interacts with the human androgen receptor similarly to dihydrotestosterone, *Endocrinology,* 126, 1165, 1990.

135. **Gower, D. B.,** Biosynthesis of the corticosteroids, in *Biochemistry of Steroid Hormones,* Makin, H. L. J., Ed., Blackwell Scientific, Oxford, 1975, 47.

136. **George, F. W., Johnson, L., and Wilson, J. D.,** The effect of a 5α reductase inhibitor on androgen physiology in the immature male rat, *Endocrinology,* 125, 2434, 1989.

137. **Chen, H., Chandrashekar, V., and Zirkin, B. R.,** Can spermatogenesis be maintained quantitatively in intact adult rats with exogenously administered dihydrotestosterone? *J. Androl.,* 15, 132, 1994.

138. **Sun, Y. T., Wreford , N. G., Robertson, D. M., and de Kretser, D. M.,** Quantitative cytological studies of spermatogenesis in intact and hypophysectomized rats: identification of androgen-dependent stages, *Endocrinology,* 127, 1215, 1990.

139. **Cameron, D. F. and Nazian, S. J.,** Eradication of Leydig cells during puberty: daily sperm production, testosterone and structure of the Sertoli/spermatid interaction, *16th Annu. Meet. Am. Soc. Androl., J. Androl. Suppl.,* 61 (Abstr.), 40, 1991.

140. **Hamilton, D. W.,** Steroid function in the mammalian epididymis, *J. Reprod. Fertil.,* 13 (Suppl.), 89, 1971.

141. **Evans, R. R. and Johnson, A. D.,** The metabolic activity of the bovine epididymis. III. Cholesterol and esterified cholesterol metabolism, *J. Reprod. Fertil.,* 43, 527, 1975.

142. **Dinakar, N., Arora, R., and Prasad, M. R. N.,** Effects of microquantities of 5α-dihydrotestosterone on the epididymis and accessory glands of the castrated Rhesus monkey, Macaca mulatta, *Int. J. Fertil.,* 19, 133, 1974.

143. **Back, D. J.,** The presence of metabolites of 3H-testosterone in the lumen of the cauda epididymis of the rat, *Steroids,* 25, 413, 1975.

144. **Turner, T. T., Jones, C. E., Howards, S. S., Ewing, L. L., Zegeye, B., and Gunsalus, G. L.,** On the androgen microenvironment of maturing spermatozoa, *Endocrinology,* 115, 1925, 1984.

145. **Robaire, B.,** Effects of unilateral orchidectomy on rat epididymal Δ4-5α-reductase and 3α-hydroxysteroid dehydrogenase, *Can. J. Physiol. Pharmacol.,* 57, 998, 1979.

146. **Mann, T.,** *Biochemistry of Semen and of the Male Reproductive Tract,* Methuen, London, 1964.

147. **Andersson, S. and Russell, D. W.,** Structural and biochemical properties of cloned and expressed human and rat steroid 5alpha-reductases, *Proc. Natl. Acad. Sci. U.S.A.,* 87, 3640, 1990.

148. **Carter, H. B. and Isaacs, J. T.,** Experimental and theoretical basis for hormonal treatment of prostatic cancer, *Invest. Urol.,* 6, 262, 1988.

149. **Udry, J. R. and Talbert, L. M.,** Sex hormone effects on personality at puberty, *J. Pers. Soc. Psychol.,* 54, 291, 1988.

150. **Archer, J.,** The influence of testosterone on human aggression, *Br. J. Psychiatry,* 82, 1, 1991.

151. **Wilson, J. D.,** Syndromes of androgen resistance, *Biol. Reprod.,* 46, 168, 1992.

152. **Parkes, A. S.,** The internal secretion of the testis, in *Marshall's Physiology of Reproduction,* Parkes, A. S., Ed., Longman, London, 1966, 412.

153. **Forbes, G.,** The effects of anabolic steroids on lean body mass: the dose response curve, *Metabolism,* 69, 776, 1985.

154. **Sinnett-Smith, P. A., Palmer, C. A., and Buttery, P. J.,** Androgen receptors in skeletal muscle cytosol from sheep treated with trenbolone acetate, *Horm. Metab. Res.,* 19, 110, 1987.

155. **Bardin, C. W., Swerdloff, R. S., and Santen, R. J.,** Androgens: risks and benefits, *J. Clin. Endocrinol. Metab.,* 73, 4, 1991.

156. **Wu, F. C. W.,** Testicular steroidogenesis and androgen use and abuse, in *Baillière's Clinical Endocrinology and Metabolism, The Testes,* Vol. 6/2, de Kretser, D. M., Ed., Baillière Tindall, London, 1992, 373.

157. **Schally, A. V., Arimura, A., Baba, Y., Nair, R. M. G., Matsuo, H., Redding, T. W., Debeljuk, L., and White, W. F.,** Isolation and properties of the FSH- and LH-releasing hormone, *Biochem. Biophys. Res. Commun.,* 43, 393, 1971.

158. **Amoos, M., Burgus, R., Blackwell, R., Vale, W., Fellows, R., and Guillemin, R.,** Purification, amino-acid composition and N-terminus of the hypothalamic luteinizing hormone-releasing factor (LRF) of ovine origin, *Biochem. Biophys. Res. Commun.,* 44, 205, 1971.

159. **Knobil, E.,** The neuroendocrine control of the menstrual cycle, *Recent Prog. Horm. Res.,* 36, 53, 1980.

160. **Krey, L. C., Butler, W. R., and Knobil, E.,** Surgical disconnection of the medial basal hypothalamus and pituitary function in the Rhesus monkey. I. Gonadotropin secretion, *Endocrinology,* 96, 1073, 1975.

161. **Barraclough, C. A. and Wise, P. M.,** The role of catecholamines in the regulation of pituitary luteinizing hormone and follicle-stimulating hormone secretion, *Endocr. Rev.,* 3, 91, 1982.

162. **Hall, P. F.,** On the stimulation of testicular steroidogenesis in the rabbit by interstitial cell-stimulating hormone, *Endocrinology,* 78, 690, 1966.

163. **McFarland, K. C., Sprenge, R., Phillips, H. S., Kohler, M., Rosemblit, N., Nicolics, K., Segaloff, D. L., and Seeberg, P. H.,** Lutropin-choriogonadotropin receptor: an unusual member of the G protein coupled receptor family, *Science,* 245, 494, 1989.

164. **Koo, Y. B., Ji, I., Slaughter, R. G., and Ji, T. H.,** Structure of the luteinizing hormone receptor gene and multiple exons of the coding sequence, *Endocrinology,* 128, 2297, 1991.

165. **Aubry, M., Collu, R., Ducharme, J. R., and Crine, P.,** Biosynthesis of a putative gonadotropin receptor component by rat Leydig cells, *Endocrinology,* 111, 1219, 1982.

166. **Habener, J. F.,** Cyclic AMP response element binding proteins: a cornucopia of transcription factors, *Mol. Endocrinol.,* 4, 1087, 1990.

167. **Freeman, D. A. and Ascoli, M.,** Desensitization of steroidogenesis receptors in cultured Leydig tumor cells: role of cholesterol, *Proc. Natl. Acad. Sci. U.S.A.,* 79, 7796, 1982.

168. **Parvinen, M.,** Regulation of the seminiferous epithelium, *Endocr. Rev.,* 3, 404, 1982.

169. **Robertson, D. M., Prisk, M., and McWaster, J. W.,** Serum FSH-suppressing activity of human recombinant inhibin A in male and female rats, *J. Reprod. Fertil.,* 91, 321, 1991.

170. **Farnworth, P. G., Robertson, D. M., de Kretser, D. M., and Burger, H. G.,** Effects of 31kDa bovine inhibin on FSH and LH in rat pituitary cells in vitro: actions under basal conditions, *Endocrinology,* 119, 233, 1988.

171. **Cheng, C. Y., Frick, J., Gunsalus, G. L., Musto, N. A., and Bardin, C. W.,** Human testicular androgen binding protein shares immunodeterminants with serum testosterone-estradiol-binding globulin, *Endocrinology,* 114, 1395, 1984.

172. **Rich, K. A., Bardin, C. W., Gunsalus, G. L., and Mather, J. P.,** Age-dependent pattern of androgen binding protein (ABP) secretion from rat Sertoli cells in primary culture, *Endocrinology,* 113, 2284, 1983.

173. **Griswold, M. D.,** Protein secretions of Sertoli cells, *Int. Rev. Cytol.,* 110, 133, 1988.

174. **Hall, P. F. and Mita, M.,** Influence of FSH on glucose transport by cultured Sertoli cells, *Biol. Reprod.,* 31, 863, 1984.

175. **Mita, M. and Hall, P. F.,** Metabolism of round spermatids from rats lactate as the preferred substrate, *Biol. Reprod.,* 26, 445, 1982.

176. **Clermont, Y. and Harvey, S. G.,** Duration of the cycle of the seminiferous epithelium of normal hypophysectomized and hypophysectomized-hormone treated albino rats, *Endocrinology,* 76, 80, 1965.

177. **Huang, H. F. S., Marshall, G. R., Rosenberg, R., and Nieschlag, E.,** Restoration of spermatogenesis by high levels of testosterone in hypophysectomized rats after long-term regression, *Acta Endocrinol.,* 116, 433, 1987.

178. **Cunningham, G. R. and Huckins, C.,** Persistence of complete spermatogenesis in the presence of low intra-testicular concentration of testosterone, *Endocrinology,* 105, 177, 1979.

179. **Sun, Y. T., Irby, D. C., Robertson, D. M., and de Kretser, D. M.,** The effects of exogenously administered testosterone on spermatogenesis in intact and hypophysectomized rats, *Endocrinology,* 125, 1000, 1989.

180. **Cameron, D. F. and Muffly, K. E.,** Hormonal stimulation of spermatid binding to Sertoli cells in vitro, in *The Male Germ Cell: Spermatogonium to Fertilization,* 11th North American Testis Workshop, 35 (Abstr.), 60, 1991.

181. **Buzek, S. W. and Sanborn, B. M.,** Nuclear androgen receptor dynamics in testicular peritubular and Sertoli cells, *J. Androl.,* 11, 514, 1990.

182. **Fabbri, A.,** The role and regulation of testicular opioids, *Trends Endocrinol. Metab.,* 1, 117, 1990.

183. **Fabbri, A., Tsai-Morris, C. H., and Luna, S.,** Opiate receptors are present in the rat testis. Identification and localization in Sertoli cells, *Endocrinology,* 117, 2544, 1985.

184. **Skinner, M. K., Fetterolf, P. M., and Anthony, C. T.,** Purification of a paracrine factor, PModS, produced by testicular peritubular cells that modulates Sertoli cell function, *J. Biol. Chem.,* 263, 2884, 1988.

185. **Skinner, M. K., Takacs, K., and Coffey, R. J.,** Transforming growth factor-α gene expression and action in the seminiferous tubule, peritubular cell-Sertoli cell interaction, *Endocrinology,* 124, 845, 1989.

186. **Aoki, A. and Fawcell, D. W.,** Is there a local feedback from the seminiferous tubules affecting activity of the Leydig cells? *Biol. Reprod.,* 19, 144, 1978.

187. **Bergh, A.,** Development of stage-specific paracrine regulation of Leydig cells by the seminiferous tubules, *Int. J. Androl.,* 8, 80, 1985.

188. **Lin, T., Calkins, J. K., Morris, P. L., Vale, W., and Bardin, C. W.,** Regulation of Leydig cell function in primary culture by inhibin and activin, *Endocrinology,* 125, 2134, 1989.

189. **Cailleau, J., Vermeire, S., and Verhoeven, G.,** Independent control of the production of insulin-like growth factor I and its binding protein by cultured testicular cells, *Mol. Cell. Endocrinol.,* 69, 79, 1990.

190. **Verhoeven, G. and Cailleau, J.,** Influence of coculture with Sertoli cells on steroidogenesis in immature rat Leydig cells, *Mol. Cell. Endocrinol.,* 71, 239, 1990.

191. **Bronson, F. H. and Heidemann, P. D.,** Seasonal regulation of reproduction in mammals, in *The Physiology of Reproduction,* Vol. 2, Knobil, E. and Neill, J. D., Eds., Raven Press, New York, 1993, 541.

192. **Binkley, S.,** Structures and moleculars involved in generation and regulation of biological rhythms in vertebrates and invertebrates, *Experientia,* 49, 648, 1993.

193. **Binkley, S., Hryshchshyn, M., and Reilly, K.,** N-Acetyltransferase activity responds to environmental lighting in the eye as well as in the pineal gland, *Nature,* 281, 479, 1979.

194. **Berria, M., Joseph, M. M., and Mead, R. A.,** Role of prolactin and luteinizing hormone in regulating timing of implantation in the spotted skunk, *Biol. Reprod.,* 40, 232, 1989.

195. **Lincoln, G. A. and Short, R. V.,** Seasonal breeding: nature's contraceptive, *Recent Prog. Horm. Res.,* 36, 1, 1980.

196. **Lincoln, G. A. and Peet, M. J.,** Photoperiodic control of gonadotrophin secretion in the ram: a detailed study of the temporal changes in plasma levels of follicle-stimulating hormone, luteinizing hormone and testosterone following an abrupt switch from long to short days, *J. Endocrinol.,* 74, 355, 1977.

197. **Barenton, B. and Pelletier, J.,** Prolactin, testicular growth and LH receptors in the ram following light and 2-Br-α-ergocryptine treatments, *Biol. Reprod.,* 22, 781, 1980.

198. **Pudney, J. and Lacy, D.,** Correlation between ultrastructure and biochemical changes in the testis of the American grey squirrel, *Sciurus carolinensis,* during the reproductive cycle, *J. Reprod. Fertil.,* 49, 5, 1977.

Chapter 12

INTRATESTICULAR FACTORS IN TESTICULAR ENDOCRINE FUNCTION

Varadaraj Chandrashekar

CONTENTS

INTRODUCTION

The ultimate function of the testis is to produce spermatozoa that are capable of fertilizing the eggs. In addition, the testis secretes testosterone. This testicular steroid has been shown to be an important hormone for induction and maintenance of spermatogenesis and male sexual behavior, and it is required for the physiological function of the male reproductive structures. The testis also synthesizes a number of other steroids and peptides/proteins. The major focus of this chapter is to present a condensed treatise on the influence of intratesticular factors on the Leydig cell function. First, a brief account of the testicular cellular architecture and its function is presented.

STEROID PRODUCTION BY THE TESTIS

Before describing the biosynthesis of testosterone, it is best to review the cell biology of the testis.

CELL BIOLOGY OF THE TESTIS

Seminiferous tubules constitute the major portion of the testis. Within the seminiferous tubules there is a number of Sertoli cells that give structural support to the germ cells. At the basal surface of these Sertoli cells there is another type of cell called the peritubular myoid cells. These peritubular cells surround the seminiferous tubules. In the interstitium, between the seminiferous tubules, the Leydig cells reside (Figure 1).

Sertoli cells are the major secretory components of the seminiferous tubules. It is believed that Sertoli cells, in addition to their secretion of estrogen, produce a number of peptides/proteins that modulate spermatogenesis and steroidogenesis (Table 1). Although there is a blood-testis barrier and the majority of Sertoli cell products are secreted into the lumen of seminiferous tubules, some of these products are secreted into the peripheral blood. Leydig cells synthesize and secrete steroids including testosterone. There are indications that Leydig cells also secrete a number of paracrine factors (Table 2). The peritubular cell secretions are believed to be important for the maintenance of the Sertoli cell function.[1]

BIOSYNTHESIS OF TESTICULAR STEROIDS

The pattern of pathways for the biosynthesis of testosterone in the mammalian testis is similar to those that occur in the adrenal cortex, ovaries, and placenta.

By glycolysis and fatty acid oxidation, acetate (acetyl coenzyme A) is formed and is the starting material for the synthesis of testosterone. By a number of intermediate steps, acetate is converted to a 27-carbon-containing cholesterol. From cholesterol, by removal of carbons and hydroxylation, a 21-carbon-containing pregnenolone is formed. This conversion is believed to occur in the mitochondria and the rest of the reactions takes place extramitochondrially. There are two major pathways for the biosynthesis of testosterone: Δ^4 and Δ^5 pathways. It has been suggested that in the human testis the Δ^5 pathway is prevalent,[2] whereas the major pathway in the rat testis is the Δ^4 pathway.[3]

In the Δ^4 pathway pregnenolone is converted to progesterone (Figure 2). A key enzyme complex, Δ^5-3β-hydroxysteroid dehydrogenase (3β-HSD)-isomerase, is responsible for this conversion. Then, progesterone is transformed to 17α-hydroxyprogesterone by the 17-hydroxylase enzyme. Another enzyme, 17,20-desmolase, acts on 17α-hydroxyprogesterone and converts it to a C-19 steroid called androstenedione. Androstenedione is a weak androgen.

In the Δ^5 pathway pregnenolone is converted to 17α-hydroxypregnenolone by the 17-hydroxylase enzyme (Figure 2). Desmolase enzyme transforms 17α-hydroxypregnenolone to a C-19 steroid hormone dehydroepiandrosterone (DHEA). In the next step of this pathway, DHEA is converted to androstenedione by a 3β-HSD-isomerase enzyme complex. Androstenedione formed in both the steroid pathways is converted to testosterone by 17α-hydroxysteroid dehydrogenase. DHEA may also be converted to androstenediol by the action of 17α-hydroxysteroid dehydrogenase. Androstenediol is transformed by 3β-HSD-isomerse to testosterone. Testosterone is the major androgen produced within the testis.

Small amounts of estrogens (C-18 steroids) are also produced by the testis. Estrogens are formed from androgens. An aromatase enzyme complex converts testosterone to estradiol-17β. Androstenedione is converted to estrone by the aromatase enzyme complex. Estrone is then transformed to estradiol-17β by 17α-hydroxysteroid dehydrogenase. Estriol, produced in large amounts by the stallion testis, is formed from estradiol-17β. Human and rat testes produce estradiol-17β.

The major enzymes that are responsible for the conversion of pregnenolone to testosterone are located in Leydig cells. However, some of these enzymes that are present in other testicular cells may also contribute to the biosynthesis of testosterone. Furthermore, in the rat, the aromatase enzyme complex is present in Sertoli cells,[4] suggesting that testosterone is converted to estrogen in Sertoli cells. Nevertheless, indirect evidence implies that the Leydig cells may also be a source of estrogen, but most of plasma estrogen comes from extratesticular transformation of nonestrogenic steroids.[5] Most recently, it has been shown that germ cells express aromatase activity in the mouse testis.[6]

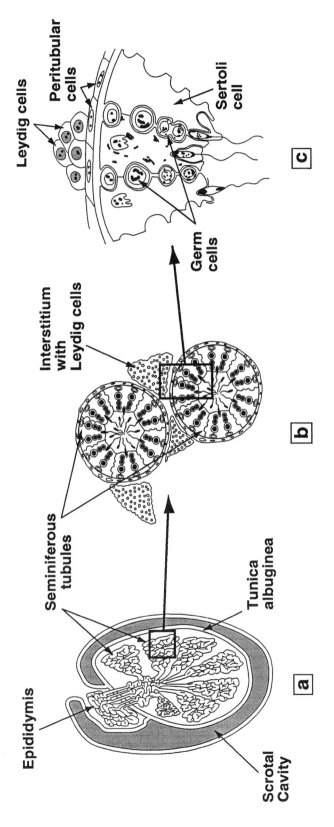

FIGURE 1. Diagrammatic representation of cellular architecture of the mammalian testis. (**a**) Arrangement of cellular architecture of the mammalian testis. (**a**) Arrangement of seminiferous tubules in the testis. (**b**) Cross-section of two seminiferous tubules. (**c**) Details of cell arrangement in the testis.

TABLE 1
Selected Sertoli Cell Factors

Factors	Function
Androgen binding proteins	Transport of androgens
Transferrin	Transport of iron
Ceruloplasmin	Transport of copper
Growth factors	
Transforming growth factor-α	Stimulation of growth
Transforming growth factor-β	Inhibition of growth
Insulin-like growth factor-I	Induction and maintenance of endocrine/paracrine effect
Interleukin-1	Stimulation of growth
Inhibin	Endocrine/paracrine effect
Lactate	Energy metabolite
Estrogen	Endocrine effect
Luteinizing hormone-releasing hormone	Endocrine/paracrine effect

TABLE 2
Selected Leydig Cell Factors with
Endocrine/Paracrine/Autocrine Function

Androgens
Proopiomelanocortin-derived peptides:
    β-Endorphin
    α-Melanophore-stimulating hormone
    Adrenocorticotropic hormone
Corticotropin-releasing hormone
Growth hormone-releasing hormone
Inhibin
Insulin-like growth factor-I

HORMONAL CONTROL OF SPERMATOGENESIS

It has been shown in gonadotropin-deficient men that treatment with luteinizing hormone (LH) or follicle-stimulating hormone (FSH) increases sperm production to some extent, but administration of FSH alone to men with normal secretion of LH leads to normal production of spermatozoa.[7] Because LH induces testosterone secretion, it can be inferred that in humans, FSH and testosterone are required for normal spermatogenesis.

Based on the extensive studies on the effect of hormones on spermatogenesis in hypophysectomized rats, it has been shown that testosterone and FSH are essential for the initiation of spermatogenesis and that testosterone is required for the maintenance of spermatogenesis.[8,9] Recent findings have confirmed that, in the absence of FSH, testosterone can maintain spermatogenesis in the rat.[10,11] However, in hypophysectomized adult rats, treatment with a recombinant FSH has been shown to maintain spermatogenesis and prevent germ cell degeneration, suggesting a role of FSH in sperm production.[12] It is known that hypophysectomy reduces more than 90% of intratesticular testosterone. Yet a small amount of testosterone is present within the testis. Therefore, this small quantity of testosterone may act with FSH to influence the process of spermatogenesis. Furthermore, a number of other hormones/factors are present in the mammalian testis, suggesting the concerted effect of different testicular factors in the process of spermatogenesis.[13,14] A detailed account of the hormonal effect on spermatogenesis is found elsewhere.[13,14]

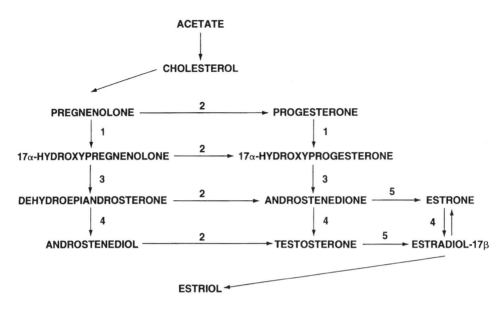

FIGURE 2. Essential steps in the biosynthesis of testosterone in the testis. Key enzymes involved in steroidogenesis are (1) 17α-hydroxylase; (2) Δ^5-3β-hydroxysteroid dehydrogenase-isomerase; (3) steroid C-17–20-desmolase; (4) 17β-hydroxysteroid dehydrogenase; and (5) aromatase enzyme complex.

HORMONAL CONTROL OF TESTICULAR FUNCTION

The major control of the testicular endocrine function is by the pituitary gland. LH, FSH, and prolactin secreted by the anterior lobe of the pituitary gland are responsible for the steroidogenic function of the testis. Results of the selected studies pertaining to Leydig cell function are discussed below.

It is well documented that LH modulates Leydig cell endocrine function. Hypophysectomy leads to a decrease in plasma testosterone levels and administration of LH restores testosterone secretion.[5] This and other evidence indicate that LH is the primary hormone that controls testosterone secretion by the testis.[5,15,16] However, FSH injections to immature hypophysectomized rats result in an increase in LH-stimulated androgen secretion by the Leydig cells,[17] and FSH treatment increases the number of LH receptors.[17] Administration of a highly purified FSH preparation to immature hypophysectomized rats increases testosterone secretion.[18] Because FSH binds to Sertoli cells but not to Leydig cells, it may be inferred that the stimulatory effect of FSH on Leydig cell function is mediated via Sertoli cells.[19]

Another pituitary hormone that influences steroidogenic capacity of the Leydig cells is prolactin. Naturally occurring increases in circulating levels of testosterone in men during sleep are preceded by elevations in plasma concentrations of prolactin.[20] Treatment of hypophysectomized rats with prolactin potentiates the effect of LH in testosterone production and increases the activity of 3β-HSD in rats[21] and 17α-hydroxysteroid dehydrogenase in mice,[22] and in adult male rats it increases testosterone secretion.[23,24] These studies indicate that prolactin influences testicular endocrine function. Furthermore, the ability of LH to induce testosterone secretion is attenuated in rats actively immunized against prolactin,[24] the presence of specific binding sites for prolactin on Leydig cells,[25] and the dependency of testicular LH receptor maintenance on prolactin,[26] strongly suggest that prolactin might be required for testosterone synthesis.

In seasonally breeding mammals, gonads become inactive during the nonreproductive period. This change is related to the duration of light exposure per day. Exposure of adult male Syrian golden hamsters to short photoperiods of less than 12 h of light per day results in a reduction of testicular weight associated with decreases in circulating levels of FSH, LH, and prolactin.[27,28] These photoperiod-related alterations also drastically decrease plasma testosterone levels, FSH, LH, and prolactin receptor contents.[29] It is known that exposure of hamsters to short photoperiod induces degeneration and a reduction in the number of Leydig cells in the testis.[30] It is suspected that the reduction in testosterone secretion following exposure to short photoperiod is due to the decreased circulating concentrations of gonado-tropins and prolactin, which in turn are related to alterations in hypothalamic function and impairment in the mechanism of gonadotropin-releasing hormone release.[31] It has been shown that prolonged treatment with prolactin via an ectopic pituitary transplant under the kidney capsule counteracts the effect of short photoperiod on testicular regression, in Syrian hamsters.[32] The plasma levels of 17α-hydroxyprogesterone, androstenedione, and testosterone are decreased after 12 weeks of exposure of adult golden hamsters to short photoperiod.[27] These data suggest decreases in the action or synthesis of 17α-steroid hydroxylase, C-17–20-desmolase, and 17β-hydroxysteroid dehydrogenase enzymes in the testis. However, plasma progesterone levels were unaffected by the short photoperiod, suggesting that the steroid-ogenic lesion occurs beyond the synthesis of progesterone.

It is also known that administration of FSH to another seasonal breeder, Djungarian (Siberian) hamsters, maintained on a short photoperiod resulted in increased testicular weight 7 days later, whereas LH treatment was ineffective in stimulating the weight of the testis.[33] These data suggest the importance of FSH in testicular function. Recently we have shown that the testosterone response to LH treatment in short photoperiod-exposed adult male Djungarian hamsters previously injected with FSH was increased, but not in prolactin-treated animals[34] (Figure 3). This indicates that FSH modulates LH action in testosterone secretion and that prolactin may have only a small role in the biosynthesis of androgen in this hamster. There is evidence demonstrating that growth hormone (GH) may have some influence on testicular endocrine function. In our laboratory we have evaluated the effects of GH on testicular function in adult transgenic mice expressing the hGH gene with the mouse metallothionein-I as a promoter, as well as in GH-deficient dwarf mice. We have found that adult male transgenic mice bearing the hGH gene are hypoprolactinemic.[35] Although the basal testosterone levels are similar in transgenic mice relative to the normal mice, administration of prolactin to transgenic mice resulted in increased testosterone response to the LH treatment (Figure 4), indicating a synergistic effect of hGH with exogenously administered prolactin in the biosynthesis of testosterone.[36] In Ames GH-deficient male dwarf mice, the testosterone response to the increased secretion of LH by exogenously administered luteinizing hormone-releasing hormone (LHRH) was attenuated.[37] Furthermore, pretreatment of these mice with GH resulted in an increased secretion of androstenedione and testosterone by the isolated testis treated with human chorionic gonadotropin (hCG).[37] These data suggest that GH possibly plays a role in the biosynthesis of androgen.

In addition to the major role of the pituitary gland in the control of testicular function, there are a number of *in vitro* studies suggesting a close interrelationship between Leydig, peritubular myoid, and Sertoli cells with regard to androgen secretion. This concept of para-crine influence of testicular function is still in its infancy. In addition to gonadotropins, prolactin, and steroids, there are reports suggesting that a number of substances including gonadotropin-releasing hormone-associated peptide (GAP),[38] LHRH,[39] corticotropin-releasing factor (CRF),[40] growth hormone-releasing hormone (GHRH),[41] serotonin,[42] vasopressin as well as oxytocin,[43,44] proopiomelanocortin-derived peptides,[44,45] and a number of growth fac-tors, including insulin-like growth factor I (IGF-I),[1] interleukin-1,[1] inhibin,[1,46] and atrial natri-uretic factor (ANF),[47,48] are present in the testis. These substances may play a vital role in the biosynthesis of testosterone. The cell origin and possible influence of these substances on testicular endocrine function will be discussed in the following sections.

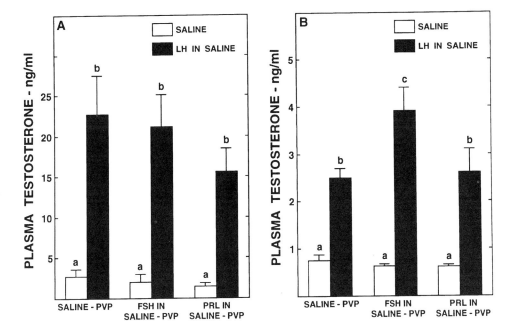

FIGURE 3.   Plasma testosterone levels in adult male Djungarian hamsters exposed to either a long photoperiod (**A**) or a short photoperiod (**B**) for 12 weeks. These animals were previously injected with the vehicle (SAL-PVP = 50% polyvinylpyrrolidone in saline), FSH, or prolactin (PRL) for 7 days. On day 8 these hamsters were treated with either saline or LH. Vertical lines represent the SEM. Values with different letters are at a significance level of at least $p < .05$. Note that values on the Y axis are different in panels **A** and **B**. (From Chandrashekar, V., Majumdar, S. S., and Bartke, A., *Biol. Reprod.,* 50, 82, 1994. With permission.)

FACTORS SECRETED BY THE TESTIS

SERTOLI CELL PRODUCTS

Sertoli cells secrete more than 80 peptides/proteins and their production is regulated by FSH. It has been shown that the number of FSH receptors on the Sertoli cells are highest at stages XII to II and the number of these receptors is low in stages VI to VII.[49,50] Therefore, the effects of FSH may vary at different regions of the seminiferous epithelium depending on the stage of spermatogenesis.

The most extensively studied Sertoli cell protein is the androgen-binding protein (ABP). It is believed that the major functions of this protein are: (1) testosterone transportation within Sertoli cells, (2) maintenance of high levels of testosterone in seminiferous tubules and epididymis, and (3) transport of testosterone from testes to epididymis.[1]

Sertoli cells secrete transferrin and ceruloplasmin for the transportation of iron and copper to germ cells.[1] It is suggested that transferrin plays an important role in germ cell growth. A number of growth factors are present in the testis. Transforming growth factors (TGF-α and TGF-β) are secreted by both the Sertoli and peritubular cells.[1,51] These growth factors play an important role in the growth of testicular cells. Another well-recognized and studied growth factor, somatomedin C (IGF-I), has been identified in cultured Sertoli cells[1] and has been shown to be produced by peritubular, Sertoli, and Leydig cells.[1,51]

The hormone inhibin is secreted by Sertoli cells. Ovarian granulosa cells also produce a similar peptide called "folliculostatin." Inhibin of testicular and ovarian origin is capable of suppressing FSH, but not LH.[46] It has been demonstrated that Sertoli cells produce an LHRH-like substance.[39,52]

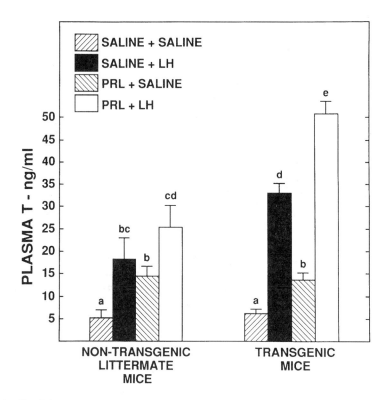

FIGURE 4. Circulating testosterone (T) levels in adult male transgenic mice expressing the hGH gene and in nontransgenic mice treated with saline-PVP (50% polyvinylpyrrolidone in saline) or prolactin (PRL) in saline-PVP and injected with saline or LH. Vertical lines represent the SEM. Values with different letters are at a significance level of at least $p < .05$. (From Chandrashekar, V., Bartke, A., and Wagner T. E., *Biol. Reprod.*, 44, 135, 1991. With permission.)

The paracrine influence of these Sertoli cell factors will be discussed in the section "Sertoli Cell-Leydig Cell Interactions."

Although Leydig cells are the major source of steroid synthesis in the testis, Sertoli cells have the capability of synthesizing steroids. Sertoli cells isolated from prepubertal animals produce estrogen.[53] However, adult Sertoli cells are less capable of producing estrogen, but during development, the estrogen produced by these cells acts on Leydig cells and inhibits androgen synthesis.[54] *In vitro* studies have shown that the Sertoli cells from adult rats can convert progesterone to testosterone, androstenedione, and 3-α-hydroxy-5-α-androstan-17-one.[55] These conversions are stimulated by FSH. Sertoli cells have FSH receptors but Leydig cells are devoid of these receptors. Therefore, it can be assumed that Sertoli cells have the potential to synthesize steroids under the influence of FSH. This is corroborated by the findings that administration of a highly purified FSH preparation increases testosterone secretion in immature hypophysectomized rats.[18] However, it should be noted that administration of an FSH antiserum to rats failed to affect plasma testosterone levels.[56] The action of FSH is mediated by the adenylate cyclase-protein kinase system and FSH increases RNA and protein synthesis in Sertoli cells.[4]

The receptors for β-endorphin are present on Sertoli cells.[57] In studies utilizing opiate antagonists, it has been shown that opiates inhibit Sertoli cell function.[58] However, β-endorphin and adrenocorticotropic hormone (ACTH)-like factors are located in the cytoplasm of Leydig cells.[59] This suggests that these peptides are produced in Leydig cells and have autocrine and paracrine functions in the testis. We have shown that β-endorphin modulates androgen secretion in rats[60] (Figure 5).

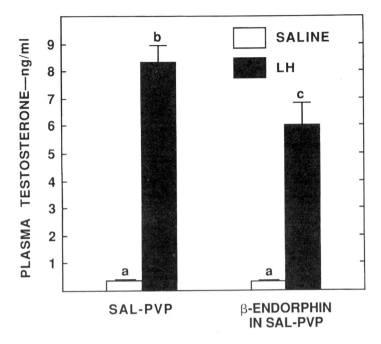

FIGURE 5. Effect of intratesticular injections of saline-polyvinylpyrrolidone (SAL-PVP) or β-endorphin in SAL-PVP on plasma testosterone levels in hypophysectomized rats treated with saline or LH. Vertical lines represent SEM. Different letters indicate significantly different values (at least $p < .05$). (From Chandrashekar, V. and Bartke, A., *Biol. Reprod.*, 47, 1, 1992. With permission.)

Because insulin is essential for the growth of Sertoli cells and IGF-I has been shown to induce DNA and/or protein synthesis in Sertoli cells, it is conceivable that insulin and IGF-I may play a vital role in Sertoli cell function.[61]

A number of steroids influence Sertoli cell function. It has been demonstrated that these cells bear testosterone and estrogen receptors.[62] Androgens regulate the number of FSH receptors on Sertoli cells. It is also known that testosterone and FSH function synergistically to stimulate the synthesis of FSH receptor.[63] However, testosterone suppresses the estrogen receptors on Sertoli cells,[62] suggesting that androgens may control estrogen receptors of these tubular cells. The major effects of FSH on the Sertoli cell function are mimicked by testosterone. Other steroids such as cortisol and progesterone can increase ABP concentrations in cultured Sertoli cells. Ingestion of a vitamin A-free diet causes loss of all germinal elements except spermatogonia, and deficiency of this vitamin also affects the Sertoli cell function in rats,[64] suggesting the importance of this vitamin in male reproduction.

PERITUBULAR MYOID CELL SECRETIONS

In addition to the secretion of IGF-I, epidermal growth factor (EGF)-like growth factor, TGF-α and TGF-β, peritubular myoid cells also produce a nonmitogenic factor termed PMods that controls the Sertoli cell differentiation and function.[51] The myoid cells influence the production of ABP[51] and transferrin[51] by the Sertoli cells. Because Sertoli cells influence the Leydig cell endocrine function, it is tempting to speculate that the peritubular cell secretions indirectly influence the testosterone secretion by the testis.

LEYDIG CELL SECRETIONS

Although testosterone is the major steroid produced by the Leydig cells, they can also synthesize and secrete a number of other steroids. The Leydig cells also produce proopiomelanocortin-derived peptides such as β-endorphin, ACTH, and α-melanophore-stimulating hormone (α-MSH).[45,59] Inhibin and IGF-I are secreted by both Sertoli and Leydig cells of the testis.[1,51] Recent studies have shown that Leydig cell produce CRF[40] and GHRH.[41] The role of these Leydig cell substances in steroidogenesis will be discussed in the following section.

SERTOLI CELL-LEYDIG CELL INTERACTIONS

Although it is known that pituitary gonadotropins and intratesticular steroids regulate Sertoli cell and Leydig cell functions, the following studies have suggested the paracrine effect of nonsteroidal testicular substances on Leydig cell steroidogenesis. Most studies pertaining to the Sertoli cell-Leydig cell interactions are done under *in vitro* conditions.

Since the observations of Aoki and Fawcett[65] showing the disruption of spermatogenesis at the site of intratesticular Silastic implants containing antispermatic agents and the hypertrophy of the Leydig cells around the tubules with disrupted spermatogenesis in the rat, a number of *in vitro* studies have been undertaken. It was shown that FSH increases Leydig cell testosterone secretion in "crude" porcine Leydig cell preparation but has no effect on purified Leydig cells in culture.[66] They also showed that FSH stimulates the activity of the Leydig cells cocultured with Sertoli cells, whereas the purified Leydig cells fail to respond to FSH stimulation. This suggests that the effect of FSH on Leydig cell steroidogenesis is mediated by Sertoli cell secretion(s). Similarly, rat Leydig cells cocultured with seminiferous tubules or with Sertoli cells enhanced both basal and LH-stimulated testosterone secretion and aromatase activity of Leydig cells.[67] These studies clearly suggest that a factor(s) secreted by the Sertoli cells influences Leydig cell function. A protein that is immunologically different from LH has been isolated from Sertoli cell-enriched culture medium that stimulates Leydig cell steroidogenesis.[68] This Sertoli cell substance seems to be different from the macromolecular factor present in the rat interstitial fluid.[69] This substance is not yet available to test its effects *in vivo*.

The hormone called inhibin is produced mainly by Sertoli cells,[1] but Leydig cells may also secrete this hormone.[70] Inhibin increases LH-induced testosterone secretion *in vitro*.[71]

Sertoli cells also secrete an LHRH-like substance and LHRH receptors are exclusively present on the Leydig cells.[39,72] There is a controversy with regard to the steroidogenic effect of LHRH. This peptide may have no effect on androgen secretion. However, a limited number of studies in the rat indicate that LHRH stimulates testosterone secretion.[39,52]

Some studies have shown that TGF-β secreted by Sertoli cells inhibits Leydig cell steroidogenesis *in vitro*.[73,74] However, IGF-I secreted by Sertoli and Leydig cells stimulates testosterone secretion in culture, and both these cell types bear IGF-I receptors.[75] In experimental animals, GH deficiency affects the onset of puberty and subnormal testosterone response to hCG treatment.[76] Because GH effects are mediated via IGF-I, it is possible that IGF-I may influence the Leydig cell function.

In addition to its immunological function, interleukin-1 inhibits steroid secretion by cultured Leydig cells.[77] Interleukin-1 is present in the testis and it is believed that it is secreted by Sertoli cells.[78]

Like Sertoli cells, Leydig cells also produce a number of other nonsteroidal substances. Leydig cells secrete proopiomelanocortin-derived peptides and influence testosterone secretion. For example, β-endorphin suppresses testosterone secretion *in vitro*,[79] and the testosterone response to LH treatment is attenuated in rats pretreated with β-endorphin. However, Sharpe and Cooper[44] have suggested that opiates are not involved in the paracrine control of the Leydig cell function. Corticotropin-releasing hormone is believed to be secreted by the Leydig cells and it inhibits testosterone secretion.[40] Infusions of two catecholamines, epinephrine and norepinephrine, also inhibit testosterone secretion.[80] Oxytocin is another intratesticular substance produced by the Leydig cells.[81] Oxytocin has been shown to inhibit testosterone secretion in culture.[82] Although the origin of testicular vasopressin-like peptide is unknown,[83] it stimulates testosterone secretion in purified Leydig cell culture.[44] The ANF gene is expressed in the rat testis[48] and Leydig cells contain receptors for ANF. ANF has been shown to increase steroidogenesis by the mouse Leydig cells *in vitro*.[47] The origin of this factor is not known.

It is imperative to keep in mind that most of the results discussed in this chapter are obtained from *in vitro* studies. Therefore, it is not clear whether the *in vitro* effects of intratesticular factors also occur *in vivo*. Due to a number of different types of cells present within the testis, it is difficult to assess the role of a particular factor on the function of a single type of cell *in vivo*. However, selective destruction of cells by chemical means or by neutralizing the effect of a particular factor by specific antibodies may indicate whether these intratesticular factors have any specific effect on steroidogenic function of the Leydig cells.

ACKNOWLEDGMENT

Investigations in our laboratory were supported by NIH grant HD-20033.

REFERENCES

1. **Skinner, M. K.,** Cell-cell interactions in the testis, *Endocr. Rev.*, 12, 45, 1991.
2. **Yanaihara, T. and Troen, P.,** Studies of the human testis. I. Biosynthetic pathways for androgen formation in human tissue in vitro, *J. Clin. Endocrinol. Metab.*, 34, 783, 1972.
3. **Samuels, L. T., Bussman L., Matsumoto K., and Huseby, R. A.,** Organization of androgen biosynthesis in the testis, *J. Steroid Biochem.*, 6, 292, 1975.
4. **Dorrington, J. H., Roller, N. F., and Fritz, I. B.,** Effects of follicle-stimulating hormone on cultures of Sertoli cell preparations, *Mol. Cell. Endocrinol.*, 3, 70, 1975.
5. **Hall, P. F.,** Testicular steroid synthesis, organization and regulation, in *The Physiology of Reproduction,* Knobil, E. and Neill, J. D., Eds., Raven Press, New York, 1988, 975.
6. **Nitta, H., Bunick, D., Hess, R.A., Janulis, L., Newton, S. C., Millette, C. F., Osawa, Y., Shizuta, Y., Toda, K., and Bahr, J. M.,** Germ cells of the mouse testis express P450 aromatase, *Endocrinology,* 132, 1396, 1993.
7. **Matsumoto, A. M.,** Hormonal control of spermatogenesis, in *The Testis,* 2nd ed., Burger H. and deKretser, D. M., Eds., Raven Press, New York, 1989, 181.
8. **Steinberger E.,** Hormonal control of mammalian spermatogenesis, *Physiol. Rev.*, 51, 1, 1971.
9. **Zirkin, B. R., Santulli, R., Awoniyi, C. A., and Ewing, L. L.,** Maintenance of advanced spermatogenic cells in the adult rat testis: quantitative relationship to testosterone concentration within the testis, *Endocrinology,* 124, 3043, 1989.
10. **Awoniyi, C. A., Sprando, R. L., Santulli, R., Chandrashekar, V., Ewing, L. L., and Zirkin, B. R.,** Restoration of spermatogenesis by exogenously administered testosterone in rats made azoospermic by hypophysectomy or withdrawal of luteinizing hormone alone, *Endocrinology,* 127, 177, 1990.
11. **McLachlan, R. I., Wreford, N. G., Tsonis, C., de Kretser, D. M., and Robertson, D. M.,** Testosterone effects on spermatogenesis in the gonadotropin-releasing hormone-immunized rat, *Biol. Reprod.*, 50, 271, 1994.
12. **Russell, L. D., Corbin, T. J., Borg, K. E., De Franca, L. R., Grasso, P., and Bartke, A.,** Recombinant human follicle-stimulating hormone is capable of exerting a biological effect in the adult hypophysectomized rat by reducing the numbers of degenerating germ cells, *Endocrinology,* 133, 2062, 1993.
13. **Spiteri-Grech, J. and Nieschlag, E.,** Paracrine factors relevant to the regulation of spermatogenesis—a review, *J. Reprod. Fertil.*, 98, 1, 1993.
14. **Weinbauer, G. F. and Nieschlag, E.,** Hormonal control of spermatogenesis, in *Molecular Biology of the Male Reproductive System,* de Kretser, D., Ed., Academic Press, New York, 1993, 99.
15. **Dufau, M. L., Veldhuis, J., Fraioli, F., Johnson, M. H., and Catt, K. J.,** Mode of bioactive LH secretion in man, *J. Clin. Endocrinol. Metab.*, 57, 993, 1983.
16. **Hall, P. F. and Eik-Nes, K. B.,** The influence of gonadotropins in vivo upon the biosynthesis of androgens by homogenate of rat testis, *Biochim. Biophys. Acta*, 71, 438, 1963.
17. **Chen, Y. D., Payne, A. H., and Kelch, K. P.,** FSH stimulation of Leydig cell function in the hypophysectomized immature rat, *Proc. Soc. Exp. Biol. Med.*, 153, 473, 1976.

18. **Grimek, H. J., Nuti, L. S., Nuti, K. M., and McShan, W. H.,** Effect of neuraminidase treatment on the biological activity of highly purified ovine FSH and LH in hypophysectomized immature male rat, *Endocrinology*, 98, 105, 1976.

19. **de Kretser, D. M. and Kerr, J. B.,** The cytology of the testis, in *The Physiology of Reproduction,* Knobil, E. and Neill, J. D., Eds., Raven Press, New York, 1994, 1177.

20. **Rubin, R. T., Poland, R. E., and Tower, B. B.,** Prolactin-related testosterone secretion in normal adult men, *J. Clin. Endocrinol. Metab.*, 42, 112, 1976.

21. **Hafiez, A. A., Philpott, J. E., and Bartke, A.,** The role of prolactin in the regulation of testicular function: the effect of prolactin and luteinizing hormone on 3β-hydroxysteroid dehydrogenase activity in the testes of mice and rats, *J. Endocrinol.*, 50, 619, 1972.

22. **Musto, N., Hafiez, A. A., and Bartke, A.,** Prolactin increases 17α-hydroxysteroid dehydrogenase activity in the testis, *Endocrinology*, 91, 1106, 1972.

23. **Belanger, A., Auclair, C., Seguin, C., Caron, S., and Labrie, F.,** Prolactin stimulation of testicular steroid biosynthesis in the male rat, *J. Androl.*, 2, 80, 1981.

24. **Chandrashekar, V. and Bartke, A.,** Influence of endogenous prolactin on the luteinizing hormone stimulation of testicular steroidogenesis and the role of prolactin in adult male rats, *Steroids*, 51, 559, 1988.

25. **Aragona, C., Bohnet, H. G., and Friesen, H. G.,** Localization of prolactin binding in prostate and testis, *Acta Endocrinol.*, 84, 402, 1977.

26. **Zipf, W. B., Payne, A. H., and Kelch, R. P.,** Prolactin, growth hormone and luteinizing hormone in the maintenance of testicular luteinizing hormone receptors, *Endocrinology*, 103, 595, 1978.

27. **Chandrashekar, V. and Bartke, A.,** The influence of short photoperiod on testicular and circulating levels of testosterone precursors in the adult golden hamster, *Biol. Reprod.*, 40, 300, 1989.

28. **Turek, F. W., Elliott, J. A., Alvis, J. D., and Menaker, M.,** Effect of prolonged exposure to nonstimulatory photoperiods on the activity of the neuroendocrine-testicular axis of golden hamsters, *Biol. Reprod.*, 13, 475, 1975.

29. **Bartke, A. and Dalterio, S.,** Effects of prolactin on the sensitivity of the testis to LH, *Biol. Reprod.*, 15, 90, 1976.

30. **Hardy, M. P., Mandis-Handagama, S. M. L. C., Zirkin, B. R., and Ewing, L. L.,** Photoperiodic variation of Leydig cell numbers in the testis of the golden hamster: a possible mechanism for their renewal during recrudescence, *J. Exp. Zool.*, 244, 269, 1987.

31. **Steger, R. W., Bartke, A., and Goldman, B. D.,** Alterations in neuroendocrine function during photoperiod induced testicular atrophy and recrudescence in the golden hamster, *Biol. Reprod.*, 26, 437, 1982.

32. **Bartke, A., Smith, M. S., and Delterio, S.,** Reversal of short photoperiod-induced sterility in male hamsters by ectopic pituitary homografts, *Int. J. Androl.*, 2, 257, 1979.

33. **Milette, J. J., Schwartz, N. B., and Turek, F. W.,** The importance of follicle stimulating hormone in the testicular growth in photostimulated Djungarian hamsters, *Endocrinology*, 122, 1060, 1988.

34. **Chandrashekar, V., Majumdar, S. S., and Bartke, A.,** Assessment of the role of follicle-stimulating hormone and prolactin in the control of testicular endocrine function in adult Djungarian hamsters (Phodopus sungorus) exposed to either short or long photoperiod, *Biol. Reprod.*, 50, 82, 1994.

35. **Chandrashekar, V., Bartke, A., and Wagner, T. E.,** Endogenous human growth hormone (GH) modulates the effect of gonadotropin-releasing hormone on pituitary function and the gonadotropin response to the negative feedback effect of testosterone in adult male transgenic mice bearing human GH gene, *Endocrinology*, 123, 2717, 1988.

36. **Chandrashekar, V., Bartke, A., and Wagner, T. E.,** Interactions of human growth hormone and prolactin on pituitary and Leydig cell function in adult transgenic mice expressing the human growth hormone gene, *Biol. Reprod.*, 44, 135, 1991.

37. **Chandrashekar, V. and Bartke, A.,** Induction of endogenous insulin-like growth factor-I secretion alters the hypothalamic-pituitary-testicular function in growth hormone-deficient adult dwarf mice, *Biol. Reprod.*, 48, 544, 1993.

38. **Seeburg, P. H., Mason, A. J., Stewart, T. A., and Nikolics, K.,** The mammalian GnRH gene and its pivotal role in reproduction, *Recent Prog. Horm. Res.*, 43, 69, 1987.

39. **Sharpe, R. M.,** Intratesticular factors controlling testicular function, *Biol. Reprod.*, 30, 29, 1984.

40. **Fabbri, A., Tinajero, J. C., and Dufau, M. L.,** Corticotropin-releasing factor is produced by rat Leydig cells and has a major local antireproductive role in the testis, *Endocrinology*, 127, 1541, 1990.

41. **Ciampani, T., Fabbri, A., Isidori, A., and Dufau, M. L.,** Growth hormone-releasing hormone is produced by rat Leydig cell in culture and acts as a positive regulator of Leydig cell function, *Endocrinology*, 131, 2785, 1992.

42. **Tinajero, J. C., Fabbri, A., Ciocca, D. R., and Dufau, M. L.,** Serotonin secretion from rat Leydig cells, *Endocrinology*, 133, 3026, 1993.

43. **Adashi, E. Y. and Hsueh, A. J. W.,** Direct inhibition of testicular androgen biosynthesis revealing antigonadal activity of neurohypophysial hormones, *Nature*, 293, 650, 1981.

44. **Sharpe, R. M. and Cooper, I.,** Comparison of the effects on purified Leydig cells of four hormones (oxytocin, vasopressin, opiates and LHRH) with suggested paracrine roles in the testis, *J. Endocrinol.*, 113, 89, 1987.

45. **Valenca, M. M. and Negro-Vilar, A.,** Proopiomelanocortin-derived peptides in testicular interstitial fluid: characterization and changes in secretion after human chorionic gonadotropin or luteinizing hormone-releasing hormone analog treatment, *Endocrinology*, 118, 32, 1986.

46. **Grady, R. R., Charlesworth, M. C., and Schwartz, N. B.,** Characterization of the FSH-suppressing activity in follicular fluid, *Recent Prog. Horm. Res.*, 38, 409, 1982.

47. **Mukhopadhyay, A. K., Schumacher, M., and Leidenberger, F. A.,** Steroidogenic effect of atrial natriuretic factor in isolated mouse Leydig cells is mediated by cyclic GMP, *Biochem. J.*, 239, 463, 1986.

48. **Vollmar, A. M., Friedrich, A., and Schulz, R.,** Atrial natriuretic peptide material in rat testis, *J. Androl.*, 11, 471, 1988.

49. **Kangasniemi, M., Kaipia, A., Toppari, J., Perheentupa, A., Huhtaniemi, I., and Parvinen, M.,** Cellular regulation of follicle-stimulating hormone (FSH) binding in rat seminiferous tubules, *J. Androl.*, 11, 336, 1990.

50. **Kangasniemi, M., Kaipia, A., Mali, P., Toppari, J., Huhtaniemi, I., and Parvinen, M.,** Modulation of basal and FSH-dependent cyclic AMP production in rat seminiferous tubules staged by an improved transillumination technique, *Anat. Rec.*, 227, 62, 1990.

51. **Skinner M. K.,** Sertoli cell-peritubular myoid cell interactions, in *The Sertoli Cell,* Russell, L. D. and Griswald, M. D., Eds., Cache River Press, Clearwater, FL, 1993, 478.

52. **Sharpe, R. M. and Cooper, I.,** The mode of action of LHRH agonists on the rat Leydig cell, *Mol. Cell. Endocrinol.*, 27, 199, 1982.

53. **Dorrington, J. H., Fritz, I. B., and Armstrong, D. T.,** Site at which follicle stimulating hormone regulates estradiol-17-beta biosynthesis in Sertoli cell preparations in culture, *Mol. Cell. Endocrinol.*, 6, 117, 1976.

54. **Chen, Y. D., Shaw, M. S., and Payne, A. H.,** Steroid and FSH action on LH receptors and LH-sensitive testicular responsiveness during sexual maturation of the rat, *Mol. Cell. Endocrinol.*, 8, 291, 1977.

55. **Tcholakian, R. K. and Steinberger, A.,** In vitro metabolism of testosterone by cultured Sertoli cell and the effect of FSH, *Steroids*, 33, 495, 1979.

56. **Madhwa Raj, H. G. and Dym M.,** The effects of selective withdrawal of FSH or LH on spermatogenesis in the immature rat, *Biol. Reprod.*, 14, 489, 1976.

57. **Fabbri, A., Tsai-Morris, C. H., Luna, S., Fraioli, F., and Dufu, M. L.,** Opiate receptors are present in the rat testis. Identification and localization in Sertoli cells, *Endocrinology*, 117, 2544, 1985.

58. **Chen, C. L. C., Margioris, A. N., Liotta, A. S., Morris, P. L., Boitani, C., Mather, J. P., Krieger, D. T., and Bardin, C. W.,** Pro-opiomelanocortin-derived peptides of Leydig cell origin may be modulators of testicular function, in *Gonadal Protein and Peptides and Their Biological Significance,* Sairam, M. R. and Atkinson, L. E., Eds., World Scientific, Philadelphia, PA, 1984, 339.

59. **Tsong, S. D., Phillips, D. M., Bardin, C. W., Halmi, N., Liotta, A. J., Margioris, A., and Krieger, D. T.,** ACTH and beta-endorphin-related peptides are present in multiple sites in the reproductive tract of the male rat, *Endocrinology*, 110, 2204, 1982.

60. **Chandrashekar, V. and Bartke, A.,** The influence of β-endorphin on testicular endocrine function in adult rats, *Biol. Reprod.*, 47, 1, 1992.

61. **Mita, M., Borland, K., Price, J. M., and Hall, P. F.,** The influence of insulin and insulin-like growth factor-I on hexose transport by Sertoli cells, *Endocrinology*, 116, 987, 1985.

62. **Nakhla, A. M., Mather, J. P., Janne, P. A., and Bardin, C. W.,** Estrogen and androgen receptors in Sertoli, Leydig, myoid, and epithelial cells: effects of time in culture and cell density, *Endocrinology*, 115, 121, 1984.

63. **Tsutsui, K. and Ishii, S.,** Hormonal regulation of follicle-stimulating hormone receptors in the testes of Japanese quail, *J. Endocrinol.*, 85, 511, 1980.

64. **Rich, K. A. and de Kretser, D. M.,** Effect of differing degrees of destruction of the rat seminiferous epithelium on levels of serum follicle stimulating hormone and androgen binding protein, *Endocrinology*, 101, 959, 1977.

65. **Aoki, A. and Fawcett, D. W.,** Is there a local feedback from the seminiferous tubules affecting activity of the Leydig cells? *Biol. Reprod.*, 19, 144, 1978.

66. **Benahamed, M., Reventos, J., Tabone, E., and Saez, J. M.,** Cultured Sertoli cell-mediated FSH stimulatory effect on Leydig cell steroidogenesis, *Am. J. Physiol.*, 248, E176, 1985.

67. **Carreau, S., Papadopoulos, V., and Drosdowsky, M. A.,** Stimulation of adult rat Leydig cell aromatase activity by a Sertoli cell factor, *Endocrinology*, 122, 1103, 1988.

68. **Cheng, C. Y., Zwain, I., and Bardin, C. W.,** Purification of a biological factor from Sertoli cell-enriched culture medium that stimulates Leydig cell steroidogenesis, 72nd Endocrine Society Annual Meeting, Atlanta, GA, 1990, abstr. #1347.

69. **Hedger, M. P., Robertson, D. M., de Kretser, D. M., and Risbridger, G. P.,** The quantification of steroidogenesis-stimulating activity of testicular interstitial fluid by an in vitro bioassay employing adult rat Leydig cells, *Endocrinology*, 127, 1967, 1990.

70. **Risbridger, G. P., Clements, J., Robertson, D. M., Drummond, A. E., Muir, J., Berger, H. G., and de Kretser, D. M.,** Immuno- and bioactive inhibin and inhibin alpha subunit expression in rat Leydig cell cultures, *Mol. Cell. Endocrinol.*, 66, 119, 1989.

71. **Hsueh, A. J. W., Dahl, K. D., Vaughan, J., Tucker, E., Rivier, J., Bardin, C. W., and Vale, W.,** Heterodimers and homodimers of inhibin subunits have different paracrine action in the modulation of LH-stimulated androgen biosynthesis, *Proc. Natl. Acad. Sci. U.S.A.,* 84, 5082, 1987.

72. **Sharpe, R. M., Doogan, D. G., and Cooper, I.,** Factors determining whether the direct effects of an LHRH agonist on Leydig cell function in vivo are stimulatory or inhibitory, *Mol. Cell. Endocrinol.*, 32, 57, 1983.

73. **Sharpe, R. M.,** Intratesticular control of steroidogenesis, *Clin. Endocrinol.*, 33, 787, 1990.

74. **Lin, T., Blaisdell, J., and Haskell, J.,** Transforming growth factor-beta inhibits Leydig cell steroidogenesis in primary culture, *Biochem. Biophys. Res. Commun.*, 146, 387, 1987.

75. **Lin, T., Haskell, J., Vison, N., and Terracio, L.,** Direct stimulatory effects of IGF-I on Leydig cell steroidogenesis in primary culture, *Biochem. Biophys. Res. Commun.*, 137, 950, 1986.

76. **de Reviers, H. M. T., de Reviers, M. M., Monet-Kuntz, C., Perreau, C., Fontaine, I., and Viguier-Martinez, C.,** Testicular growth and hormonal parameters in the male Snell dwarf mouse, *Acta Endocrinol.*, 115, 399, 1987.

77. **Hales, D. B.,** Interleukin-1 inhibits Leydig cell steroidogenesis primarily by decreasing 17-alpha-hydroxylase/C17-20 lyase cytochrome P450 expression, *Endocrinology*, 131, 2165, 1992.

78. **Syed, V., Soder, O., Arver, S., Lindh, M., Khan, S., and Ritzen, E. M.,** Ontogeny and cellular origin of an interleukin-1-like factor in the reproductive tract of male rats, *Int. J. Androl.*, 11, 437, 1988.

79. **Knotts, L. K. and Glass, J. D.,** Effects of photoperiod, beta-endorphin, and naloxone on in vitro secretion of testosterone in white-footed mouse (Peromyscus leucopus) testes, *Biol. Reprod.*, 39, 205, 1988.

80. **Damber, J. E. and Janson, P. O.,** The effects of LH, adrenaline and noradrenaline on testicular blood flow and plasma testosterone concentration in anaesthetized rats, *Acta Endocrinol.*, 88, 390, 1978.

81. **Guldenaar, S. E. F. and Pickering, B. T.,** Immunochemical evidence for the presence of oxytocin in rat testis, *Cell Tissue Res.*, 240, 485, 1985.

82. **Adashi, E. Y., Tucker, E. M., and Hsueh, A. J. W.,** Direct regulation of rat testicular steroidogenesis by neurohypophysial hormones, *J. Biol. Chem.*, 259, 5440, 1984.

83. **Kasson, B. G. and Hsueh, A. J. W.,** Arginine vasopressin as an intragonadal hormone in brattleboro rats: presence of a testicular vasopressin-like peptide and functional vasopression receptor, *Endocrinology*, 118, 23, 1986.

Chapter 13

ENDOCRINOLOGY IN THE AGED

Raj Purushothaman and John E. Morley

CONTENTS

INTRODUCTION

The population of the world is rapidly aging. In 1990 12.4% of the U.S. population was over 65 years old and this is expected to rise to 21.2% by the year 2030. This increase in older persons is occurring not only in developed nations, but also in the developing nations of the world. By the end of the century, it is predicted that India and China will have more than 270 million persons over the age of 60. The most long-lived population in the world is the Japanese, with an average life expectancy of 76 years for males and nearly 82 years for females (Figure 1). Life expectancy in the United States is 72.1 years for males and 78.9 years for females. At present the state with the most long-lived population is Hawaii.

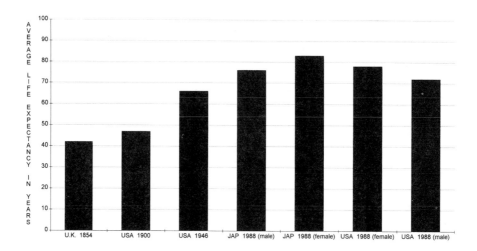

FIGURE 1. Graph showing average life expectancies since the middle of the last century. JAP = Japan.

As one gets older there is a blurring of distinction between health and the disease process. This is particularly true when one considers endocrine disorders, where the age-related decline in glandular function is often difficult to distinguish from the classical endocrine disease seen in younger individuals. Table 1 shows the effects of aging on endocrine disorders.

TABLE 1
Effects of Aging on Endocrine Disorders

1. Aging may mimic endocrine deficiency.
2. Leads to altered normal ranges.
3. Decreased functional reserve of endocrine organs.
4. Decreased receptor and postreceptor responsiveness.
5. Decreased T suppressor lymphocytes and associated increase in circulating antibodies.
6. Increasing age predisposes to have more than one endocrine disease.
7. Endocrine diseases present atypically, which can lead to missed diagnoses.
8. Increased prevalence of neoplasia and ectopic hormone production.

With advancing age, there are major alterations in hormone production, their action, and their metabolism. Whether these changes play a role in senescence is not yet established. The degree of age-related alteration in hormones is variable and, in part, age dependent. Changes in glucose hemostasis, sexual function, and bone metabolism are more apparent, compared to changes that occur in pituitary function and in thyroid hormone secretion. In older persons, nutritional status and coexisting disease need to be taken into consideration when one has to interpret endocrine tests.

With advancing age, there is a decrease in T suppresser lymphocytes and an increase in circulating antibodies. As a result, there is an increased propensity to develop autoimmune disease with aging. A study in centenarians has suggested that failure to develop high titers of antimicrosomal antibodies with aging may be a marker for longevity.

Increasing age also predisposes the elderly to have more than one endocrine disease.[1] There are also changes in the response at receptor and postreceptor levels, which can result in atypical presentations.[2] When endocrine diseases present atypically, this can lead to missed diagnoses or even to mismanagement.

It is not uncommon for certain changes to be attributed to aging, not to an endocrine disease, by both the patient and the physician. Some of the common presentations frequently missed in older persons are weight loss, fatigue, delirium, and depression. Table 2 lists the endocrine and metabolic causes of weight loss, depression, and dementia. Major diseases can alter basal and stimulated hormone levels. This is the case particularly for thyroid function tests in a severely ill patient.

TABLE 2
Endocrine and Metabolic Causes of Weight Loss,
Dementia, and Depression

	Endocrine Causes	Metabolic Causes
Weight Loss	Hyperthyroidism	
	Pheochromocytoma	
	Hyperparathyroidism	
	Diabetes mellitus	
Dementia	Hypothyroidism	Hypoxemia
	Diabetes mellitus	Electrolytic disturbance
	Hypoglycemia	Malnutrition
	Hypoparathyroidism	Hyperlipidemia
	Hyperparathyroidism	
	Hypoadrenalism	
Depression	Hypothyroidism	Malnutrition
	Diabetes mellitus	Pernicious anemia
	Cushing's disease	Hypokalemia
	Addison's disease	Folic acid deficiency
	Impotence	
	Apathetic thyrotoxicosis	

Malignant diseases can produce nonendocrine manifestations, due to ectopic hormone production. Ectopic adrenocorticotropic hormone (ACTH) is produced by small cell carcinoma of the lungs and a parathormone-like peptide is produced by squamous carcinoma of the lungs. Cancer occurs with increasing frequency in the elderly, and awareness of ectopic hormone production and its correct interpretation can lead to early detection of neoplasm. In addition, measurment of these hormone levels may result in the early detection of a recurrence of a cancer, an example being measurement of human chorionic gonadotrophic levels in testicular tumor. Ectopic production of bombesin or calcitonin due to lung cancer may lead to cancer anorexia.[3]

With increasing health awareness and use of health foods, changes secondary to ingestion of β-carotene (which causes yellow discoloration of the body, except the conjunctiva) could lead to a mistaken diagnosis of hypothyroidism in the elderly. Ginseng tea, a product which is claimed to improve health, energy, and vigor, causes hypertension. Elderly patients also often believe that arthritis can be cured by ingestion of cod liver oil capsules, which can lead to hypercalcemia and associated complications.

Salt and water balance is controlled mainly by arginine vasopressin (AVP). There is a relatively higher tendency for hypo- and hypernatremia in the older person, compared to the younger age group. There is a diminished response to thirst and osmotic changes in older persons.[4] In addition, older persons have impaired response to dehydration, which could be due to water deprivation or heat stress. Secondary to a rise in plasma osmolality, the sensitivity of AVP secretion is variably reported to increase with age[5] or be lower than in the young.[6-9] Basal levels of AVP are also variable in older persons, when compared to the young.[10] Due to a reduction both in the glomerular filtration rate and in the secretion rate of AVP, and possibly due to other urological problems, many older persons complain of polyuria and nocturia.[11] In younger persons there is normally an increase in nocturnal AVP levels, but this rise is not present in older subjects.[12] This explains nocturnal diuresis in middle aged and older persons. See Table 3 for posterior pituitary hormonal changes in the elderly.

TABLE 3
Posterior Pituitary Hormonal Changes in the Elderly

1. Relatively higher tendency for hyponatremia and hypernatremia.
2. Diminished response to thirst and osmotic changes.
3. Impaired response to dehydration.
4. Basal levels of AVP are variable, compared to young.
5. Decreased nocturnal AVP levels, which explains nocturnal diuresis in older persons.
6. Lower levels of AVP in patients with Alzheimer's disease.

Patients with Alzheimer's disease are at risk of developing dehydration during periods of water deprivation. In patients with Alzheimer's disease there are reduced cholinergic neurons in the central nervous system, and vasopressin is under direct cholinergic control. It has been demonstrated that there are lower levels of vasopressin in patients with Alzheimer's disease.[13] Following head injury, subdural hematoma, cerebellar tumor, chest infection, and meningitis, there is inappropriate secretion of AVP. Many drugs also cause an inappropriate secretion of AVP, resulting in hyponatremia. Other biochemical features of this syndrome include low blood urea nitrogen, low creatinine, decreased serum osmolality, and increased urinary osmolality. Careful consideration needs to be given in the treatment of hyponatremia, secondary to the syndrome of inappropriate secretion of ADH. Overzealous treatment could lead to neuroencephalopathy, with convulsions, coma, and eventual death.

In older persons, there is also an increase in the level of atrial natriuretic peptide, which can further alter water balance. In the young old (65–80), norepinephrine levels increase but epinephrine levels are unchanged. There is a decrease in β-adrenergic receptor responsiveness and a smaller decrease in receptor binding. In persons older than 80 years, there is an increase in epinephrine as well as norepinephrine levels. Table 4 lists the hormonal changes commonly present in older persons.

Although with aging there are major changes in the thyroxine (T_4) production rate and plasma clearance rate, these balance out, resulting in no change in serum T_4 levels. Serum triiodothyronine (T_3) levels decline slightly with age. This does not appear to be due to the euthyroid sick syndrome. Mooradian et al.[14] found an age-related decrease in the thyroid hormone responsiveness at both the mRNA level and the enzyme activity of hepatic cytosolic maleate dehydrogenase.

Diminished functional reserve of endocrine target organs can lead to the need for smaller replacement doses of hormones. For example, inappropriately high doses of T_4 in the elderly could precipitate angina or cardiac failure. Also in older persons, T_4 could accelerate the development of osteoporosis. Severe anorexia and weight loss are reported among elderly patients following treatment with calcitonin for Paget's disease.[15]

Multiple medication use is very common in older persons. Polypharmacy can have its own effects on hormone levels. Drugs such as rifampin and phenytoin increase metabolism of T_4, which results in a need for slightly higher replacement doses of T_4. Cimetidine, in addition to causing gynecomastia, has other antiandrogenic effects. Beta blockers prevent the conversion of T_4 to T_3 and in high doses act as a local anesthetic preventing entry of thyroid hormone into the cells. This can result in spurious elevation of T_4 and T_3 levels, leading to misdiagnosis of hyperthyroidism in older persons. Many cough mixtures contain iodine, which interfere with radioactive iodine uptake. High doses of vitamin C can interfere with the measurement of glucose in the blood. Theophylline causes weight loss, tachycardia, and tremors and may mimic the clinical signs of hyperthyroidism (Table 5).

TABLE 4
Hormonal Changes in Older Persons

Hormone	Effect
Pituitary hormones	
Growth hormone	Decreased
Prolactin	Mild increase
TSH (basal)	Normal
ACTH (basal)	Normal
Gonadotropins	
Males	Low LH
	High FSH
Females	Increased
Thyroid hormone	
Thyroxine	Normal
Triiodothyronine	Mild decrease
Sex hormone	
Males	Testosterone—normal or decreased
	Bioavailable testosterone or free testosterone—decreased
Females	Estradiol—unchanged
Adrenal hormones	
Cortisol	Normal
Aldosterone	Decreased
Norepinephrine	Increased
Epinephrine	Unchanged in young old
	Increased in old-old
Parathyroid hormone	
PTH	Increased
Calcitonin	Decreased
1,25(OH)2 vitamin D	Normal or decreased

TSH, thyroid-stimulating hormone; ACTH, adrenocorticotropic hormone; LH, luteinizing hormone; FSH, follicle-stimulating hormone; PTH, parathyroid hormone; "young old," 65–80 years; "old-old," older than 80.

TABLE 5
Drugs and Hormonal Effects in the Elderly

Drug	Effect of Aging
Rifampin	Increased metabolism of thyroid hormone
Phenytoin	Increased metabolism of thyroid hormone
Cimetidine	Antiandrogenic effect; gynecomastia
Beta blocker—normal dose	Affects conversion of T_4 to T_3
Beta blocker—high dose	Local anesthetic effect; prevents entry of thyroid hormone into the cells; causes hyperthyroxinemia
High-dose vitamin C	Interferes with serum glucose measurement
Theophylline	Causes weight loss, tachycardia, and tremors; may mimic hyperthyroidism
Cough mixtures	Iodine interferes with radioactive iodine uptake

Special care needs to be taken regarding compliance in the elderly. Memory problems associated with aging can result in poor compliance. Devices such as calendar pill boxes and clear, written instructions are often essential in obtaining appropriate compliance in older persons. Finally, the general principle of geriatric therapeutics should always be remembered: "start low and go slow."

THEORIES ON AGING

There are multiple theories concerning the factors responsible for the aging process. One theory suggests that aging is the result of environmental insults and the production of free radicals.[16] The chemical and physical alterations in biomolecules result in the formation of intermediate products, which increase free-radical availability. The response of T cells to free-radical damage depends on environmental and inherited factors. DNA repair is an effective way to protect against radiation damage, but other constitutive or inducible defense mechanisms can also modify biological response, and these processes generally become less effective with age. Ionizing radiation or other external stresses such as ultraviolet light, heat, chemotherapeutic agents, chemical carcinogens, and tumor promoters interact with nucleic acids, proteins, and membrane phospholipids, facilitating free-radical-mediated oxidation. The possibility that antioxidants may slow the aging process and reduce carcinogenesis and atherosclerosis is under intensive study at the present time. Clinical and epidemiological studies, to date, have suggested that the biochemical promises do not mean lives will be saved.

Singh and colleagues attempted to show the role played by DNA damage as a central theme to aging, but their results were contradictory.[17] Using novel techniques, they were able to obtain and directly measure basal levels of DNA single-strand breaks and alkali labile sites from human peripheral blood lymphocytes. These samples were obtained from people younger than 60 years and group older than 60 years of age. They were able to show that while the average changes with age were small, the mean increase in damage was only 12%, but the increase in a subpopulation of highly damaged lymphocytes was of the order of fivefold. However, this increase was seen in only 3 of 17 older subjects. Further work needs to be done to establish a relationship between DNA damage and aging.

Platt[18] found that DNA damage and repair may be crucial to senescence. There is a direct relationship between the repair capacity and the maximum life span of a given species. The division potentials of normal human diploid fibroblast cells *in vitro* is well documented, and this has been established as a model for cellular aging. Fibroblasts taken from young individuals have a greater doubling capacity, compared to fibroblasts derived from older individuals.

Mitochondrial DNA (mtDNA) has a high propensity for mutational error, but past theories of aging based on somatic mutation neglected mtDNA as a factor. Negly et al.[19] suggested a theory of aging based on the accumulative effect of mutation on human mtDNA. Their theory was based on the occurrence of mtDNA mutations with aging and their functional effect and on the effects of human mtDNA mutations seen in the mitochondrial cytopathies. Heteroplasmy was a feature of this concept, representing a combination of normal mtDNA and mutant mtDNA at the cellular and mitochondrial level. This in turn resulted in a "tissue mosaic" of total bioenergetic deficits. Evidence for this concept was based on two changes: (1) in the tissues of aged individuals, there was a focal loss of staining for mitochondrially encoded enzymes, such as cytochrome oxidase, and (2) by application of the polymerase chain reaction to the DNA template from individuals of different ages, they found that there was an age-related increase in deletional mutations in mtDNA.

One theory of aging gives neural and endocrine involvement a central stage in the pathogenesis of senescence in mammals and other multicellular species.[20] The data collected by Finch[20] supports the hypothesis that age-related changes are generally caused by specific physiological factors that are extrinsic to cells, and that successful manipulation can retard or reverse specific age-related changes, thereby retarding their life span. According to Finch, their findings have converted time in the analysis of senescence from an independent variable to a dependent variable.

In the past it was generally accepted and assumed that the thymus underwent progressive and irreversible involution. This led to the assumption that in the aged, thymic changes were responsible for the deterioration of immune function and, ultimately, for the increased incidence of infection, neoplasia, and autoimmune disease. This is only partially true, because it has been demonstrated that age-related thymic involution is not an intrinsic and irreversible process.[21] Even in old age, various neuroendocrine or nutritional manipulations can result in regrowth of the thymus.[21] With thymal reconstitution there is generally an improvement and recovery of peripheral immune function. In the young there is normally a neuroendocrine-thymic interaction, but with advancing age, there is disruption of such interactions, which leads to most of the age associated dysfunction. These and other findings have led, as an alternative, from a purely immune or neuroendocrine theory to a neuroendocrine immune hypothesis of aging.

In 1992 Kristal and Yu proposed that age-related deterioration was primarily due to structural and functional modifications of cellular constituents.[22] Whereas free-radical theory proposes damage to cellular constituents as the cause of aging, a second discovery proposes damage induced by nonenzymatic glycation and other Maillard reactions and subsequent modification of macromolecules. It is more than likely that the age-related deterioration is produced by the sum of the damage induced by free-radicals, glycation, and Maillard reactions and their interactions.[22] Manso proposed that oxygen radicals produced during cellular combustion contribute to aging by way of cumulative microlesions throughout life.[23]

Food restriction in rats, mice, and hamsters retards the aging process.[24] Food restriction leads to a decrease in physiological age, prolongs life expectancy, and retards age-related changes in the physiological process. Food restriction also delays or prevents most age-associated disease processes and produces its antiaging effects by reducing the intake of energy rather than through the alteration of intake of a specific nutrient.

The thermodynamics of irreversible processes that occur in cells considered open systems was reviewed by Toussaint and his colleagues.[25] They concluded that cells operating in a steady state optimize the free energy production by lowering their entropy production to a minimum. Some instability can occur which leads a cell from one steady state to another, characterized by a lower production of entropy.[25] Along with this there is a possibility that the level of errors or entropy of the system will increase. If the process continues, the cell goes from one state to another, eventually a critical level is reached, and the cell cannot cope any more and will die. Cells subsist in certain states, which are the results of genetic contribution and an optimization of cellular functions. This theory reconciles the two major theories of aging, namely the programmed and stochastic theories.[26] The programmatic theory simply states that aging is an inherent genetic process. The stochastic theory proposes that aging represents random damage from the environment. Cellular manifestations of aging include reduced life span of the cells,[26] decreased responsiveness of cells to growth signals with loss of cellular receptors to growth factors, and in turn increased responsiveness to growth inhibitors. These changes are demonstrated prominently in photodamaged cells.[26] Aging fibroblasts show altered membrane composition, with increased production of extracellular matrix and increased activity of catalase.[26]

Theories of aging are numerous, and as yet there is no convincing evidence as to whether age changes are programmed or due to accumulation of random changes in constituent cells.[27] Several theories and hypotheses have been postulated with regard to aging, ranging from the free-radical theory to immunological and genetic theories. The major theories of aging are summarized in Table 6.

AGE-RELATED HORMONAL EFFECTS

GROWTH HORMONE AND INSULIN-LIKE GROWTH FACTOR I

It is now widely established that there is an age-related decline in circulating levels of growth hormone (GH) and insulin-like growth factor I (IGF-I) (somatomedin-C). Apparently, there is a decrease in both the number and life of somatotrophs.[28] Sleep-related pulsatile growth hormone secretion decreases with age.[29] Florini et al.[30] found a significant correlation

TABLE 6
Theories on Aging

Cellular theory	Defective DNA repair and DNA damage
	Mitochondrial DNA theory
	Free-radical damage
System-based theory	Neuroendocrine theory
	Immune theory
Programmed theory	An inherent genetic process
Stochastic theory	Random damage from environment
Environmental damage	Radiation damage; genetic mutation; food restriction

between daily growth hormone secretion and IGF-I levels but failed to find a fall in integrated GH levels with advancing age. Vermeulen[31] found a decrease in GH peaks that was predominantly responsible for the declining somatomedin-C levels seen with advancing age. There is a more marked fall in basal GH levels in older females and this appears to be related to estrogen deficiency. Administration of estrogen increased both resting[32] and stimulated GH levels.[33] The response to growth hormone-releasing hormone (GHRH) has been found to be attenuated with advancing age, in some, but not all studies.[34] The response to insulin-induced hypoglycemia is decreased with advancing age.[35] There is also a decrease in the response to apomorphine with increasing age.[36] Injection of arginine seems to increase GH response in older persons, equivalent to that seen in younger subjects.[37] These studies and animal studies have suggested that with aging, there is an increase in somatostatin activity and a decrease in GHRH release from the hypothalamus. In addition, reduced effectiveness at the pituitary level leads to a decline in the overall function of the hypothalamo-pituitary-GH axis. IGF-I levels are reduced in both sexes and this reduction is correlated with 24 h of GH release.[31,38-40] Even lower levels of IGF-I have been reported in nutritionally impaired elderly persons in chronically institutionalized situations.[41] Increased adipose tissue results in a blunted response to provocative stimuli[42] and the levels of IGF-I levels. The significance of altered GH and IGF-I levels with advancing age is unclear, but it is well established that with both aging and GH deficiency, there is an associated increase in adipose tissue and a reduction in muscle, bone mass, the size of the liver, spleen, and kidney, and altered blood flow and reduced glomerular filtration rate occurs. This led to the concept of the so-called GH menopause.

Two studies have investigated the effect of recombinant GH on healthy older persons.[43,44] Both studies produced an unacceptable level of side effects in less than one year. Major side effects included the development of carpal tunnel syndrome and gynecomastia. GH therapy increased IGF-I and decreased body fat. However, it is clear that GH is not a hormonal fountain of youth. Preliminary studies have suggested that both IGF-I and gonadotropin-releasing factor (GRF), and its nonpeptide analogues, can be safely given to older persons. There is, however, little evidence that they will be more efficacious than GH in reversing the aging process.

Alternative uses that have been postulated for these agents include their use as adjunctive therapy in severely malnourished older persons and those demonstrating marked frailty. GH has been demonstrated to enhance nitrogen retention and improve weight gain in severely malnourished older persons.[45] To date no studies in these groups have demonstrated decreased mortality or improved functional status. Results of the ongoing studies on the effect of GH on muscle weakness are yet to be published.

PROLACTIN

Prolactin is the only hormone under inhibitory control. One study showed basal prolactin levels were slightly decreased in elderly females.[46] Another study, however, showed a mild but significant increase in circulating prolactin levels with advancing age in males,[47] which parallels the diminished dopaminergic activity seen with advancing age. The significance of an increased level of prolactin in elderly diabetics is not well established.

THYROID-STIMULATING HORMONE

There are no major age-related changes in the basal levels of thyroid-stimulating hormone (TSH) in the elderly, although one study showed that about 3.5% of men and about 17.4% of older women have elevated serum TSH levels, suggesting incipient hypothyroidism.[48-50] Following TRH stimulation in one study, it was found that the TSH response was decreased in elderly men but not in elderly women.[51] T_4 and T_3 production and T_4 clearance rate decrease with age, in the absence of thyroidal or nonthyroidal illness.[52] The T_3 resin uptake (T_3 Ru), which measures the hormone binding sites on the circulating proteins, does not change with age. In the normal elderly, there is no change in the circulating free T_4 levels. There is a decline in radioactive iodine uptake starting in middle age.[53] There is an increase in the nodularity of the thyroid gland with aging.

Despite the inconsistencies in various studies on the hypothalamo-pituitary-thyroid axis, it appears that there is a resetting of the whole axis in the elderly. This seems to be more of an adaptation process, and does not cause hypothyroidism with advancing age. Studies are needed to evaluate the availability of the thyroid hormone and the tissue responsiveness in older humans.

ADRENAL CORTEX

With advancing age, there is a slight decrease in the weight of the adrenal gland. The cortex degenerates secondary to fibrosis and a decrease in epithelial cells. With increasing age there is a reduction in the cortisol secretion rate; however, its metabolic clearance rate is also decreased, so that plasma level of cortisol remains unchanged.[54-56] With advancing age there is no change in the circadian rhythm of cortisol secretion.[57] The adrenal gland maintains its ability to produce cortisol in response to exogenous ACTH administration throughout life, but because of decreased clearance rate, there is a suggestion of diminished adrenal responsiveness.[58] ACTH levels tend to be greater in response to CRF and insulin-induced hypoglycemia.[59] Older persons have a higher level of cortisol when depressed.[60] There is also failure to adequately suppress the hypothalamic-pituitary-adrenal axis, following dexamethasone administration, in depressed older persons. These findings are similar to those in younger persons.

There is a decreased plasma secretion and clearance rate of aldosterone and a decreased plasma concentration and urinary excretion of aldosterone. Aldosterone and plasma renin activity levels show diminished response with aging.[61] In women age 70 and above, one third failed to show any rise in renin activity to salt restriction. There is a linear decline in renin concentration throughout life, and as a result, older patients are at increased risk of developing hyperkalemia.

With advancing age, there is an increase in norepinephrine levels with a near normal epinephrine level. This can predispose to the development of isolated systolic hypertension.[62] Hypertension *per se* becomes increasingly common after the age of 65. This is a significant risk factor for strokes, heart failure, and coronary heart disease.[63] The increase in norepinephrine in the aged appears to be due to both an increase in norepinephrine in the plasma and its decreased clearance rate.[64] Age and body fat play an important role in producing increased norepinephrine responsiveness to both upright posture and oral glucose ingestion.[65] In addition to a reduced lymphocyte adenylate cyclase response,[66] there is also reduced response by way of heart rate, secondary to isoproterenol.[67] There is a small decrease in the proportion of β-adrenergic receptors in the high-affinity state,[68] and also a reduction in receptor affinity.[69] α-Adrenergic receptor function in platelets has been variably reported as decreased,[70] increased,[71] or nonaltered.[72] In persons over the age of 80 an increase in epinephrine levels, as well as norepinephrine levels, has been reported to occur.

ADRENAL ANDROGENS

Compared to glucocorticoids, alterations in adrenal androgen production with age are more marked. Urinary 17-ketosteroid excretion is reduced in both sexes. Dihydroepiandrosterone (DHEA) levels decline linearly from as early as 20 years to 96 years of age.[73,74] Stimulation of the adrenal gland with exogenous ACTH results in a markedly decreased DHEA response. Selective cell death in the zona reticularis may account for the selective reduction in DHEA with preservation of glucocorticoid secretion. Other 17α-hydroxylated compounds such as 17α-pregnenolone and 17α-OH-progesterone are reduced with aging, as is pregnenolone sulfate. DHEA and DHEA sulfate are inversely associated with mortality from coronary heart disease.[75] DHEA causes weight loss without decreasing food intake.[76] Low levels of DHEA and DHEA sulfate are associated with hypercholesterolemia[77] and hypertension.[78] At least in animals, DHEA has a protective effect against diabetes mellitus, immune disorders, and tumorogenesis. Pregnenolone and its sulfated form are potent memory enhancers in animals.

HORMONES ASSOCIATED WITH WATER METABOLISM

Elderly persons who are either house bound or institutionalized are at marked risk for the development of either hyper- or hyponatremia. They also have an impaired response to fluid deprivation.[79] Animal[80] and human[81] studies suggest that this is due to a failure of opioid drinking drive. Impaired release of peripheral angiotensin-II may play a role in the development of dehydration. The aging kidneys adapt slowly to salt restriction with advancing age. This is due to reduced nephrons and a fall in renin and aldosterone levels.[82] Older persons are more prone to develop volume depletion in the event of a febrile illness. Basal AVP levels are increased in older subjects for a given level of osmolality.[83] The normal nocturnal increase in vasopressin fails to materialize in older persons, which may explain the nocturnal diuresis seen in the elderly.[84] Ethanol infusion in younger subjects produced inhibition of AVP, whereas older subjects had breakthrough secretions. Baroreceptor-mediated release of AVP is impaired in older humans.

Hyponatremia in an institutionalized setting is often due to the syndrome of inappropriate secretion of antidiuretic hormone. Hyponatremia may present as anorexia, depression, agitation, fatigue, and confusion.

Ohashi et al.[85] showed increased levels of atrial natriuretic factor (ANF) in older persons. These levels were lower than those seen in patients with cardiac failure.[86] The role of ANF in water balance of older persons is yet to be determined.

MALE SEX HORMONES

In the young, testosterone is secreted episodically in response to pulsatile release of LH. Levels of free and bioavailable testosterone decrease with aging and the circadian rhythm is abolished.[87] There is also decreased LH pulse frequency and possibly amplitude with aging. In the elderly there is an increased binding of testosterone in the plasma. There is a decreased rate of secretion, matched by a decreased rate of testosterone clearance, with aging. Anatomically, there is a reduction in testicular weight, and histologically, in the total number of Leydig cells.[88] Alcohol consumption, even in moderate amounts, tends to reduce testosterone levels. There is impaired response to exogenous human chorionic gonadotropin with increasing age. The decrease in testosterone is less than would be expected by the declining production rate. This is because of an increase in sex hormone-binding globulin (SHBG) levels.[89] There is an increased efficacy of testosterone to inhibit LH with advancing age. Most older persons develop secondary hypothalamo-pituitary failure rather than primary hypogonadism. FSH levels increase with age, suggesting a fall in inhibin level.

Estradiol levels are unchanged with age. This results in an increase in the estradiol/testosterone ratio. There is a decrease in the clearance ratio of estradiol with no alteration in its production rate. Because testosterone is bound with greater avidity to SHBG than estradiol, the ratio of the estradiol to bioavailable testosterone is increased.

The sperm count decreases with aging and a decrease in sperm motility occurs. Sperm morphology in older men is also altered.[90] Despite the changes in sperm with aging, extremely old males have been demonstrated to be capable of fathering children. The decrease in testosterone in old age is associated with a decrease in libido. Impotence, which occurs in approximately half of males by 70 years of age, is predominantly due to vascular disease and medication use. Testosterone appears to play a minimal role in the impotence seen in older males but is related to the decrease in libido seen with aging.

Testosterone replacement therapy has been reported to increase upper arm muscle strength, enhance calcium metabolism, increase hematocrit, and decrease LDL cholesterol in three studies in older persons.[91-93] It may also improve balance. Animal studies have suggested that testosterone may improve memory, and correlative studies have suggested a role for testosterone in age-related memory decline. Prostrate-specific antigen increases minimally in older humans when treated with testosterone. Short-term therapy appears to be safe and produces a number of positive effects in elderly men.

FEMALE SEX HORMONES

In most women, there is failure of ovarian function by the fifth or sixth decade. In the United States, the average age for menopause is about 51. Menopause plays a significant role in the remaining years of a woman's life. About 80% of women experience symptoms due to ovarian failure. Osteoporosis, vasomotor symptoms, and sex tissue atrophy are some of the prominent symptoms of menopause. At this stage, estrone replaces estradiol as the major circulating estrogen.[94] Progesterone levels are not altered with advancing age. After menopause the plasma clearance rate of estrone decreases by 30%,[95] whereas there is a 20% reduction in the clearance rate of estrone. The major source of postmenopausal estrogen is the adrenal gland, with most of the estrone being produced by peripheral aromatization of androstenedione.[95] Both LH and FSH levels increase after menopause, FSH levels tending to be higher than LH levels.[94] This may be due to a longer clearance rate of FSH. At approximately 70 years of age there is a decrease in LH levels in females, suggesting that a secondary hypogonadism is superimposed on the primary hypogonadism of menopause.

HYPOPITUITARISM

There is no change in the pituitary weight with aging, as suggested by autopsy studies.[96] With advancing age, there is reduced vascularity, increase in connective tissue, and increase in chromophobe and basophil cells. Little is known about the effects of aging and hypopituitarism in the elderly.

Typical presentation would be fatigue, weight loss, hypoglycemia (especially on fasting), anemia, hypogonadism, and orthostatic hypotension. All these features can occur in the elderly, but these presentations can be subtle and easily missed. Belchetz[97] reported five patients between ages 70 and 90 with hypopituitarism. Clinical features included anemia, hypotension, and pale skin. All patients had normal skull x-rays, all the pituitary hormones were reduced, and response to releasing hormones was poor. Critical illness can mimic hypopituitarism and, for this reason, tests to detect hypopituitarism should be carried out after the patient's illness has settled down.

THYROID DISEASES

HYPOTHYROIDISM

Hypothyroidism is much more common in women older than 50 years of age than in younger women and men.[98] In this group, there is often no goiter. In some cases spontaneous hypothyroidism that occurs in the elderly might be due to thyroiditis that occurred earlier in life, and this is associated with progressive destruction of gland tissue. Secondary hypothyroidism is rather rare, with an incidence of less than 2.5%.

It is easy to miss the diagnosis of hypothyroidism in the elderly, because of the insidious onset and atypical presentation. The commonest cause of hypothyroidism is chronic autoimmune thyroiditis. Other causes are thyroid ablation and antithyroid drugs for Graves' disease. Up to 20% of older persons have increased titers for thyroglobulin and antimicrosomal antibodies.[99] A combination of high antimicrosomal antibodies and a raised TSH level between 5 and 20 µ/L in patients with subclinical hypothyroidism is highly predictive that they will progress to permanent thyroid failure.[100]

Common symptoms of hypothyroidism include cold intolerance, constipation, dry skin, and lassitude. But these symptoms could easily be missed as part of the normal aging process. Symptoms may develop over a long period of time. Other features include fatigue, weight gain, poor concentration, slowness in activities, and psychomotor retardation. Less common presentations include myopathy, hyponatremia, anemia, and raised creatinine phosphokinase (CPK) levels.[101] On examination, patients have bradycardia, dry coarse skin, husky voice, nonpitting edema, loss of eyebrows, and myxedematous faces. They may also have delayed tendon reflexes, particularly ankle jerk. Concomitant diseases, such as congestive heart failure, may present with pitting edema. Hair texture can change. Raised CPK levels could easily be confused with myocardial infarction. In addition, there are elevated levels of serum glutamic oxaloacetic transaminase and lactic dehydrogenase. Other biochemical abnormalities include raised levels of cholesterol and triglycerides, which can lead to coronary artery disease. Johnston et al.[102] found that mean serum cholesterol was increased significantly in patients whose serum TSH was greater than 20 µ/L. On replacement there was a significant drop in serum cholesterol and a decrease in serum TSH. There was a poor correlation between decrease in cholesterol and increase in either T_3 or T_4 levels.

Reinke's edema is a condition affecting the vocal cords. It is commonly associated with cigarette smoking and vocal abuse. In the past, hypothyroidism was associated with it as an etiological factor. White et al.,[103] however, found no etiological association in the development of Reinke's edema and hypothyroidism. Treatment involves replacement therapy with L-thyroxine. In older persons, because of low metabolism, patients usually do not complain of angina prior to treatment. Following treatment they are more prone to angina and even myocardial infarction. Replacement therapy therefore needs extreme care. It is usual to start the dose of L-thyroxine at 25 µg and increase it by 25 µg at 4 weekly intervals to a maintenance dose of 75 to 100 µg. In older persons with heart disease or chronic obstructive pulmonary disease (COPD), slightly lower replacement doses may be associated with symptomatic improvement.

Myxedema coma is a fatal complication of hypothyroidism in older persons. The clinical picture includes hypothermia, altered mental status, and coma. Precipitating events include surgery, hypothermia, infection, hypoglycemia, and sedative drugs. Other features include bradycardia, reduced cardiac output, and reduced circulating volume. Treatment of myxedema coma involves treatment of the precipitating event and other supportive measures. Congestive cardiac failure and decrease in blood volume should be treated with caution. Use of steroids is controversial. These patients also need careful rewarming. For proven cases of myxedema coma, L-thyroxine is useful.[104,105]

THYROTOXICOSIS

The exact incidence of hyperthyroidism in the elderly is not known, but it is much lower than the incidence of hypothyroidism. One study suggested that about 70% of all persons with hyperthyroidism are over the age of 70.[106] The term denotes clinical and physiological findings, when tissues are exposed to the excessive thyroid hormone. Graves' disease is the commonest cause of hyperthyroidism in the elderly. Other causes are multinodular goiter and thyrotoxicosis secondary to a single nodule. Drugs like amiodarone can cause both hypo- and hyperthyroidism.

Symptoms such as heat intolerance, diarrhea, weight loss, and restlessness, commonly seen in the younger age group, are seen less commonly in the elderly. They are more likely to complain of lassitude and fatigue. Other symptoms include palpitation, muscle weakness, and shortness of breath. At least 30% will complain of anorexia, and constipation is not an uncommon symptom. Almost one third of patients present with atrial fibrillation. Patients with preexisting angina complain of worsening angina pectoris. Congestive cardiac failure is another clinical presentation.[107] When patients present with complaints of fatigue, depression, and weight loss without the signs and symptoms of adrenergic hyperstimulation, it is called apathetic hyperthyroidism. Elderly patients with thyrotoxicosis are sometimes difficult to diagnose clinically, and this is made even more difficult because they do not have features of ophthalmopathy, as seen in the young.

Thyroid function tests should be carried out in patients with a history of weight loss, palpitation, arrhythmias, myopathy, or dementia, and with psychiatric symptoms. The usual findings are raised levels of T_4 and T_3 and subnormal levels of TSH. However, the TSH level has poor sensitivity and specificity for the diagnosis of hyperthyroidism in older persons. Circulating autoantibodies may falsely raise TSH levels, producing false negative test results.[108]

The treatment of choice for Graves' disease in the elderly is usually radioactive ablation of the thyroid gland. Prior to this, a short course of antithyroid drug is preferable. This measure ensures the gland is deplete of preformed thyroid hormone. Failure to do so can precipitate a "thyroid crisis." Also, the use of beta blockers has a protective action against the cardiovascular complications of hyperthyroidism. Management of multinodular goiter is different in the sense that it may require more than one course of radioactive iodine. Surgery is less of an alternative in the elderly. Whatever the mode of treatment, regular thyroid function tests should be carried out to pick up early cases of hypothyroidism, which is the commonest outcome following the treatment of hyperthyiodism.

ADRENAL DISORDERS

In the elderly, there is no change in the adrenal weight, but histologically, there are cortical changes. Main features are loss of steroid-containing lipids and increased fibrosis and fragmentation of mitochondria.[109] Up to 50% of adrenal glands at autopsy show nodular hyperplasia. With aging, there is no change in cortisol level,[55] and this is due to diminished clearance rate.

The elderly have a raised cortisol level[60] when depressed. There is no change in response of cortisol for insulin-induced hypoglycemia, compared to the younger patients.[110] In addition, the response to ACTH in the elderly is unaltered.[111]

ADDISON'S DISEASE

Addison's disease is not an uncommon disease in the elderly, but it is more than likely that its diagnosis depends on the clinician's awareness. Like any other endocrine disease in the elderly, nonspecific presentation is common. Depending on the awareness, diagnosis depends on biochemical tests. Features include hyponatremia, hyperkalemia, raised BUN, and normal or low blood sugar levels. Symptoms of fatigue, lethargy, and hypotension with or without orthostasis should suggest a diagnosis of Addison's disease. Approximately 10% of patients with Addison's disease are in the elderly age group.[112]

Common causes are tuberculosis, hemorrhage into the adrenal gland, autoimmune causes, and metastatic disease. Diagnostic tests are similar to those used in younger subjects. Treatment is usually replacement therapy with prednisone or hydrocortisone and fludrocortisone.

Complications, due to glucocorticoids, are usually rare in the doses used. With fludrocortisone, edema, hypertension, and hypokalemia are common.

CUSHING'S SYNDROME

Causes of Cushing's syndrome are adrenal hyperplasia or adrenal neoplasia, which include adenoma or carcinoma, and prolonged use of glucocorticoids or ACTH. Ectopic production of ACTH due to bronchogenic carcinoma, carcinoid of thymus, and bronchial adenoma are the other causes. Of the above, adrenal carcinoma and ectopic production of ACTH are more likely to occur in the elderly, closely followed by iatrogenic causes. Cushing's syndrome is relatively uncommon in the elderly, and it is estimated that about 8% of patients with adrenal carcinoma are over the age of 60.[113]

The typical habitus seen in the younger age group is not commonly seen in the elderly. Clinical and biochemical suspicion is more likely to reward with a diagnosis. If an individual has hypertension, diabetis, osteoporosis, hypokalemia, and low levels of eosinophils in the peripheral blood, a diagnosis of Cushing's syndrome should be considered. In patients with ectopic production of ACTH, hypokalemia, hypochloremia, and metabolic alkalosis are more commonly seen.

Diagnosis depends on demonstration of increased cortisol levels and a dexamethasone suppression test that fails to suppress endogenous cortical secretion. Elderly patients with dementia, alcohol abuse, or obesity, and certain drugs such as phenytoin, can also cause nonsuppression. Ectopic production of ACTH is seen much more commonly in males, and plasma levels can exceed more than 200 pg/ml. Chest x-ray may reveal either a bronchogenic carcinoma or a thymoma.

RENIN-ANGIOTENSIN-ALDOSTERONE AXIS

There is a decrease in both the secretion and clearance rate of aldosterone in the elderly. Concentration of renin is also lower. If salt is restricted in elderly patients, they are less likely to show an increase in their aldosterone level. They also fail to show a rise in renin activity in response to salt restriction or on standing.

Tsundo et al.[114] were able to show that changes in renin secretion with aging were not due to a decrease in plasma renin substrate concentration. They also showed that, there were no effects in the total and inactive renin concentration with aging. In contrast, there is a marked linear decrease in active renin concentration throughout life. So it is more than likely that in the elderly, there is decreased conversion of inactive renin to active renin. The end result is that older persons are more prone to develop hyperkalemia secondary to hyporeninemic hypoaldosteronism.

MENOPAUSE

Menopause occurs between 40 to 60 years of age.[115] At least 80% of women experience symptoms due to ovarian failure. Around the age of 40 to 50 years most women have vasomotor symptoms. During the later half of their life, osteoporosis and its sequelae are experienced.

Variation in menstrual cycle begins to appear by the age of 35 and above. The follicles decrease in number and circulating estrogen levels decrease. FSH and LH levels increase due to the feedback mechanism. At this stage, estrone is the main circulating hormone produced from aromatization of adrenal androstenedione.[116] Estrogen modulates the synthesis of angiotensinogen, clotting factors, apoproteins for HDL and LDL, and a decrease in the bile flow.

Clinical features, such as sex tissue atrophy, osteoporosis, and hot flashes, are mainly due to estrogen deprivation. Normally, estrogen has an influence on central thermoregulation. In menopause, the same central thermoregulatory center misperceives core overheating and activates the autonomic cooling mechanism, accounting for the hot flashes. Other symptoms include mood changes, irritability, sleep disturbances, vaginal atrophy, vaginal dryness, dyspareunia, bleeding, itching, frequent urinary tract infection, and delayed sexual arousal.

Treatment is with estrogen replacement therapy, which is very effective for control of vasomotor symptoms. Recently, estrogen replacement has been associated with better memory function.[117] Long-term treatment with estrogen, reduces the rate of osteoporosis and also has a cardiovascular protective role. Known side effects include increased blood pressure, gallbladder disease, hypercoagulable states, and endometrial carcinoma. Small doses of progesterone may have a protective effect. Patients with a history of thrombosis should be excluded from estrogen replacement therapy.

Oral estrogens are metabolized in the liver and hence lower levels are available for the target tissues. Topical and transdermal estrogens bypass the liver and produce fewer side effects.[118] Topical estrogens help in the management of local symptoms. Clonidine and medroxyprogesterones are the drugs of choice for patients with contraindication to the use of estrogens.

DISEASES OF PARATHYROID GLAND

Like other endocrine glands, age-related changes affect the parathyroid gland. There is an age-related rise in parahormone levels, attributable to reduced calcium absorption. There is also a resistance to PTH action by target organs and reduced renal clearance. Serum calcium levels are slightly lower in women but, in later life, the levels equate.[119] Lower levels of 25(OH) vitamin D levels are found in older persons.[120] Low levels of 1,25(OH)2 vitamin D are particularly noted in nursing home patients.[120-122] Measurements of ionized calcium would be more reliable in the elderly than total calcium levels.

HYPERPARATHYROIDISM

Hyperparathyroidism is much more common in women than in men. It is most common between 50 and 70 years of age.[123] Most often diagnosis is made accidentally after laboratory results are available. Sometimes patients present with psychiatric and neuromuscular manifestations. Atypical symptoms such as constipation, confusion, dehydration, anorexia, weight loss, and renal stones are also seen. Psychiatric manifestations are more common in elderly patients than in the young.[124] Hypertension and chondrocalcinosis are fairly frequent. Fatigue, muscle weakness, and parasthesia are other symptoms.

Diagnosis depends on finding hypercalcemia in the presence of raised PTH levels. Other laboratory features of the disease are hypophosphatemia, hypomagnesimia, raised alkaline phosphatase, hyperuricemia, and possibly anemia. Measurements of urinary calcium would be ideal. Hypercalcemia, secondary to the use of thiazide diuretic or lithium, and certain types of malignancy should be excluded.

Treatment is usually surgical removal of the adenoma, which is the most common cause of hyperparathyroidism in the elderly. Surgical treatment is usually associated with improved memory function and reversal of anorexia. In those with high surgical risk, an alternative would be treatment with estrogen therapy.[125] For those with mild to moderate elevation of PTH levels, early surgery is increasingly suggested because of improved functional outcome.[126]

HYPOPARATHYROIDISM

Hypoparathyroidism is not a common problem in the elderly, unless it is part of multiple endocrine gland failure of an autoimmune etiology. Sometimes it can occur secondary to thyroid surgery and irradiation. Signs and symptoms are due to hypocalcemia, and treatment involves use of calcitriol and oral calcium.

CONCLUSION

By the end of the fifth decade, the functional ability of various organs in the body declines, and this includes organs of the endocrine system. Levels of certain hormones in the plasma decrease with increasing age, although plasma concentration of certain hormones remain unchanged. All these changes may reflect either depressed rate of secretion or decline in both secretion and degradation. Hence, diagnosis and management of endocrine disorders in older persons can sometimes be daunting. With a good history, clinical examination, and currently available laboratory techniques, management of endocrine problems in the elderly should no longer be a problem for the geriatrician.

REFERENCES

1. **Trence, D.L., Morley, J.E., and Handwerger, B.S.,** Poly-glandular autoimmune syndrome, *Am. J. Med.,* 77, 107, 1984.
2. **Mooradian, A.D. and Scarpace, P.J.,** The response of isoproterenol stimulated adenylate cyclase activity after administration of L triiodothyronine is reduced in aged rats, *Horm. Metab. Res.,* 21, 638, 1989.
3. **Morley, J.E. and Levine, A.S.,** Pharmacology of eating behavior, *Annu. Rev. Pharmacol. Toxicol.,* 25, 127, 1985.
4. **Philips, P.A., Ledingham, J.G.G., Rolls, B., Crowe, M.J., and Wollner, L.,** Reduced thirst perception after water deprivation in a healthy elderly man, *N. Engl. J. Med.,* 311, 7536, 1984.
5. **Helderman, J.H., Vestal, R.E., Rowe, J.W., Tobin, J.D., Andres, R., and Robertson, G.R.,** The response of arginine vasopressin to intravenous ethanol and hypertonic saline in man. The impact of aging, *J. Gerontol.,* 33, 39, 1978.
6. **Phillips, P.A., Bretherton, M., Risvanis, J., Casley, D., Johnston, C., and Grayl, L.,** Effects of drinking on thirst and vasopressin in a dehydrated elderly man, *Am. J. Physiol.,* 264, R 877, 1993.
7. **Phillips, P.A., Bretherton, M., Johnston, C.I., and Gray, L.,** Reduced osmotic thirst in healthy elderly men, *Am. J. Physiol.,* 261, R 166, 1991.
8. **Mc Lean, K.A., O'Neill, P.A., Davies, I., and Catania, J.,** Changes in the response to saline load with age, *Clin. Sci.,* 81, 6, 1991.
9. **Duggan, J., Catania, J., O'Neill, P.A., and Davies, I.,** Response to dehydration in long term care elderly patients, *Clin. Sci.,* 82, 27, 1992.
10. **Helderman, J.H.,** The impact of normal aging on the hypothalamic neurohypophyseal renal axis, in *Endocrine Aspects of Aging,* Korenman, S.G., Ed., Elsevier Biomedical, New York, 1982, 108.
11. **Faull, C.M., Holmes, C., and Baylis, P.H.,** Water balance in elderly people: Is there a deficiency of vasopressin? *Age Ageing,* 22, 114, 1993.
12. **Aspund, R. and Aberg, H.,** Diurnal variation in the levels of antidiuretic hormone in the elderly, *J. Intern. Med.,* 229, 131, 1991.
13. **North, W.G., Harbaugul, R., and Reeder, T.,** An evaluation of human neurophysin production in Alzheimer's disease, *J. Am. Geriatr. Soc.,* 37, 843, 1989.
14. **Mooradian, A.D., Deebaji, L., and Wong, N.C.W.,** Age related alteration in the response of hepatic lipogenic enzymes to altered thyroid states in the rat, *J. Endocrinol.,* 128, 79, 1991.
15. **Morley, J.E., Krahn, D.O., Gosnell, B.A., Billington, C.J., and Levine, A.S.,** Interrelationships between calcitonin and other modulators of feeding behavior, *Psychol. Pharmacol. Bull.,* 20, 463, 1984.
16. **Greenstock, C.L.,** Radiation and aging: free-radical damage, biological response and possible antioxidant intervention, *Med. Hypothesis,* 41(5), 473, 1993.
17. **Singh, N.P., Danner, D.B., Tice, R.R., Pearson, J.D., Brant, L.J., Morrell, C.H., and Schneider, E.L.,** Basal DNA damage in individual human lymphocytes with age, *Mutat. Res.,* 256(1), 1, 1991.
18. **Platt, D.,** Aging—from the molecule to the organism, *Z. Rheumatol.,* 51(6), 280,1992.
19. **Negley, P., Mackay, I.R., Baumes, A., Maxwell, R.J., Vaillant, F., Wang, X., Zhang, C., and Linnane, A.W.,** Mitochondrial DNA mutation associated with aging and degenerative diseases, *Ann. N.Y. Acad. Sci.,* 673, 92, 1992.
20. **Finch, C.E.,** A FRAR course on laboratory approaches to aging, *Aging,* 5(4), 272, 1993.
21. **Fabris, N.,** Biomarkers of aging in the neuroendocrine immune domain, *Ann. N. Y. Acad. Sci.,* 663, 335, 1992.
22. **Kristal, B.S. and Yu, B.P.,** An emerging hypothesis: synergistic induction of aging by free-radicals and Maillard reactions, *J. Gerontol.,* 47(4), B 107, 1992.

23. **Manso, C.,** Aging and free-radicals, *Acta Med. Portuguesa,* 5(2), 87, 1992.

24. **Masoro, E.J.,** Retardation of aging process by food restriction: an experimental tool, *Am. J. Clin. Nutr.,* 55 (Suppl. 6), 1250s, 1992.

25. **Toussaint, O., Raes, M., and Remacle, J.,** Aging as a multistep process characterized by a lowering of entropy production leading the cell to a sequence of defined stages, *Mech. Aging Dev.,* 61(1), 45, 1991.

26. **Yaar, M. and Gilchrist, B.A.,** Cellular and molecular mechanism of cutaneous aging, *J. Dermatol. Surg. Oncol.,* 16(10), 915, 1990.

27. **Blair, K.A.,** Aging: physiological aspects and clinical implications, *Nurse Practitioner,* 15(2), 14, 1990.

28. **Sin, Y.K., Xix-P., Fenoglio, C.M., et al.,** The effects of age on the number of pituitary cells immuno reactive to growth hormone and prolactin, *Hum. Pathol.,* 15, 169, 1984.

29. **Prinz, P.N., Weitzman, E.D., Cunningham, G.R., et al.,** Plasma growth hormone during sleep in young and aged men, *J. Gerontol.,* 38, 519, 1983.

30. **Florini, J., Prinz, P.N., Vitiello, M.V., et al.,** Somatomedine C levels in healthy young and old men: relationship to peak and 24 hour integrated levels of growth hormone, *J. Gerontol.,* 40, 2, 1985.

31. **Vermeulen, A.,** Nyctohumerol growth hormone profiles in young and aged men: correlation with somatomedine-c levels, *J. Clin. Endocrinol. Metab.,* 64, 884, 1987.

32. **Weideman, E., Schwartz, E., and Frantz, A.G.,** Acute and chronic estrogen effects upon serum somatomedine activity, growth hormone and prolactin in man, *J. Clin. Endocrinol. Metab.,* 42, 942, 1976.

33. **Frantz, A.G. and Rabkin, M.T.,** Effects of estrogen and sex difference on secretion of human growth hormone, *J. Clin. Endocrinol. Metab.,* 25, 1470, 1965.

34. **Shibasaki, T., Shizume, K., Nakahara, M., et al.,** Age related changes in plasma growth hormone response to growth hormone releasing factor in man, *J. Clin. Endocrinol. Metab.,* 58, 212, 1984.

35. **Laron, Z., Doron, M., and Amikam, B.,** Plasma growth hormone in old age, *Harefuah,* 73, 375, 1967.

36. **Lal, S., Nair, N.P.V., Thavndagi, I., et al.,** Growth hormone response to apomorphine, a dopamine receptor agonist, in normal aging and in dementia of the Alzheimer's type, *Neurobiol. Aging,* 10, 227, 1989.

37. **Dudl, R.J., Ensinek, J.W., Palmer, H.E., et al.,** Effect of age on growth hormone secretion in man, *J. Clin. Endocrinol. Metab.,* 67, 11, 1973.

38. **Rudman, D., Kutner, M.H., Rogers, C.M., et al.,** Impaired growth hormone secretion in the adult population:relation to age and adiposity, *J. Clin. Invest.,* 67, 1361, 1981.

39. **Tan, K. and Baxter, R.C.,** Serum insulin like growth factor 1 levels in adult diabetic patients: the effect of age, *J. Clin. Endocrinol. Metab.,* 63, 651, 1986.

40. **Bennett, A.E., Wahner, M.W., Riggs, B.L., et al.,** Insulin like growth factors 1 and 2: aging and bone density in women, *J. Clin. Endocrinol. Metab.,* 59, 7012, 1984.

41. **Rudman, D., Nagraji, H.S., Mattson, D.E., et al.,** Hyposomatomedinemia in the nursing home patients, *J. Am. Geriatr. Soc.,* 34, 427, 1986.

42. **Williams, T., Berelowitz, M., Joffe, S.N., et al.,** Impaired growth hormone response to growth hormone releasing factor in obesity, *N. Engl. J. Med.,* 311, 1403, 1984.

43. **Cohn, L., Feller, A.G., Draper, M.U., Rudman, I.W., and Rudman, D.,** Carpal tunnel syndrome and gynecomastia during growth hormone treatment of elderly men with low circulating IGF-1 concentration, *Clin. Endocrinol.,* 39, 417, 1993.

44. **Holloway, L., Butterfield, G, Hintz, R.L., Gesandhert, N., and Marcus, R.,** Effects of recombinant human growth hormone on metabolic indices, body composition and bone turnover in healthy elderly women, *J. Clin. Endocrinol. Metab.,* 79, 470, 1994.

45. **Kaiser, F.E., Silver, A.J., and Morley, J.E.,** The effect of recombinant human growth hormone on malnourished older individuals, *J. Am. Geriatr. Soc.,* 39, 235, 1991.

46. **Vekemann, M. and Robin, C.,** Influence of age on serum prolactin levels in men and women, *Br, J. Med.,* 4, 738, 1975.

47. **Sawin, C.T., Carlson, H.E., Geller, A., Castelli, W.D., and Bacharach, P.,** Serum prolactin and aging: basal values and changes with estrogen use and hypothyroidism, *J. Gerontol.,* 44, 131, 1989.

48. **Sawin, C.T., Chopra, D., Azizi, F., Mannix, J.E., and Bacharach, P.,** The aging thyroid: increased prevalence of elevated serum thyrotropin in the elderly, *J. Am. Med. Assoc.,* 242, 247, 1979.

49. **Jeffreys, P.M., Farran, M.E.A., Hoffenberg, R., Fraser, P.M., and Hodkinson, H.M.,** Thyroid function tests in the elderly, *Lancet,* 1, 924, 1972.

50. **Rosenthal, M.J., Hun, W.C., Garry, P.J., and Goodwin, J.S.,** Thyroid function in the elderly. Microsomal antibodies as a discriminant for therapy, *J. Am. Med. Assoc.,* 258, 209, 1987.

51. **Kaiser, F.E.,** Variability of respose to TRH in normal elderly, *Age Ageing,* 16, 345, 1987.

52. **Robushi, G., Safran, M., Brarerman, C.E., et al.,** Hypothyroidism in the elderly, *Endocrinol. Rev.,* 8, 142, 1987.

53. **Gaffney, G.W., Gregerman, R.I., and Shock, N.W.,** Relationship of age to the thyroidal accumulation, renal excretion and distribution of radioiodide in euthyroid man, *J. Clin. Endocrinol. Metab.,* 22, 786, 1962.

54. **Samuels, L.T.,** Factors affecting the metabolism and distribution of cortisol as measured by levels of 17-hydroxycorticosteroids in blood, *Cancer,* 10, 746, 1957.

55. **West, C.D., Brown, H., Simmons. E.L., Carter, D.B., Kumaje, L.F., and Englebert, E.L.,** Adrenocorticol function and cortisol metabolism in old age, *J. Clin. Endocrinol. Metab.,* 21, 1197, 1961.

56. **Romanoff, L.P., Morris, C.W., Welch, P., Rodriguez, R.M., and Pincus, G.,** The metabolism of cortisol 4c-14 in young and elderly men. Secretion rate of cortisol and daily excretion of tetra hydrocortisone and cortalon (20 alpha and 20 beta), *J. Clin. Endocrinol. Metab.,* 21, 1413, 1961.

57. **Jenson, H.K. and Blichert-Toft, M.,** Serum corticotrophin, plasma cortisol and urinary secretion of 17 ketogenic steroids in the elderly age group: 66-94 years, *Acta Endocrinol. (Copenhagen),* 66, 25, 1971.

58. **Friedman, M., Green, M.F., and Shrland, D.G.,** Assessment of hypothalamic-pituitary-adrenal function in the geriatric age group, *J. Gerontol.,* 24, 292, 1969.

59. **Pavlov, E.P., Hrman, S.M., Chronsos, G.P., Iouriznx, D.L., and Blackman, M.R.,** Response of plasma adrenocorticotrophin, cortisol and dehydroepiandrosterone to ovine corticotrophin releasing hormone in healthy aging men, *J. Clin. Endocrinol. Metab.,* 62, 762, 1986.

60. **Greden, J.F., Flegel, P., Haskett, R., et al.,** Age effects in serial hypothalamic pituitary-adrenal monitoring, *Psychoneuroendocrinology,* 11, 195, 1986.

61. **Tsunoda, K., Abe, K., Goto, T., Yasujima, M., Sato, M., Seino, M., and Yashinaga, K.,** Effects of age on the renin-angiotensin-aldosterone system in normal subjects. Simultaneous measurement of active and inactive renin, renin substrate and aldosterone in plasma, *J. Clin. Endocrinol. Metab.,* 62, 384, 1986.

62. **Tuck, M.L., Griffiths, R.F., Jhonson, L., Stern, N., and Morley, J.E.,** Hypertension in the elderly, *J. Am. Geriatr. Soc.,* 36, 630, 1988.

63. **Tuck, M. and Sowers, J.R.,** Hypertension and aging, in *Endocrine Aspects of Aging,* Korenman, S.G., Ed., Elsevier Biomedical, New York, 1982, 81.

64. **Esler, M., Jackman, G., Bobik, A., et al.,** Determination of nor-epinephrine apparent release rate and clearance in humans, *Life Sci.,* 25, 1461, 1979.

65. **Schwartz, R.S., Jeager, L.F., and Veith, R.C.,** The importance of body composition to the increase in plasma norepinephrine appearance rate in elderly men, *J. Gerontol.,* 42, 546, 1987.

66. **Krall, J.F., Connnell, M., Weisbart, R., et al.,** Age related elevation of plasma catecholamine concentration and reduced responsiveness of lymphocyte adenylate cyclase, *J. Clin. Endocrinol. Metab.,* 52, 863, 1981.

67. **Lakata, E.G.,** Alteration in the cardiovascular system that occurs in advanced age, *Fed. Proc.,* 38, 163, 1979.

68. **Kent, R.S., Delean, A., and Lefkowitz, R.J.,.** A quantitative analysis of beta adrenergic receptor interaction: resolution of high and low affinity states of the receptor by computer modelling of ligand binding data, *Mol. Pharmacol.,* 17, 14, 1980.

69. **Feldman, R.D., Limbird, L.E., Nadean, J., et al.,** Alteration in leukocyte beta receptor affinity with aging. A potential explanation for altered beta-adrenergic sensitivity in the elderly, *N. Engl. J. Med.,* 310, 815, 1984.

70. **Brodde, O.E., Anlaug, M., Graben, N., et al.,** Age dependent decrease of alpha 2-adrenergic receptor number in human platelets, *Eur. J. Pharmacol.,* 81, 345, 1982.

71. **Yokoyama, M., Kueni, A., Sakamoto, S., et al.,** Age associated increments in human platelet alpha-adrenoceptor capacity. Possible mechanism for platelet hyperactivity to aging man, *Thromb. Res.,* 34, 287, 1984.

72. **Elliot, J.M. and Grahame Smith, D.G.,** The binding characteristics of [3 H] dihydroergocriptin on intact human platelets, *Br. J. Pharmacol.,* 76, 121, 1982.

73. **Yamaji, T. and Ibayashi, H.,** Plasma dehydroepiandrosterone sulfate in normal and pathological conditions, *J. Clin. Endocrinol. Metab.,* 29, 273, 1969.

74. **Oventreich, N., Brind, J.C., Rizer, R.L., and Vogelman, J.M.,** Age changes in sex difference in serum dehydroepiandrosterone sulfate concentration throughout adulthood, *J. Clin. Endocrinol. Metab.,* 59, 531, 1984.

75. **Barrett-Conner, E., Khaw, K.T., and Yen, S.C.C.,** A prospective study of dehydroepiandrosterone sulfate: mortality and cardiovascular disease, *N. Engl. J. Med.,* 315, 1519, 1986.

76. **Coleman, D.L., Leites, E.M., and Applezweig, N.,** Therapeutic doses of dehydroepiandrosterone metabolites in diabetic mutant mice, *Endocrinology,* 115, 239, 1984.

77. **Lopez, S.A.,** Metabolic and endocrine factors in aging, in *Risk Factors for Senility,* Rothchild, H. and Chapman, C.F., Eds., Oxford University Press, New York, 1984, 205.

78. **Nowaczynski, W., Fragachan, F., Silah, J., et al.,** Further evidence of altered adrenocortical function in hypertension: Dehydroepiandrosterone excretion rate, *J. Physiol. (London),* 56, 650, 1984.

79. **Phillips, P.A., Rolls, B.J., Ledingham, J.C.G., et al.,** Reduced thirst after water deprivation in healthy elderly men, *N. Engl. J. Med.,* 311, 753, 1984.

80. **Silver, A.J., Flood, J.F., and Morley, J.E.,** Effects of aging on fluid ingestion in mice, *J. Gerontol.,* 46, B 117, 1991.

81. **Silver, A.J. and Morley, J.E.,** The role of the opioid system in the hypodypsia associated with aging, *J. Am. Geriatr. Soc.,* 40, 556, 1992.

82. **Epstein, M. and Hollenberg, N.K.,** Age as a determinant of renal sodium conservation in normal man, *J. Lab. Clin. Med.,* 87, 411, 1976.

83. **Helderman, J.H.,** The impact of normal aging on the hypothalamic-neurohypophysial renal axis, in *Endocrine Aspects of Aging,* Korenman, S.G., Ed., Elsevier Biomedical, New York, 1982, 9.

84. **Asplund, R. and Abug, H.,** Diurnal variation in the levels of ADH in the elderly, *J. Intern. Med.,* 229, 131, 1991.

85. **Ohashi, M., Fujia, N., Nawata, H., et al.,** High plasma concentration of human atrial natriuretic polypeptide in aged men, *J. Clin. Endocrinol. Metab.,* 64, 81, 1987.

86. **Saito, Y., Nakao, K., Nishimura, K., et al.,** Clinical application of atrial natriuretic polypeptide in patients with congestive heart failure. Beneficial effects on left ventricular function, *Circulation,* 76, 115, 1987.

87. **Korenman, S.G., Morley, J.E., Mooradian, A.D., Davis, S.S., Kaiser, F.E., Silver, A.J., Viosca, S.P., and Garza, D.,** Secondary hypogonadism in older men: its relationship to impotence, *J. Clin. Endocrinol. Metab.,* 71, 963, 1990.

88. **Morley, J.E.,** Endocrine factors in geriatric sexuality clinics, *Geriatr. Med.,* 7, 85, 1991.

89. **Tenover, J.S., Matsumoto, A.M., Plymate, S.R., et al.,** The effects of aging in normal men on bioavailable testosterone and luteinizing hormone secretion: response to clomiphene citrate, *J. Clin. Endocrinol. Metab.,* 65, 1118, 1987.

90. **Natoli, A., Riondino, G., and Brancati, A.,** Studio delta Funizone ammonia e spermato genitica nel corso della senecenza muschille, *G. Gerontol.,* 20, 1103, 1972.

91. **Tenover, J.S.,** Effects of testosterone supplimention in the aging male, *J. Clin. Endocrinol. Metab.,* 75, 1092, 1992.

92. **Morley, J.E., Perry, H.M., III, Kaiser, F.E., Kraenzle, D., Jensen, J., Houston, K.A., Mattamal, M., and Perry, H.M., Jr.,** Effects of testosterone replacement therapy in old hypogonadal males, *J. Am. Geriatr. Soc.,* 41, 149, 1993.

93. **Sih, R., Kaiser, F.E., Morley, J.E., Sawardekar, M.A., Patrick, P., and Perry, H.M.,** Testosterone increases strength in older hypogonadal men, *J. Am. Geriatr. Soc.,* 42, A 25, 1994

94. **Kaiser, F.E. and Morley, J.E.,** The menopause and beyond, in *Geriatric Medicine,* Cassel, C.R. and Reisenberg, D., Eds., Springer-Verlag, New York, 1990, 279.

95. **Judd, H.L. and Korenman, S.G.,** Effects of aging on reproductive function in women, in *Endocrine Aspects of Aging,* Korenman, S.G., Ed., Elsevier Biomedical, New York, 1982, 163.

96. **Andres, R. and Tobin, J.D.,** Endocrine systems, in *Handbook of the Biology of Aging,* Finch, C.E. and Hayflick, L., Eds., Van Nostrand Reinhold, New York, 1977, 367.

97. **Belchetz, P.E.,** Idiopathic hypopituitarism in the elderly. *Br. Med. J.,* 291, 241, 1985.

98. **Sawin, C.T., Castelli, W.D., Hershman, J.M., et al.,** The aging thyroid. Thyroid deficiency in the Framingham study, *Arch. Intern. Med.,* 145, 1386, 1985.

99. **Levy, E.G.,** Thyroid disease in the elderly, *Med. Clin. North Am.,* 75, 151, 1991.

100. **Rosenthal, M.J., Hunt, W.C., Garre, P.J., and Goodwin, J.S.,** Thyroid failure in the elderly. Microsomal antibodies as discriminant for therapy, *J. Am. Med. Assoc.,* 258, 209, 1987.

101. **Kavorian, G.D., Wong, N.C.W., and Mooradian, A.D.,** Unusual manifestations of hypothyroidism in an elderly patient, *Geriatr. Med. Today,* 6, 28, 1985.

102. **Johnston, J., McLelland, A., and O'Reilly, D.S.,** The relationship between serum cholesterol and serum thyroid hormone in male patients with suspected hypothyroidism, *Ann. Clin. Biochem.,* 30, 256, 1993.

103. **White, A., Sim, D.W., and Maran, A.G.,** Reinke's edema and thyroid function, *J. Laryngol. Otol.,* 105(4), 291, 1991.

104. **Nicoloff, J.T.,** Thyroid storm and myxedema coma, *Med. Clin. North Am.,* 69(5), 1005, 1985.

105. **Nicoloff, J.T. and Lopresti, J.S.,** Myxedema coma: a form of decompensated hypothyroidism, *Endocrinol. Metab. Clin. North Am.,* 22(2), 279, 1993.

106. **Palmer, K.T.,** A prospective study into thyroid disease in a geriatric unit, *N.Z. Med. J.,* 86, 323, 1977.

107. **Bartels, E.C. and Kingsley, J.W.J.,** Hyperthyroidism in patients over 65, *Geriatrics,* 4, 333, 1949.

108. **Kaiser, F.E. and Morley, J.E.,** Endocrine changes in the elderly, in *Geriatric Surgery: Comprehensive Care of the Elderly Patients,* Katlic, M.R., Ed., Urban & Schwanzenberg, Baltimore, 1990, 115.

109. **Wolfsen, A.R.,** Aging and the adrenals, in *Endocrine Aspects of Aging,* Korenman, S.G., Ed., Elsevier Biomedical, New York, 1982, 55.

110. **Cartlidge, N.E.F., Black, M.M., Hall, M.R.P., et al.,** Pituitary function in the elderly, *Gerontol. Clin.,* 12, 65, 1970.

111. **West, C.D., Brown, H., Simons, E.L., et al.,** Adrenocortical function and cortisol metabolism in old age, *J. Clin. Endocrinol. Metab.,* 21, 1197, 1961.

112. **Irwin, W.J. and Barnes, E.W.,** Addison's disease, ovarian failure and hypothyroidism, *Clin. Endocrinol. Metab.,* 4, 379, 1975.

113. **Hunter, A.M. and Kayhoe, D.E.,** Adrenal cortical carcinoma: clinical features of 138 patients, *Am. J. Med.,* 41, 572, 1966.

114. **Tsundo, K., Abe, K., Goto, T., et al.,** Effects of age on the renin-angiotensin-aldosterone system in normal subjects: simultaneous measurement of active and inactive renin, renin substrate and aldosterone in plasma, *J. Clin. Endocrinol. Metab.,* 62, 384, 1986.

115. **Mooradian, A.D., Mosley, J.E., and Korenman, S.G.,** Endocrinology in aging, *Disease-a-Month,* 34, 395, 1988.

116. **Judd, H.L., Shamonki, I.M., Frumar, A.M., and Lagasse, L.D.,** Origin of serum estradiol in post menopausal women, *Obstet. Gynecol.,* 59: 680, 1982.

117. **Robinson, D., Friedman, L., Marcus, R., Tinklenburg, J., and Yesavage J.,** Estrogen replacement therapy and memory in older women, *J. Am. Geriatr. Soc.,* 9, 919, 1994.

118. **Chetkowski, R.J., Meldrum, D.R., Steingold, K.A., et al.,** Biologic effects of transdermal estradiol, *N. Engl. J. Med.,* 314, 1615, 1986.

119. **Keating, F.R., Jones, J.D., Elveback, C.R., et al.,** The relation of age and sex to distribution of values in healthy adults of serum calcium, inorganic phosphorus, magnesium, alkaline phosphatase, total proteins, albumin and blood urea, *J. Lab. Clin. Med.,* 73, 825, 1969.

120. **Aknes, L., Rodland, O., Odegaard, O.R., Bakke, K.J., et al.,** Serum levels of Vit D metabolites in the elderly, *Acta Endocrinol.,* 121, 27, 1989.

121. **Riggs, B.C., Gallaher, J.C., Celce, H.F., Edis, A.J., and Lambert, P.W.,** A syndrome of osteoporosis, increased immunoreactive parathyroid hormone and inappropriately low dihydroxy Vitamin D, *Mayo Clin. Proc.,* 53, 701, 1978.

122. **Dandona, P., Menon, R.K., Shenoy, R., Houlder, S., et al.,** Low 1,25-dihydroxy Vit D, secondary hyperparathyroidism and normal osteocalcin in elderly subjects, *J. Clin. Endocrinol. Metab.,* 63, 459, 1986.

123. **Heath, H., Hodgson, S., and Kennedy, M.,** Primary hyperparathyroidism: incidence, morbidity and potential economic impact in a community, *N. Engl. J. Med.,* 302, 189, 1980.

124. **Sier, H.C., Hartnell, J., Morley, J.E., et al.,** Primary hyperparathyroidism and delirium in the elderly, *J. Am. Geriatr. Soc.,* 36, 157, 1988.

125. **Selby, P.L. and Peacock, M.,** Ethinyl estradiol and nor-ethindrone in the treatment of primary hyperparathyroidism in post-menopausal women, *N. Engl. J. Med.,* 314, 1481, 1986.

126. **Barzel, U.,** Parathyroid surgery in elderly patients, *Ann. Intern. Med.,* 98, 114, 1983.

Chapter 14

NEUROENDOCRINE-IMMUNE INTERACTIONS: THE ROLE OF HPA/IL-1 FUNCTION IN DISEASE SUSCEPTIBILITY

Julio Licinio and Esther M. Sternberg

CONTENTS

INTRODUCTION

It is now well established that neurohormones affect the activity of the immune system, and that immune mediators, such as cytokines, affect neuroendocrine function. At this time more than 30 cytokines have been isolated and cloned. Each cytokine acts via specific receptors, which are either single- or multi-unit elements. An even greater number of neurohormones and neuropeptides has been identified in the central nervous system (CNS). The possible interactions between each cytokine and each neuropeptide are myriad. As a general rule, cytokines are synthesized, or have their secretion increased, during states of system illness.

Cytokines, acting via cytokine receptors, affect brain functions to promote adaptation to inflammatory stress and to inhibit functions that are biologically disadvantageous during states of inflammation or infection. Hence, most cytokines stimulate functions required for an adequate response to infection or to inflammatory stress: those functions include fever, increased sympathetic output, and hypothalamic-pituitary-adrenal (HPA) axis activation, which ultimately provides the necessary negative feedback to inhibit inflammation. On the other hand, most cytokines inhibit functions that are not essential during inflammatory stress; those vegetative functions inhibited by cytokines include food intake and reproduction. In this chapter, rather than exhaustively review all the effects of cytokines on neuroendocrine function and vice versa, we will keep our focus on the pathophysiological relevance of the interactions between the prototypical Th-1 cytokine, interleukin-1 (IL-1), and the major stress-responsive neuroendocrine system, the HPA axis. Our rationale for focusing on these two systems is that of all neuroendocrine-immune interactions, the mutual relationship between IL-1 and HPA function has been the most intensively studied; furthermore, disruptions of IL-1/HPA interactions lead to disease susceptibility.[1,2]

THE MOLECULES OF THE IL-1/HPA NETWORK

IL-1 is a 17-kDa peptide, which is bioactive on most cells of the body, except erythrocytes.[3] There are three forms of IL-1: IL-1α and IL-1β, both of which bind to receptors and exert action, and IL-1 receptor antagonist (IL-1ra), the first pure endogenous antagonist to be discovered. IL-1ra binds to IL-1 receptors with the same affinity as IL-1α or IL-1β but does not elicit receptor activation even at very high concentrations.[4,5] There are four possible binding sites for IL-1: the type I IL-1 receptor (IL-1RI), which has a long intracellular domain and transduces a signal; the type II IL-1 receptor (IL-1RII), which has a very short intracellular domain and does not transduce a signal, functioning as decoy for bioactive IL-1; soluble receptors; and autoantibodies. The HPA axis consists of three major molecules: corticotropin-releasing hormone (CRH), proopiomelanocortin (POMC), and cortisol. CRH is a 41-amino acid peptide that has a dual role as both the major regulator of pituitary corticotroph activity and a neurotransmitter with profound behavioral effects. CRH causes the pituitary to release adrenocorticotropic hormone (ACTH).[6,9] This in turn results in release of corticosteroids, which have a key role in immunity.[10,11] Basal levels of cortisol are necessary for optimal immune function; however, high endogenous levels of this hormone, such as those achieved during IL-1 stimulation of the HPA axis in the context of inflammation or infection, cause immunosuppression, effectively shutting off the immune response that initiated the cycle.

HOW DO PERIPHERAL IMMUNE MEDIATORS AFFECT THE BRAIN?

Cytokines that stimulate HPA function by inducing CRH gene expression and secretion include IL-1, IL-6, tumor necrosis factor-α (TNF-α), and IL-2. The mechanism by which peripheral immune mediators affect brain function has been the subject of intense investigation. The most common question for investigators in this field is: How do such large molecules exert their effects accross the blood brain barrier? Several mechanisms have been proposed to answer this question. Although there is evidence to suggest that cytokines, such as IL-1, can cross the blood-brain barrier (BBB),[12-14] and may therefore directly stimulate the hypothalamus, those cytokines also induce prostaglandin production in endothelial cells in CNS vasculature, and thereby exert their effect indirectly through prostanoids.[15] Evidence for the importance of this indirect mechanism is the inhibitory effect of prostaglandin inhibitors, such as indomethacin, on many functional effects of cytokine-CNS interactions. However, active transport across the BBB is not the only mechanism by which cytokines may directly stimulate the hypothalamus because peptides, such as IL-1, can cross at circumventricular organs, such as the organum vasculosum laminae terminalis (OVLT), where the barrier is relatively permeable. Furthermore, during conditions of systemic inflammation when cytokines may be released, the integrity of the BBB may be diminished, allowing greater access of cytokines to the CNS. Table 1 lists the four mechanisms by which peripheral inflammatory signals can reach the brain. Those mechanisms are not mutually exclusive and may coexist in different combinations during various pathophysiological scenarios.

TABLE 1
Mechanisms By Which Peripheral Inflammatory Mediators May
Signal the Central Nervous System

1. Acting in peripheral organs that are innervated and can send a signal to the brain
   (e.g., liver, spleen).
2. Acting at the level of brain vasculature, with secondary signals being generated
   (e.g., prostaglandins, nitric oxide).
3. Entering the brain in areas where there are gaps in the blood-brain barrier (BBB)
   (e.g., OVLT).
4. Crossing the BBB via specific (putative) transport mechanisms.

LOCALIZATION OF IMMUNE MEDIATORS IN THE BRAIN

Cytokines are localized in brain. The best-defined cytokine pathway in the brain involves IL-1 and IL-1 receptor.[16-19] Even though it is clear that the genes encoding for the IL-1 system are expressed in the brain, there is some controversy in the field as to whether there is significant constitutive IL-1 in brain and whether IL-1 has a role in the normal functioning of the brain, or if it only functions as a response to injury, stress, infection, or inflammation. Furthermore, it is not clear whether the IL-1 in uninflamed brain is localized in neurons or in glia. Various groups have reported discrepant results on the localization of IL-1 in the brain. Bandtlow et al.[16] have reported constitutive localization in the hippocampus; however, in their studies on IL-1β gene expression in brain, neither Gatti and Bartfai[20] nor Yabuuchi et al.[21] found any IL-1β gene expression in hippocampus. These differences in the findings of IL-1β mRNA in brain may be due to technical variations among laboratories or could be caused by confounding factors, such as stress at the time of death, infection, circadian variations, or age of the animal.

Even though there are discrepancies, a substantial body of evidence indicates that several components of the IL-1 system are present in normal brain. IL-1β has been localized by immunohistochemistry in human brain.[17] Additionally, the following IL-1 molecules or their mRNAs have been identified in rodent brain: IL-1α,[22] IL-1β,[16,21] IL-1ra,[18] and IL-1 receptor[23,24] (Figure 1). Those data indicate that endogenous IL-1 molecules may have a physiological role in brain.

PHYSIOLOGICAL ROLES FOR IL-1 IN THE BRAIN

The most well-substantiated evidence for a role of IL-1 in normal physiology comes from the studies of Opp and Krueger,[25,26] which show that inhibition of IL-1 activity by neutralizing antibodies or by IL-1ra affects normal sleep, rebound sleep after sleep deprivation, and sleep induced by inflammatory mediators. Additionally, endogenous IL-1 in the brain may contribute to the regulation of neuronal cell death and survival. Indeed, *in vitro* studies have shown that IL-1 can be neurotoxic or neuroprotective, depending on the neuronal stage or maturation stage.[27] In adulthood it seems that IL-1 can be profoundly neurotoxic. Relton and Rothwell[28] have shown that inhibition of IL-1 activity can reduce neuronal death by 50% in an animal model of ischemia caused by middle cerebral artery occlusion, and can also reduce neuronal cell death by 70% in a model of acute neurodegeneration caused by excitotoxic damage resulting from administration of an NMDA receptor agonist in the striatum. Recent evidence seems to indicate that IL-1β converting enzyme (ICE) may have a role in apoptosis and cell death. ICE cleaves biologically inactive pro-IL-1β into bioactive IL-1β.[29,30] Yuan et al. have postulated that ICE is the mammalian analogue of the *C. elegans* cell death gene CED-3.[31] That group has shown that the vaccinia virus protein crm-A, an ICE inhibitor, protects against

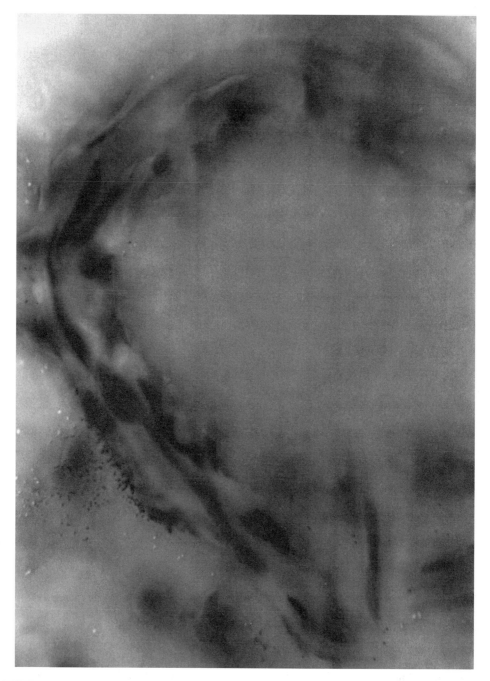

FIGURE 1.   Brightfield photomicrograph showing results of *in situ* hybridization histochemistry for the type I IL-1 receptor mRNA in an arteriole in the adult rat brain. *In situ* hybridization was performed with a ^{35}S-labeled, species-specific, antisense riboprobe as described in Ref. 23 (cDNAs were generously provided by Drs. C. Liu and R. P. Hart, Rutgers University, Newark, NJ). Note deposit of silver grain (black dots in the picture) in lower left of photomicrograph.

apoptosis.[32] There are questions as to whether ICE itself is required for apoptosis because transgenic mice with a knock out for ICE have normal apoptosis *in vivo* during development and adulthood; those mice also have normal apoptosis *in vitro*.[33] It seems that ICE is a member of a family of proteases that is involved in apoptosis. It has been recently shown that a newly discovered ICE homologue affects apoptosis.[34] Inhibition of that homologue abolishes all manifestations of apoptosis *in vitro*, including morphological changes and production of an oligonucleosomal ladder. These data seem to indicate that ICE-like molecules have a role in apoptosis.

CYTOKINES, HPA AXIS ACTIVATION, AND DISEASE SUSCEPTIBILITY

Independent of the role they have in normal brain physiology, cytokine-mediated activation of the HPA axis is relevant to the susceptibility to disease. When inflammatory mediators fail for any reason to activate the HPA axis there is increased susceptibility to and severity of inflammatory disease.[1] Investigation of various animal models of inflammation have shown a genetic blunting of HPA axis responses in association with increased susceptibility to inflammatory disease.[35] Table 2 illustrates how various animal models of autoimmune disease are characterized by a disruption in the immune-neuroendocrine axis.

TABLE 2
Defects in HPA/IL-1 Interactions in Autoimmunity-Prone Strains

Strain	Disease	Response of HPA Axis to IL-1	Defective Production of Glucocorticoid-Inducing Cytokines
OS chicken	Hashimoto-like thyroiditis	Defective	Normal production of glucocorticoid-increasing factors
UCD200	Scleroderma	Protracted return to baseline	Not determined
(NZB × W)F1	Lupus	Defective at 2 months of age	Yes (IL-1, IL-6, TNF-α)
MRL/*lpr*	Lupus	Defective at 2 months of age	Yes (IL-1, IL-6)
NOD	IDDM	Not determined	Yes (IL-1, IL-6, TNF-α)
BB rat	IDDM	Not determined	Yes (IL-1)
Lewis rat	Susceptible to experimental autoimmunity	Yes	Not determined

Modified from Wick, G., Hu, Y., Schwarz, S., and Kroemer, G., *Endocr. Rev.,* 14, 539, 1993. With permission.

Lewis (LEW/N) rats are highly susceptible to inflammatory disease, compared to the relatively inflammatory-disease-resistant histocompatible strain, Fischer (F344/N).[36,37] LEW/N rats develop inflammatory diseases related to the specific proinflammatory stimulus to which they are exposed. Their overall susceptibility to inflammation is related to their inability to produce HPA axis activation in response to peripheral inflammatory mediators or to other stimuli. LEW/N rats have a profound blunting of hypothalamic CRH responses to a variety of proinflammatory and stress stimuli, leading to a lack of ACTH and corticosterone responses to peripheral inflammatory mediators. This defect is not observed at baseline and can be seen only after challenge with proinflammatory stimuli.[36] Compared to F344/N rats, LEW/N HPA axis responses are markedly reduced in response to bacterial streptococcal peptidoglycan polysaccharide (streptococcal cell walls, SCW), which induces an arthritis in LEW/N rats resembling human rheumatoid arthritis. LEW/N rats exhibit similar diminished HPA axis responses to other stimuli including IL-1, quipazine (a serotonin agonist), adrenergic and cholinergic agonists, as well as to a variety of physical and psychological stress situations.[38,39] The observed differential LEW/N hypo- and F344/N hyper- HPA axis responsiveness occurs very early in ontogeny and persists throughout adulthood.[40]

Finding that inflammation is associated with disruptions of HPA activity does not in itself prove that there is a causal relation between these two events. This is particularly true in the light of the fact that inflammation per se affects HPA function and is a stressor. Thus, confirmation that alterations in the immune-neuroendocrine axis lead to susceptibility to inflammatory disease has been based on a series of experiments in which interruption of immune-neuroendocrine feedback caused susceptibility to inflammation. Treatment of F344/N rats with the glucocorticoid antagonist RU 486, or the serotonin 5-HT2 antagonist LY53857, renders these otherwise inflammatory-resistant rats highly susceptible to the pro-inflammatory and lethal effects of SCW.[36] Inflammatory-resistant rat strains also become susceptible to inflammation after surgical interruptions of the axis by adrenalectomy or hypophysectomy. Hypophysectomy predisposes to the lethal effects of salmonella,[41] whereas adrenalectomy without glucocorticoid replacement predisposes to the lethal and inflammatory effects of myelin basic protein in induction of experimental allergic encephalomyelitis.[42] In animals experimentally rendered susceptible to inflammation by interruption of the immune-neuroendocrine axis, or replacement treatment with intermediate or therapeutic doses of glucocorticoids results in suppression of the manifestations of disease.

In conclusion, interruptions of immune-neuroendocrine communication pathways, whether based on genetic factors in LEW/N rats, or as result of a surgical or pharmacological manipulations in otherwise resistant strains, increase susceptibility to inflammatory disease. Conversely, reconstitution of the immune-neuroendocrine axis reverses the inflammatory susceptibility in these strains,[36] or experimental allergic encephalomyelitis (EAE),[42] in a dose-related way.

CRH has profound biological effects. Initially discovered as a secretagogue for ACTH,[43] CRH is also a neurotransmitter, and it affects most of the key functions of the brain such as reproduction, food intake, metabolic rate, temperature regulation, memory, learning, and behavior.[44,45] The behavioral effects of CRH are related to the responsiveness to stress, and include cautious avoidance, freeze posture, focused attention, and inhibition of behaviors associated with vegetative functions, such as feeding and reproductive behaviors. CRH hypo-responsive LEW/N rats, and CRH hyperresponsive F344/N rats have behavioral responses to stress consistent with their CRH responsiveness. In an open field, LEW/N rats spend more time exploring the periphery of the field compared to F344/N and Sprage Dawley rats, which spend more time in the middle.[39] However, although this behavioral pattern is consistent with differential CRH responsiveness, other neurotransmitters, such as serotonin, may also be associated with these differences. That is particularly noteworthy given the observations that LEW/N and F344/N rats exhibit differences in several neurotransmitter systems, such as hippocampal 5-HT1A receptors and 5-HT content,[46] as well as hypothalamic benzodiazepine receptors.[47] These differences may represent a primary defect or may be secondary to their profound HPA axis responsiveness; they may also contribute to differential behavioral responses to stressful situations.

The associations between differential behavioral responses to stress and differential inflammatory disease susceptibility may be clinically relevant and might explain the long-recognized association in humans between affective disorders, such as depression, and inflammatory diseases, such as rheumatoid arthritis (RA).[1,48] Melancholic depression is characterized by HPA axis hyperactivity and atypical depression seems to be associated by HPA hyporesponsiveness.[49,50] Consequently, the association between depression and RA, rather than being secondary to chronic pain, as previously thought, could instead be caused by an underlying neuroendocrine dysregulation of central CRH function. Such a dysregulation might potentially predispose an individual to inflammatory disease, if the individual encounters an appropriate inflammatory stimulus, or alternatively to depression, if the individual encounters a major life stress. Susceptible individuals, when faced with both an inflammatory stimulus and a major life stressor might develop depression and RA; the clinical comorbidity of those two disorders is not uncommon. Decreased HPA axis responsiveness may also explain some of the clinical features of fatigue states, such as fibromyalgia and chronic fatigue syndrome, associated with varying degrees of immune activation and depressive symptoms.[51-53]

OTHER IMMUNE-NEUROENDOCRINE INTERACTIONS

Although the focus of this chapter has been the HPA axis, it is important to recognize that other neuroendocrine systems, including the hypothalamic-pituitary-gonadal (HPG) axis,[54,55] called into play or inhibited during stress, may exert similar or opposite effects on the immune response. Reproductive hormones, such as estrogen, progesterone, and prolactin are immunostimulatory rather than immunosuppressive. Additionally, sympathetic nervous system activation of immune organs such as thymus and spleen has an important role in inflammation,[56-58] and may be affected during the response to stress. Finally, chronic inflammation itself is a stressor that affects the neuroendocrine milieu. During chronic inflammation, there is a shift in the regulation of HPA regulation, which becomes mostly AVP (arginine vasopressin) driven.[59,60] This shift is also apparent in uninflamed Lewis rats.[61]

CONCLUDING REMARKS

In conclusion, the balance of susceptibility to and severity of inflammatory disease can be conceptualized as the result of a balance in which environmental proinflammatory stimuli induce inflammation through an intact immune system that is able to recognize and respond to those stimuli. The neuroendocrine stress response then exerts a negative feedback modulating effect which suppresses inflammation. If such responses are blunted or absent, inflammation will persist unchecked. Thus, in any individual, the degree of stress responsiveness to inflammatory and other stimuli plays an important modulatory role in the final degree of inflammation expressed. At the same time, other neuronal and hormonal factors called into play during stress and inflammation may have similar immunosuppressive, or opposing immunostimulatory effects. Thus, the final effect of stressors on inflammatory severity will depend on the balance of neuronal and neuroendocrine factors called into play during the organism's response to stress.

ACKNOWLEDGMENT

This work was partially supported by the Alma Foster Davis Investigator Award from NARSAD (to J.L.).

REFERENCES

1. **Sternberg, E.M., Chrousos, G.P., Wilder, R.L., and Gold, P.W.,** The stress response and the regulation of inflammatory disease, *Ann. Intern. Med.,* 117(10), 854, 1992.
2. **Wick. G., Hu, Y., Schwarz, S., and Kroemer, G.,** Immunoendocrine communication via the hypothalamo-pituitary-adrenal axis in autoimmune diseases, *Endocr. Rev.,* 14(5), 539, 1993.
3. **Dinarello, C.A. and Wolff, S.M.,** The role of interleukin-1 in disease, *N. Engl. J. Med.,* 328, 106, 1993.
4. **Hannum, C.H., Wilcox, C.J., Arend, W.P., et al.,** Interleukin-1 receptor antagonist activity of a human interleukin-1 inhibitor, *Nature,* 343, 336, 1990.
5. **Eisenberg. S.P., Evans, R.J., Arend, W.P., et al.,** Primary structure and functional expression from complementary DNA of a human interleukin-1 receptor antagonist, *Nature,* 343, 341, 1990.
6. **Berkenbosch, F., van Oers, J., del Rey, A., Tilders, F., and Besedovsky, H.,** Corticotropin-releasing factor-producing neurons in the rat activated by interleukin-1, *Science,* 238, 524, 1987.
7. **Bernton, E.W., Beach, J.E., Holaday, J.W., Smallridge, R.C., and Fein, H.G.,** Release of multiple hormones by a direct action of interleukin-1 on pituitary cells, *Science,* 238, 519, 1987.
8. **Besedovsky, H.O., del Rey, A., Sorkin, E., and Dinarello, C.A.,** Immunoregulatory feedback between interleukin-1 and glucocorticoid hormones, *Science,* 233, 652, 1986.
9. **Sapolsky, R., Rivier, C., Yamamoto, G., Plotsky, P., and Vale, W.,** Interleukin-1 stimulates the secretion of hypothalamic corticotropin releasing factor, *Science,* 238, 522, 1987.

10. **Cupps, T.R. and Fauci, A.S.,** Corticosteroid-mediated immunoregulation in man, *Immunol. Rev.,* 65, 133, 1982.
11. **Munck, A., Guyre, P.M., and Holbrook, N.J.,** Physiological functions of glucocorticoids in stress and their relation to pharmacological actions, *Endocr. Rev.,* 5, 25, 1984.
12. **Banks, W.A., Kastin, A.J., and Gutierrez, E.G.,** Interleukin-1 alpha in blood has direct access to cortical brain cells, *Neurosci. Lett.,* 163, 41, 1993.
13. **Banks, W.A., Kastin, A.J., and Durham, D.A.,** Bidirectional transport of interleukin-1 alpha across the blood-brain barrier, *Brain Res. Bull.,* 23, 433, 1989.
14. **Banks, W.A., Ortiz, L., Plotkin, S.R., and Kastin, A.J.,** Human interleukin (IL) 1a, murine IL-1a and murine IL-1b are transported from blood to brain in the mouse by a shared saturable mechanism, *J. Pharmacol. Exp. Ther.,* 259, 988, 1991.
15. **Ristimaki, A., Garfinkel, S., Wessendorf, J., Maciag, T., and Hla, T.,** Induction of cyclooxygenase-2 by interleukin-1 alpha. Evidence for post-transcriptional regulation, *J. Biol. Chem.,* 269, 11769, 1994.
16. **Bandtlow, C.E., Meyer, M., Lindholm, D., Spranger, M., Heumann, R., and Thoenen, H.,** Regional and cellular codistribution of interleukin 1 beta and nerve growth factor mRNA in the adult rat brain: possible relationship to the regulation of nerve growth factor synthesis, *J. Cell. Biol.,* 111, 1701, 1990.
17. **Breder, C.D., Dinarello, C.A., and Saper, C.B.,** Interleukin-1 immunoreactive innervation of the human hypothalamus, *Science,* 240, 321, 1988.
18. **Licinio, J., Wong, M.L., and Gold, P.W.,** Localization of interleukin-1 receptor antagonist mRNA in rat brain, *Endocrinology,* 129(1), 562, 1991.
19. **Takao, T., Tracey, D.E., Mitchell, W.M., and DeSouza, E.B.,** Interleukin-1 receptors in mouse brain: characterization and neuronal localization, *Endocrinology,* 127, 3070, 1990.
20. **Gatti, S. and Bartfai, T.,** Induction of tumor necrosis factor-alpha mRNA in the brain after peripheral endotoxin treatment: comparison with interleukin-1 family and interleukin-6, 624, 291, 1993.
21. **Yabuuchi, K., Minami, M., Katsumata, S., and Satoh, M.,** In situ hybridization study of interleukin-1 beta mRNA induced by kainic acid in the rat brain, *Brain Res. Mol. Brain Res.,* 20, 153, 1993.
22. **Rettori, V., Les Dees,W., Hiney, J.K., Lyson, K., McCann, S.M.,** An interleukin-1-alpha-like neuronal system in the pre-optic-hypothalamic region and its induction by bacterial lipopolysaccharide in concentrations which alter pituitary hormone release, *Neuroimmunomodulation,* 1, 251, 1994.
23. **Wong, M.-L. and Licinio, J.,** Localization of interleukin 1 type I receptor mRNA in rat brain, *Neuroimmunomodulation,* 1, 110, 1994.
24. **Cunningham, E.T.J., Wada, E., Carter, D.B., Tracey, D.E., Battey, J.F., and De Souza, E.B.,** In situ histochemical localization of type I interleukin-1 receptor messenger RNA in the central nervous system, pituitary, and adrenal gland of the mouse, *J. Neurosci.,* 12, 1101, 1992.
25. **Opp, M.R. and Krueger, J.M.,** Anti-interleukin-1 beta reduces sleep and sleep rebound after sleep deprivation in rats, *Am. J. Physiol.,* 266, R688, 1994.
26. **Imeri, L., Opp, M.R., and Krueger, J.M.,** An IL-1 receptor and an IL-1 receptor antagonist attenuate muramyl dipeptide- and IL-1-induced sleep and fever, *Am. J. Physiol.,* 265, R907, 1993.
27. **Brenneman, D.E., Page, S.W., Schultzberg, M., et al.,** A decomposition product of a contaminant implicated in L-tryptophan eosinophilia myalgia syndrome affects spinal cord neuronal cell death and survival through stereospecific, maturation and partly IL-1-dependent mechanisms, *J. Pharmacol. Exp. Ther.,* 266(2), 1029, 1993.
28. **Relton, J.K. and Rothwell, N.J.,** Interleukin-1 receptor antagonist inhibits ischaemic and excitotoxic neuronal damage in the rat, *Brain Res. Bull.,* 29, 243, 1992.
29. **Thornberry, N.A., Bull, H.G., Calaycay, J.R., et al.,** A novel heterodimeric cysteine protease is required for interleukin-1 beta processing in monocytes, *Nature,* 356, 768, 1992.
30. **Cerretti, D.P., Kozlosky, C.J., Mosley, B., et al.,** Molecular cloning of the interleukin-1 beta converting enzyme, *Science,* 256, 97, 1992.
31. **Yuan, J., Shaham, S., Ledoux, S., Ellis, H.M., and Horvitz, H.R.,** The C. elegans cell death gene ced-3 encodes a protein similar to mammalian interleukin-1 beta-converting enzyme, *Cell,* 75, 641, 1993.
32. **Gagliardini, V., Fernandez, P.A., Lee, R.K., et al.,** Prevention of vertebrate neuronal death by the crmA gene, *Science,* 263, 826, 1994.
33. **Li, P., Allen, H., Banerjee, S., et al.,** Mice deficient in IL-1β converting enzyme are defective in production of mature IL-1β and resistant to endototoxic shock, *Cell,* 80, 401, 1995.
34. **Lazebnik, Y.A., Kaufmann, S.H., Desnoyers, S., Poirier, G.G., and Earnshaw, W.C.,** Cleavage of poly(ADP-ribose) polymerase by a proteinase with properties like ICEl, *Nature,* 371, 346, 1994.
35. **Wick, G., Hu, Y., Schwarz, S., and Kroemer, G.,** Immunoendocrine communication via the hypothalamo-pituitary-adrenal axis in autoimmune diseases, *Endocr. Rev.,* 14, 539, 1993.
36. **Sternberg, E.M., Hill, J.M., Chrousos, G.P., et al.,** Inflammatory mediator-induced hypothalamic-pituitary-adrenal axis activation is defective in streptococcal cell wall arthritis-susceptible Lewis rats, *Proc. Natl. Acad. Sci. U.S.A.,* 86(7), 2374, 1989.

37. **Sternberg, E.M., Young, W.S., III, Bernardini, R., et al.,** A central nervous system defect in biosynthesis of corticotropin-releasing hormone is associated with susceptibility to streptococcal cell wall-induced arthritis in Lewis rats, *Proc. Natl. Acad. Sci. U.S.A.*, 86(12), 4771, 1989.

38. **Calogero, A.E., Sternberg, E.M., Bagdy, G., et al.,** Neurotransmitter-induced hypothalamic-pituitary-adrenal axis responsiveness is defective in inflammatory disease-susceptible Lewis rats: *in vivo* and *in vitro* studies suggesting globally defective hypothalamic secretion of corticotropin-releasing hormone, *Neuroendocrinology*, 55(5), 600, 1992.

39. **Sternberg, E.M., Glowa, J.R., Smith, M.A., et al.,** Corticotropin releasing hormone related behavioral and neuroendocrine responses to stress in Lewis and Fischer rats, *Brain Res.*, 570(1-2), 54, 1992.

40. **Aksentijevich, S., Whitfield, H.J.J., Young, W.S., III, et al.,** Arthritis-susceptible Lewis rats fail to emerge from the stress hyporesponsive period, *Brain Res. Dev. Brain Res.*, 65(1), 115, 1992.

41. **Edwards, C.K.I., Yunger, L.M., Lorence, R.M., Dantzer, R., Kelley, K.W.,** The pituitary gland is required for protection against lethal effects of Salmonella typhimurium, *Proc. Natl. Acad. Sci. U.S.A.*, 88(6), 2274, 1991.

42. **MacPhee, I.A.M., Antoni, F.A., and Mason, D.W.,** Spontaneous recovery of rats from experimental allergic encephalomyelitis is dependent on regulation of the immune system by endogenous adrenal corticosteroids, *J. Exp. Med.*, 169, 431, 1989.

43. **Vale, W., Spiess, J., Rivier, C., and Rivier, J.,** Characterization of a 41-residue ovine hypothalamic peptide that stimulates secretion of corticotropin and b-endorphin, *Science*, 213, 1394, 1981.

44. **Britton, D.R., Koob, G.F., Rivier, J., and Vale, W.,** Intraventricular corticotropin-releasing factor enhances behavioral effects of novelty, *Life Sci.*, 31, 363, 1982.

45. **Sutton, R.E., Koob, G.F., LeMoal, M., Rivier, J., and Vale, W.,** Corticotropin-releasing factor produces behavioural activation in rats, *Nature*, 297, 331, 1982.

46. **Burnet, P.W., Mefford, I.N., Smith, C.C., Gold, P.W., and Sternberg, E.M.,** Hippocampal 8-[3H]hydroxy-2-(di-n-propylamino) tetralin binding, *J. Neurochem.*, 59(3), 1062, 1992.

47. **Smith, C.C., Hauser, E., Renaud, N.K., et al.,** Increased hypothalamic [3H]flunitrazepam binding in hypothalamic-pituitary-adrenal axis hyporesponsive Lewis rats, *Brain Res.*, 569(2), 295, 1992.

48. **Cash, J.M., Crofford, L.J., Gallucci, W.T., et al.,** Pituitary-adrenal axis responsiveness to ovine corticotropin releasing hormone in patients with rheumatoid arthritis treated with low dose prednisone, *J. Rheumatol.*, 19(11), 1692, 1992.

49. **Gold, P.W., Goodwin, F.K., and Chrousos, G.P.,** Clinical and biochemical manifestations of depression: relation to the neurobiology of stress (Part 1 of 2 parts), *N. Engl. J. Med.*, 319, 348, 1988.

50. **Gold, P.W., Goodwin, F.K., and Chrousos, G.P.,** Clinical and biochemical manifestations of depression: relation to the neurobiology of stress (Part 2 of 2 parts), *N. Engl. J. Med.*, 319, 413, 1988.

51. **Demitrack, M.A., Dale, J.K., Straus, S.E., et al.,** Evidence for impaired activation of the hypothalamic-pituitary-adrenal axis in patients with chronic fatigue syndrome, *J. Clin. Endocrinol. Metab.*, 73(6), 1224, 1991.

52. **Sternberg. E.M.,** Hyperimmune fatigue syndromes: diseases of the stress response? *J. Rheumatol.*, 20(3), 418, 1993.

53. **Crofford, L.J., Pillemer, S.R., Kalogeras, K.T., et al.,** Hypothalamic pituitary adrenal axis perturbations in patients with fibromyalgia, *Arthritis Rheum.*, 37(2), 1583, 1994.

54. **Rivier, C., Rivier, J., and Vale, W.,** Stress-induced inhibition of reproductive functions: role of endogenous corticotropin-releasing factor, *Science*, 231, 607, 1986.

55. **Vernikos, J., Dallman, M.F., Keil, L.C., O'Hara, D., and Convertino, V.A.,** Gender differences in endocrine responses to posture and 7 days of –6 degrees head-down bed rest, *Am. J. Physiol.*, 265, E153, 1993.

56. **Felten, S.Y. and Felten, D.L.,** Innervation of lymphoid tissue, in *Psychoneuroimmunology*, 2nd ed., Ader, R., Felten, D.L., Cohen, N., Eds., Academic Press, San Diego, 1991, 27.

57. **Madden, K.S., Moynihan, J.A., Brenner, G.J., Felten, S.Y., Felten, D.L., and Livnat, S.,** Sympathetic nervous system modulation of the immune system. III. Alterations in T and B cell proliferation and differentiation *in vitro* following chemical sympathectomy, *J. Neuroimmunol.*, 49(1-2), 77, 1994.

58. **Tollefson, L. and Bulloch, K.,** Dual-label retrograde transport: CNS innervation of the mouse thymus distinct from other mediastinum viscera, *J. Neurosci. Res.*, 25, 20, 1990.

59. **Harbuz, M.S., Rees, R.G., Eckland, D., Jessop, D.S., Brewerton, D., and Lightman, S.L.,** Paradoxical responses of hypothalamic corticotropin-releasing factor (CRF) messenger ribonucleic acid (mRNA) and CRF-41 peptide and adenohypophysial proopiomelanocortin mRNA during chronic inflammatory stress, *Endocrinology*, 130, 1394, 1992.

60. **Whitnall, M.H., Perlstein, R.S., Mougey, E.H., and Neta, R.,** Effects of interleukin-1 on the stress-responsive and -nonresponsive subtypes of corticotropin-releasing hormone neurosecretory axons, *Endocrinology*, 131, 37, 1992.

61. **Patchev, V.K., Kalogeras, K.T., Zelazowski, P., Wilder, R.L., and Chrousos G.P.,** Increased plasma concentrations, hypothalamic content, and *in vitro* release of arginine vasopressin in inflammatory disease-prone, hypothalamic corticotropin-releasing hormone-deficient Lewis rats, *Endocrinology*, 131, 1453, 1992.

INDEX

A

ABP, see Androgen-binding protein

Accessory glands, androgen effects on, 209–210

ACE, see Angiotensin converting enzyme

Acetyl-CoA, see Acetyl coenzyme A

Acetyl coenzyme A, cholesterol synthesis, 199, 228

Acid-base balance
buffering systems, 67
definition of, 67
effect of corticosteroids, 70–73
organ systems involved in, 67

Acidification, urinary, see Urinary acidification

ACTH, see Adrenocorticotropic hormone

Actin, 38

Actin-binding proteins, in chromaffin cells, 4–5

Activin, effect on ovarian steroidogenesis, 109

Addison's disease
causes of, 253–254
in elderly, 253

Adenocarcinoma, vaginal, diethylstilbestrol and, 150

Adenohypophysis, 212

Adenosine, effect on urinary acidification, 75

Adrenal cortex
age-related hormonal effects, 249
embryology of, 16

Adrenal gland
age-related disorders of
Addison's disease, 253–254
Cushing's syndrome, 254
menopause, 254–255
renin-angiotensin-aldosterone axis, 254
hypothalamic-pituitary axis, see
Hypothalamic-pituitary-adrenal axis
medulla, see Adrenal medulla

Adrenal hyperplasia, congenital
cause of, 15–16
in children, treatment modalities, 23
clinical features, enzymatic deficiencies
20,22-desmolase, 22
11β-hydroxylase, 20–21
17α-hydroxylase/17,20-lyase, 21
21-hydroxylase, 17–20
3β-hydroxysteroid dehydrogenase, 21
defined, 15–16
embryology of, 16
genetic mutations of, 26
salt-wasting, 23
treatment of, 23–24

Adrenal medulla, see also Adrenal gland
chromaffin cells
catecholamine secretion from, 2
endocytosis, 5–6
exocytosis, 2–5
messengers, 4, 6–7
characteristics of, 1

cholinergic stimulation of, 6–7
stimulation of, 2–3
sympathetic nervous system and, 1
transplantation of
graft survival and function, 7–8
objectives, 7
trophic hypothesis, 8

Adrenal zona fasciculata, function of, 16

Adrenocorticotropic hormone, 16–17, 83

Adrenogenital syndrome, see Adrenal hyperplasia, congenital

Adseverin, 5

Aging, see also Elderly
adrenal gland disorders
Addison's disease, 253–254
Cushing's syndrome, 254
menopause, 254–255
renin-angiotensin-aldosterone axis, 254
effect on ovary function, 116
and endocrine disorders, 242
hormonal effects
adrenal cortex, 249–250
androgens, 250
growth hormone, 247–248
hormones associated with water metabolism, 250
insulin-like growth factor I, 247–248
male sex hormones, 250–251
progesterone, 251
prolactin, 248–249
testosterone, 250–251
thyroid-stimulating hormone, 249
and hypopituitarism, 251
and parathyroid gland disorders
hyperparathyroidism, 255
hypoparathyroidism, 255–256
theories of
antioxidants, 246
DNA damage, 246
neuroendocrine involvement, 246
overview, 248
and thyroid diseases
hypothyroidism, 251–252
thyrotoxicosis, 252–253
vitamin D absorption decreases in, 35

α_2 agonists, effect on urinary acidification, 75

Aldosterone
age-related effects, 249
effect on urinary acidification, 70–73
overproduction of, 21-hydroxylase deficiency and, 19
synthesis of, 17
corticosterone methyloxidase deficiency, 23
in 17α-hydroxylase/17,20-lyase deficient patients, 21

Alfacalcidol, see 1α-Hydroxycholecalciferol

Alopecia, resistance to vitamin D action, 47

Alveolar cells, surfactant synthesis, 82

W

X

Z